Hᴀɴᴅʙᴏᴏᴋ ᴏғ

Clinical
Trauma
Care

The First Hour

HANDBOOK OF
Clinical Trauma Care
The First Hour

Fourth Edition

DIANNE M. DANIS, RN, MS
Director, Nursing Practice Innovation
University of Wisconsin Hospital and Clinics
Madison, Wisconsin

JOSEPH S. BLANSFIELD, RN, MS, NP
Trauma Program Coordinator
Colonel, United States Army Reserve
Deputy Commander, Nursing
399th Combat Support Hospital
Bedford, Massachusetts

ALICE A. GERVASINI, PhD, RN
Trauma and Emergency Surgery Program Nurse Manager
Massachusetts General Hospital
Boston, Massachusetts

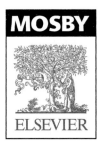

MOSBY
ELSEVIER

11830 Westline Industrial Drive
St. Louis, Missouri 63146

HANDBOOK OF CLINICAL TRAUMA CARE: THE FIRST HOUR   ISBN 13: 978-0-323-03232-2
4th edition   ISBN 10: 0-323-03232-X

Notice

Neither the Publisher nor the Authors assume any responsibility for any loss or injury and/or damage to persons or property arising out of or related to any use of the material contained in this book. It is the responsibility of the treating practitioner, relying on independent expertise and knowledge of the patient, to determine the best treatment and method of application for the patient.

The Publisher

Previous editions copyrighted 1989, 1994, 1999

ISBN 13 978-0-323-03232-2
ISBN 10 0-323-03232-X

Executive Publisher: Barbara Nelson Cullen
Executive Editor: Cindy Tryniszewski, RN, MSN
Developmental Editor: Laurie Sparks
Publishing Services Manager: John Rogers
Senior Project Manager: Kathleen L. Teal
Book Designer: Andrea Lutes

Working together to grow
libraries in developing countries
www.elsevier.com | www.bookaid.org | www.sabre.org

ELSEVIER   BOOK AID International   Sabre Foundation

Printed in the United States of America

Last digit is the print number: 9 8 7 6 5 4 3 2 1

Contributors

CAROL C. ATKINSON, MS, PNP
Trauma Nursing Coordinator
Children's Hospital
Boston, Massachusetts

MARY-LIZ BILODEAU, RN, MS, CCRN, CCNS, CS, BC
Critical Care Clinical Nurse Specialist/Acute Care Nurse Practitioner
Sumner Redstone Burn Center
Massachusetts General Hospital
Boston, Massachusetts

PAMELA W. BOURG, RN, MS
Clinical Nurse Specialist
Trauma Services
St. Anthony General Hospital
Denver, Colorado

KATHLEEN J. BURNS, RN, MS, CS
Acute Care Nurse Practitioner
Trauma Service
Massachusetts General Hospital
Boston, Massachusetts

MAUREEN M. CULLEN, RN, MS, ANP-C
Critical Care Transport Nurse
Boston MedFlight
Boston, Massachusetts
Nurse Practitioner – Emergency Room
Anna Jaques Hospital
Newburyport, Massachusetts

MARY M. CUSHMAN, RN, BSN
Trauma Coordinator
Baystate Medical Center
Springfield, Massachusetts

DEBORAH A. D'AVOLIO, PHD, ARNP-BC, ACNP, ANP
Assistant Professor, Coordinator, Acute Care Specialty
MGH Institute of Health Professions
Boston, Massachusetts

KAREN DRISCOLL, RN, MS, CCRN, CEN
Critical Care Transport Nurse
Boston MedFlight
Boston, Massachusetts

NICKI GILBOY, RN, MS, CEN, FAEN
Nurse Educator
Emergency Department
Brigham and Women's Hospital
Boston, Massachusetts

CATHY M. GRAGG, RN, BSN
Outpatient Services Unit Manager
Shepherd Center
Atlanta, Georgia

MAUREEN A. HARRAHILL, RN, MS, ACNP-BS
Trauma Program Director
Oregon Health Sciences University
Portland, Oregon

PATRICIA MAHER HARRISON, RN, MS, ACNP, CCRN
Trauma Nurse Practitioner
Department of Surgery
Boston Medical Center
Boston, Massachusetts

BENJAMIN E. HOLLINGSWORTH, RN, MS, ACNP
Trauma Nurse Practitioner
Massachusetts General Hospital
Boston, Massachusetts

SANDRA A. JUTRAS, RN, MS, LNC
Manager, Impartial Medical Unit
Department of Industrial Accidents
Commonwealth of Massachusetts
Boston, Massachusetts

Owner, Keville Medical-Legal Consulting
Amesbury, Massachusetts

DONNA W. LOUPUS, APRN, BC
Manager of Professional Nursing Practice
Shepherd Center
Atlanta, Georgia

MARY LOU LYONS, RN, MS
Clinical Nurse Specialist
Massachusetts General Hospital
Boston, Massachusetts

KAREN MACAULEY, RN, MEd
Trauma Prevention and Outreach Director
St. Christopher's Hospital for Children
Philadelphia, Pennsylvania

ANNE P. MANTON, PHD, APRN, FAAN, FAEN
Psychiatric Mental Health Nurse Practitioner
Psychiatric Center-Urgent Care
Cape Cod Hospital
Hyannis, Massachusetts

JOAN MEUNIER-SHAM, RN, MS
Associate Director
Massachusetts Pediatric Sexual Assault
Nurse Examiner Program
Massachusetts Office for Victim Assistance
Boston, Massachusetts

PATRICIA MIAN, RN, MS, APN-BC
Psychiatric Clinical Nurse Specialist
Massachusetts General Hospital
Boston, Massachusetts

ROBIN L. OHKAGAWA, RN, BSN, CPTC
Donation Coordinator
New England Organ Bank
Newton, Massachusetts

LAURIE PETROVICK, MS
Administrative Coordinator for Biostatistics
and Performance Improvement
Massachusetts General Hospital
Boston, Massachusetts

TENER GOODWIN VEENEMA, RN, PHD, MPH, MS, CPNP
Associate Professor and Program Director for
Disaster Nursing and Strategic Initiatives
Center for Disaster Medicine and Emergency
Preparedness
University of Rochester
Rochester, New York

GAIL M. WILKES, RNC, MS, AOCN
Nursing Educator, Oncology
Boston Medical Center
Boston, Massachusetts

STEPHEN P. WOOD, MS, EMT-P
Critical Care Transport Paramedic
Boston MedFlight
Boston, Massachusetts

EMS Coordinator
Beth Israel Deaconess
Medical Center
Boston, Massachusetts

REVIEWERS

ALESE BAGBY, RN, BSN, CEN
Staff Nurse, Emergency Department
Penrose Community Hospital
Colorado Springs, Colorado

MARY B. GALLAGHER, RN, MSN, CCRN
Critical Care/Trauma Clinical Educator
Abington Memorial Hospital
Abington, Pennsylvania

ANNETTE GRINDLE, RN, BSN
Nurse Educator
Heart Failure and Heart Transplant
Strong Memorial Hospital
Rochester, New York

PREFACE

Providing care to trauma patients is a demanding, yet rewarding, experience. For those of us who have made a career of trauma care and for those who are just beginning this adventure, staying current in our practice is a major challenge. With the publication of the first edition of the *Manual of Clinical Trauma Care: The First Hour* (1989), I doubt the editors and authors could foresee the impact a manual like this would have on clinicians. A focused reference with practical applications to direct caregivers is the backbone of the philosophy put forth in the first edition, and it continues through this current edition. While the format and organization of the text have not changed, the change in title from *Manual* to *Handbook* serves to emphasize the book's continuing usefulness as a compact and portable reference.

As the body of knowledge supporting current clinical strategies in managing trauma patients has grown, so has the movement of greater expectations for the clinicians to accomplish significant clinical applications during the first hours post trauma. With this new edition of the *Handbook of Clinical Trauma Care: The First Hour*, we continue to recognize the heritage of the text and concepts from previous editions. However, the reader will find that the text covers not only the first hour, but the entire early post-injury phase. The initial resuscitation of trauma patients has historically occurred in the Emergency Department, but that is no longer the only environment where resuscitations are performed. As patients move seamlessly through a system from community hospitals, to tertiary centers, directly to operating rooms and intensive care units, the vital information necessary for clinicians to achieve optimal patient outcomes is provided in this handbook.

We are very excited about this edition and believe we have provided the content that will support excellence in clinical practice. The format has been expanded to not only address the clinical practice of each system of care, but to include focused content on unique populations that are becoming a large percent of the trauma patients we see, the elderly, the obese, and those suffering from interpersonal violence, pre-existing emotional issues, and/or substance abuse. Chapter authors are content experts with established links to trauma care. It is our belief that you will find this handbook to be an asset to your daily practice and that it supports your continuing efforts to achieve the best possible clinical outcomes.

Dianne M. Danis
Joseph S. Blansfield
Alice A. Gervasini

ACKNOWLEDGMENTS

As Editors of the fourth edition of the *Handbook of Clinical Trauma Care: The First Hour,* we have many people to thank and acknowledge. We would first like to thank all of the chapter authors who have contributed their time and talents – all among the best of the best in their area of trauma expertise. We are also grateful for the assistance of our publisher, Elsevier, in helping us get the book into print: in particular Cindy Tryniszewski, RN, MSN, Executive Editor, and Developmental Editor Laurie Sparks.

In addition, we would like to acknowledge all of the editors and chapter authors who contributed to previous editions of the text. We would especially like to thank and acknowledge Susan Budassi Sheehy, co-editor of each of the first three editions. Her vision and leadership have shaped this book.

And, last, we thank each other. Without our support of each other, and our willingness to alternate the "lead" on the project, we would never have been able to navigate the multiple competing demands of work, family, professional activities, job changes, military activation, and writing a book.

CONTENTS

PART I

TRAUMA CARE SYSTEMS

CHAPTER 1

THE MODEL TRAUMA SYSTEM

LAURIE PETROVICK

Trauma is the result of an act that damages, harms or hurts; unintentional or intentional damage to the body resulting from acute exposure to mechanical, thermal, electrical, or chemical energy or from the absence of such essentials as heat or oxygen.[1]

The total cost of unintentional trauma in 2002 was estimated at $586.3 billion, of which 30% went to medical expenses and 70% for property damage, lost wages, lost productivity, and disability. In 2002, 99,500 lives were lost to traumatic injury, and trauma is the number one cause of death for persons less than 44 years of age. The majority of unintentional deaths was motor vehicle crashes (44%), followed by falls at 14%. In the United States a fatal injury occurs every 5 seconds and a disabling injury every 1½ seconds. In 2003 the average economic cost (which includes wage and productivity, medical expenses, administrative expenses, motor vehicle damage, and uninsured employer costs per death, injury, or crash) per episode was $1,120,000 for death, $45,000 for nonfatal disabling injury, and $8,200 for property damage crash. Approximately 2.6 million persons will be hospitalized for nonfatal injuries, another 34 million will be treated in the emergency department, and 87.6 million will seek treatment at their physician's office.[2] Injury is a major public health problem in the United States.

HISTORY

In 1966 the National Academy of Sciences and National Research Council published a report titled *Accidental Death and Disability: The Neglected Disease of Modern Society.* This single report identified the lack of funding, research, and concern for the trauma patient and initiated the current thinking that trauma is a disease. The report also stimulated the growth and development of trauma systems throughout the country. Illinois recognized trauma as being a serious public health issue and established a statewide trauma system in 1971, and R. Adams Cowley established the first comprehensive statewide trauma care system that included prehospital care in Maryland. In 1976 the American College of Surgeons (ACS) created the reference book *The Optimal Hospital Resources for Care of the Injured Patient.* The manual is updated every 4 years, and the last edition, *Resources for Optimal Care of the Injured Patient* from 1999, stresses the importance of trauma systems and system development. This manual is recognized nationally as the standard of care for trauma patients and for developing trauma systems. In 1987 the ACS Committee on Trauma established trauma center guidelines that lead to a verification and consultation process for designating trauma centers. Virginia was the second state to establish a state trauma system in 1985, and that system was based on the ACS Committee on Trauma guidelines.[3] In 1990 the U.S. Congress passed the Trauma Care Systems Planning and Development Act (PL 101-590), and the division of Trauma and Emergency Medical Services was established. This division provided competitive grants for states for trauma system development and produced the Model Trauma Care System Plan in

1992. Approximately $2 million in grant money has been awarded every year to state trauma system development.[4] In 1988 only two states had statewide trauma systems in place, and by 2000 the number had expanded to 35. The National Highway Traffic Safety Administration voluntarily can review the emergency medical services with a program called Technical Assistance Teams. These teams will review the emergency medical services system using standards developed by the National Highway Traffic Safety Administration.[3]

TRAUMA SYSTEMS

A trauma care system is an organized and coordinated method for the multidisciplinary treatment of all injured patients in a geographic location. This system provides properly trained health care professionals, state-of-the-art equipment, and facilities. The spectrum of care includes injury prevention, emergency medical services, emergency department care, acute and general in-hospital care, surgical intervention, and rehabilitation services. The goal of the trauma system is to decrease the incidents of trauma, ensure timely access to optimal and quality patient care, contain costs, and improve patient outcomes. A schematic of a preplanned trauma care continuum developed by the Division of Trauma and Emergency Medical Services, Bureau of Health Service Resources, is described in Figure 1-1. Trauma systems are organized by region or by state so that the unique health care requirements of the population are met and resources are used efficiently. The trauma care system should be continuous between all phases of care, including prehospital care, acute and general care facilities, trauma centers, rehabilitation, and home care.

Prehospital Care

A complete prehospital system includes the following: emergency medical services management agency, ambulance and nontransporting guidelines, triage, medical direction, and communications system. The prehospital providers must be able to provide appropriate care at the scene and must be able to transport the patient safely and quickly to the closest, most suitable facility. The most severely injured are transported to the designated trauma center, which guarantees prompt availability of trauma surgeons, diagnostic departments, and subspecialties 24 hours a day, 7 days a week, and the less severely injured are transported to appropriate acute care facilities. Overtriaging to trauma centers will congest and overburden the system. This results in an inappropriate overutilization of equipment and is not cost-effective. Undertriaging would increase the incidents of morbidity and mortality of the trauma patient. It is necessary to match appropriate medical treatment during transportation such as advanced life support or basic life support and to transport the patient to the nearest definitive care facility as quickly as possible using ground or air transportation.

A 911 or enhanced 911 system is required for a prehospital communication system, as well as trained dispatch personnel. Personnel at scene must be able to communicate with dispatch, other units, other regions, and the definitive care facility.

Medical direction is included in the prehospital system and can be in the form of off-line—meaning protocols training, triage, or skill enhancement—or online, meaning medical direction from a physician at the hospital.

Definitive Care Facilities

Trauma care facilities must provide a wide range of services in order to meet the needs of the trauma patient within the geographic area. Trauma care systems should be developed to address the special health care needs of the region or community. Coordination of care among all levels

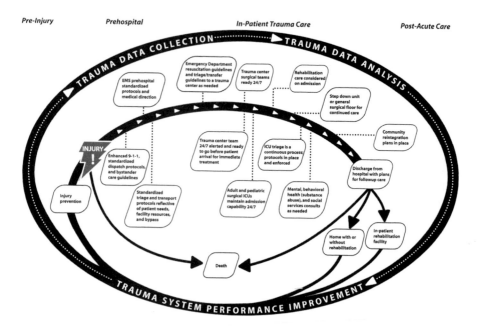

Figure I–I. Preplanned Trauma Care Continuum. *(From U.S. Department of Health and Human Services, Health Resources and Services Administration, Model Trauma System Planning & Evaluation, February 2006, p. 8. www.hrsa.gov/trauma/model.htm)*

of trauma centers, specialty facilities (burn, pediatric), and acute care facilities must be accomplished, and the system must have the appropriate mix of these institutions so that resources are not duplicated or wasted, or conversely, definitive care is not accessible in a timely manner. Not all hospitals should be trauma centers. Acute care facilities can treat 75% of trauma patients and can transfer the more severely injured patient to a higher-level trauma center. Interfacility transfers must be coordinated within the trauma care system.

Trauma system leadership must design criteria for trauma center designation or use established guidelines such as from the ACS (Box 1-1).

Rehabilitation is a major part of the trauma care system, and integration back into society is the longest and most difficult part of recovery. Rehabilitation should begin at the acute care facility and progress to a rehabilitation facility or to home care. All specialties should be available, such as physical therapy, occupational therapy, social work, psychiatric services, and substance abuse services.

Administrative Components

Administrative components consist of four areas: leadership, system development, legislation, and finances. The state has a substantial responsibility for implementing and maintaining the

| Box I–I | AMERICAN COLLEGE OF SURGEONS TRAUMA CENTER VERIFICATION LEVELS |

Level I

- Serves large cities or population-dense areas
- Tertiary facility with extensive resources and personnel
- Admits at least 1200 with 20% having injury severity score greater than 15 *or* 35 patients per surgeon with injury severity score greater than 15
- General Surgeon must be present and participate in major resuscitations, therapeutic decisions, and operations; 24-hour in-house availability is the most direct method for providing this.
- Research activities
- Prevention, outreach, and education programs
- Provides all aspects of trauma care for all injuries 24 hours a day
- Medical education programs

Level II

- Provides initial definitive care
- Works closely with a Level I institution, *or* in less densely populated areas serves as the lead trauma facility
- Same trauma surgeon involvement as Level I with the less dense population
- Available for all major traumas and evaluation of all trauma admissions and available for operative procedures and resuscitations
- Outreach, prevention, and education programs
- Transfer agreement

Level III

- Must be able to manage the initial care of the majority of injured patients
- Transfer agreements
- Trauma surgeon promptly available
- Outreach, prevention, and education programs
- Continuous general surgeon coverage
- General surgeon available for all major resuscitations

Level IV

- Rural areas
- Provide initial evaluation and assessment of injured patients
- Most require transfer to larger facility
- 24-hour emergency coverage by physician
- Specialty coverage may not be available
- Transfer most patients to larger facilities
- Operating room available for surgeon
- Prevention, outreach, and education programs

(Adapted from Committee on Trauma, American College of Surgeons: *Resources for optimal care of the injured patient: 2006,* Chicago, 2006, The College.)

trauma care system (Box 1-2). Leadership involves health care administrators and state, regional, and local political officials. The leadership must be committed to providing an inclusive and accessible trauma system that is cost-effective. Legislation is necessary to establish an oversight agency, acquire finances, designate facilities, and establish protocols and standards for all aspects of trauma care.[5]

Operational and Clinical Components

Monies must be allocated for injury prevention and educational programs. These educational programs reduce the incidence of trauma by changing behavior and reducing risk factors. The trauma system and the public health department should work closely to determine which preventive programs would provide the most positive impact in the community served by the trauma system.

A quality trauma system will have a human resources commitment and will employ the most qualified personnel throughout the continuum of care. The system also will provide educational opportunities to all providers. A strategy to retain qualified personnel is essential, as are strategies to acquire more personnel.

Information Systems and System Evaluation

Trauma systems must be evaluated objectively over time, and data must be collected from all phases of the trauma system. An established trauma system should define an inclusion criterion, which is the population for the database, and decide which data fields would be the most meaningful to collect in order to analyze system performance and outcomes. The data collected will be specific to meet the goals of the trauma system and flexible to change with the evolution of trauma practice. Data must be reliable and valid, and a system must be established that monitors incomplete, erroneous, and missing data. Analyzed data can be used to monitor care provided, monitor resource utilization, identify public health issues, perform research, and provide performance improvement activities.

Box 1-2   RESPONSIBILITY OF THE STATE IN A TRAUMA SYSTEM

1. Standards and guidelines are in place for the entire continuum of care.
2. A thorough evaluation process is in place for those hospitals that apply to be trauma centers.
3. Independent and qualified site survey teams are formed to determine if the applicant hospital meets the level of standard for trauma center certification.
4. Trauma system conducts research and provides education for health care providers, the public, and especially for the patient/victim.
5. The system continuously assesses workforce capability.
6. Appropriate trauma care and trauma system data are collected and used effectively to ensure high-level quality care delivery using performance improvement techniques.

(From U.S. Department of Health and Human Services, Health Resources and Services Administration, www.hrsa.gov/trauma/model.htm#core)

The goal of the performance improvement program for a trauma system is to improve system design and patient outcomes. A performance improvement program, which covers the continuum of care and identifies areas for improvement through data collection and analysis, is essential for the success of the trauma system. The performance improvement program should be dynamic and have the ability and authority to make changes. To solve performance improvement issues, strategies can be developed, implemented, and then reevaluated, and loop closure can be accomplished through establishing guidelines and policies, changing existing guidelines and policies, education, and purchasing equipment. The system includes monitoring mortality, morbidity, and outcomes, and meetings should be held to review results and give feedback.

Research

Research is essential for the improvement of trauma care. Quality research increases the knowledge of trauma as a disease, which then refines practice, creates better techniques, advances patient care, and improves patient outcomes.

Disaster Planning

An inclusive trauma system is of the utmost importance with disaster planning and response. The system uses common terminology and procedures in order to help with communication and coordination among state, federal agencies, and health care facilities. The plan distributes the patients in an equitable manner in order to prevent overburdening of facilities. A trauma system disaster plan includes many situations such as natural disasters, human-created disasters, terrorism, and use of weapons of mass destruction. The goal of the plan is to reduce mortality caused by the disaster and do the greatest good for the greatest number of people. The four components of a disaster plan are as follows: search and rescue, triage and initial stabilization, definitive care, and evacuation.[6]

SUMMARY

The trauma care system is an inclusive system integrating prehospital care, acute and general care, trauma centers, and rehabilitation facilities to ensure prompt and optimal treatment for all injured patients in a region or state. A successful trauma system allows all injured patients, urban or rural, to have equal access to all levels of care; reduces morbidity and mortality; has a formalized continuum of care from prehospital to rehabilitation; and has a performance improvement program to evaluate systems and outcomes using data collection and analysis.

References

1. Committee on Trauma, American College of Surgeons: *Resources for optimal care of the injured patient: 2006,* Chicago, 2006, The College.
2. National Safety Council: *Report on injuries in America,* Itasca, Ill, 2002, The Council. Available from *www.nsc.org/lrs/statinfo/99report.htm*
3. Maull KI, Esposito TJ: Trauma system design. In Mattox KL, Feliciano DV, Moore EE, editors: *Trauma,* ed 4, New York, 2000, McGraw-Hill.
4. U.S. Department of Health and Human Services Program Support Center, *Model Trauma System Planning* & Evaluation, Washington DC, February 2006, Health Resources and Services Administration, p. 1-70. *www.gov/trauma/model.htm*

Chapter 2

Prehospital Care

Stephen P. Wood

The earliest aspect of trauma care is the prehospital phase, the period from the injury occurrence through recognition of the emergency situation, response, resuscitation, triage, and transportation to definitive care. Prehospital trauma care is the foundation upon which subsequent elements of the trauma care system are built. A successful prehospital system integrates the public safety, public health, and health care systems to provide appropriate assessment, treatment, and transport of the trauma patient to an appropriate facility.

Modern civilian trauma systems have implemented many of the principles first learned by the military services during wartime. The military experience demonstrated that trauma is a time-sensitive disease event. The military achieved dramatic improvements in casualty survival by providing an organized system for trauma care. Lives were saved when care was initiated in the field (at the scene) and the time from injury to definitive surgical care was decreased. As these lessons were applied to civilian practice, prehospital emergency medical services (EMS) systems were developed that brought together education of the public and prehospital care providers, triage and practice guidelines, communications capabilities, and ground/air transport modes. Mature systems now also are engaged in quality improvement activities, clinical and systems research, public education, injury prevention, legislative activities, and public policy formation.

Prehospital Environment and Scene Safety

The prehospital environment is dynamic and can present sundry logistical situations to trauma care providers. The prehospital scene can at times be well controlled, while at other times chaotic. There can be threats of personal injury or illness not only to the patient but also to the care providers. Prehospital care providers may be exposed to a variety of adverse weather conditions, difficult terrain, biohazards and hazardous materials, extremes of noise, risk of fire, violent patients, and crowd control issues. For example, even a simple motor vehicle crash presents risks such as broken glass, downed wires, hazardous materials from the vehicle, the use of heavy extrication tools, traffic issues, and potentially combative patients. At all times, the personal safety of prehospital trauma care providers must come first.

The most important step for safety at the incident is personal preparation. Education is the key to safety preparedness. Prehospital care providers should receive ongoing continuing education in the principles of biologic hazards, hazardous materials response, and general scene safety. Additionally, prehospital care providers should practice this skill set actively. The prehospital care provider must be mentally alert and have focused communication with other team members. Standard precautions must be used at all times, including eye protection, gloves, respiratory protection, and gowns when appropriate. Personal immunization against hepatitis B and tetanus also should be current, as well as routine tuberculosis screening. Physical fitness and agility should be sufficient to permit the rescuer to perform tasks such as lifting and carrying equipment and patients, and care providers should be aware of and understand their own personal limitations. Protective, high-visibility clothing appropriate to the environmental risk should be used. For example, when caring for a patient during motor vehicle crash extrication, protection consisting of a helmet with face shield, heavy gloves, boots, and firefighting coat and pants is mandatory. All medical and rescue equipment should be checked at the beginning of each shift to ensure that it is complete and functional.

Many trauma scenes also may have criminal considerations, in which critical physical and forensic evidence may be present. Prehospital care providers should understand this and should ensure that the scene and any pertinent evidence are preserved to the best of their abilities. This frequently is accomplished with the assistance of appropriate law enforcement personnel.

INCIDENT MANAGEMENT AND WORKING AT THE SCENE

The prehospital care provider always works as part of a team. The field team is usually a heterogeneous, multiagency effort, made up of fire/rescue, law enforcement, and EMS personnel. To coordinate safely and effectively the efforts of individual units as a team, most jurisdictions implement an incident management system, also known as the incident command system (ICS). Incident management is a standard method of operating at all incidents, irrespective of incident size. The ICS was developed in the early 1970s to address the issues faced in the response to several California wildfires. The ICS was designed to be applicable to any scene management situation. The key element of the ICS is the establishment of a unified command structure. This system allows for an integrated approach to scene management and multipersonnel or multiagency communication. The incident commander, typically the senior medical or fire officer, is one of the most important positions in the ICS structure, and the commander is responsible for all aspects of the scene response. For large-scale scenes or events, several of these responsibilities can be delegated to other appropriate personnel, including duties such as planning, operations, security, triage, and safety.

On arrival at the incident location, the individual prehospital care provider should report, by radio, to the incident commander. The scene should not be approached until it has been evaluated for life-threatening hazards and access has been granted by the incident commander. The mechanism of the event then can be assessed to provide information regarding the potential number of victims, the potential severity of injury, and any special clinical issues such as burns or chemical exposure. The incident commander then must decide what resources will be required to secure the scene effectively and to provide rapid transport to the appropriate level of medical care.

Once one is working at the scene, constant vigilance is required so that risks are identified and controlled. An early determination also should be made whether the assets available on scene are sufficient to manage the situation. The unified command system ensures that appropriate triage, transport, fire suppression, and safety measures are being observed and communicated. This is especially important for air medical helicopter services and specialty rescue units, such as confined space, heavy rescue, or hazardous materials teams.

TRIAGE AND TRANSPORT

One of the most important concepts in prehospital trauma care is trauma triage. Triage is the responsibility of the individual prehospital care provider (or triage officer during mass casualty situations). The goal is to identify patients who need the specialty services of a trauma center. Trauma triage protocols and practices should be developed and monitored at the system level. A model approach to trauma triage has been promulgated by the American College of Surgeons (Figure 2–1).

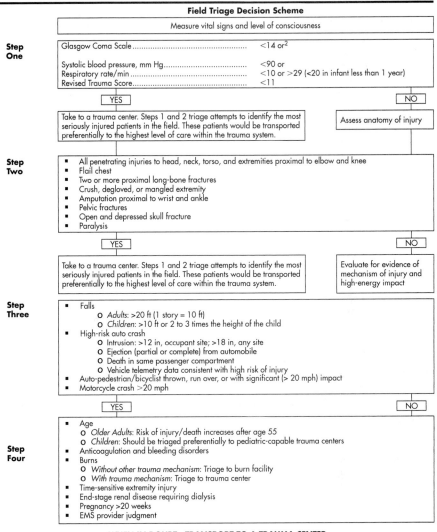

Field Triage Decision Scheme

| Measure vital signs and level of consciousness |

Step One

Glasgow Coma Scale	<14 or^2
Systolic blood pressure, mm Hg......................................	<90 or
Respiratory rate/min	<10 or >29 (<20 in infant less than 1 year)
Revised Trauma Score..	<11

YES   NO

Take to a trauma center. Steps 1 and 2 triage attempts to identify the most seriously injured patients in the field. These patients would be transported preferentially to the highest level of care within the trauma system.

Assess anatomy of injury

Step Two

- All penetrating injuries to head, neck, torso, and extremities proximal to elbow and knee
- Flail chest
- Two or more proximal long-bone fractures
- Crush, degloved, or mangled extremity
- Amputation proximal to wrist and ankle
- Pelvic fractures
- Open and depressed skull fracture
- Paralysis

YES   NO

Take to a trauma center. Steps 1 and 2 triage attempts to identify the most seriously injured patients in the field. These patients would be transported preferentially to the highest level of care within the trauma system.

Evaluate for evidence of mechanism of injury and high-energy impact

Step Three

- Falls
  - *Adults:* >20 ft (1 story = 10 ft)
  - *Children:* >10 ft or 2 to 3 times the height of the child
- High-risk auto crash
  - Intrusion: >12 in, occupant site; >18 in, any site
  - Ejection (partial or complete) from automobile
  - Death in same passenger compartment
  - Vehicle telemetry data consistent with high risk of injury
- Auto-pedestrian/bicyclist thrown, run over, or with significant (> 20 mph) impact
- Motorcycle crash >20 mph

YES   NO

Step Four

- Age
  - *Older Adults:* Risk of injury/death increases after age 55
  - *Children:* Should be triaged preferentially to pediatric-capable trauma centers
- Anticoagulation and bleeding disorders
- Burns
  - *Without other trauma mechanism:* Triage to burn facility
  - *With trauma mechanism:* Triage to trauma center
- Time-sensitive extremity injury
- End-stage renal disease requiring dialysis
- Pregnancy >20 weeks
- EMS provider judgment

WHEN IN DOUBT—TRANSPORT TO A TRAUMA CENTER

*From the publication *Resources For Optimal Care of the Injured Patient:* 2006, © Committee on Trauma, American College of Surgeons, Chicago, IL, p.14. Reprint permission by the American College of Surgeons.

Continued

A
RL/G4183036/EMS

Figure 2–1. Field triage decision scheme. *(From American College of Surgeons: Resources for optimal care of the injured patient: 2006, © Committee on Trauma, American College of Surgeons, Chicago. Reprint permission by the American College of Surgeons.)*

B

Note for Figure 1

This field triage decision scheme, originally developed by the American College of Surgeons Committee on Trauma, was revised by an expert panel representing emergency medical services, emergency medicine, trauma surgery, and public health. The panel was convened by the Centers for Disease Control and Prevention (CDC), with support from the National Highway Traffic Safety Administration (NHTSA). Its contents are those of the expert panel and do not necessarily represent the official views of CDC and NHTSA.

Figure 2–1, *cont'd,* Field triage decision scheme. *(From American College of Surgeons: Resources for optimal care of the injured patient: 2006, © Committee on Trauma, American College of Surgeons, Chicago. Reprint permission by the American College of Surgeons.)*

The greatest potential for harm comes from undertriage. *Undertriage* means that the patient's injuries were underestimated or that the patient was transported to a facility that did not have adequate resources to manage the patient. This can result in a delay in care and additional morbidity and mortality. A patient is *overtriaged* when the potential for injury is overestimated or more resources are deployed than are needed. The problem with overtriage is that it incurs additional expense to the system and diverts resources away from more seriously injured patients. Currently, no triage methodology totally avoids overtriage and undertriage. Trauma systems developers usually agree to tolerate a certain level of overtriage to protect patients and ensure that undertriage is kept to a minimum.

The provider must assess the patient's potential for serious injury and determine the best available facility to care for the patient, considering transport time and the capabilities of that particular facility. The closest facility is not always the best facility. The provider must decide whether the patient meets the criteria for entry into a trauma center, which may not be the closest facility. Determining the mode of transport also depends on the capabilities of the prehospital care providers and of the destination facility. When the destination is in question, it is best to make a conservative judgment and transport the patient to a predesignated trauma center. Early radio communication to the hospital of choice facilitates activation of the appropriate hospital personnel and opens a line of communication for online medical control.

The need for air medical transport from the scene is an additional consideration. These are helicopters or fixed-wing aircraft, typically staffed with advanced level providers with specialty training in trauma care. The use of air medical transport should be based on the mechanism of injury, severity of the patient's injuries, the need for rapid transport, physical distance from the appropriate care facility, the need for a higher level of care during transport, and other situational considerations. Some EMS systems use the criterion of travel time (e.g., greater than 20 minutes by ground) from an appropriate trauma center as one of the indications for activation of air transport. Air medical transport offers the advantages of high-level care, mobility, and speed of transport; disadvantages include the possibility of weather restrictions and lack of proximity of available landing zones. For an overview of the advantages and disadvantages of air and ground transport, see Chapter 4.

If air medical services are used, providers must know how to access the program and should have attended a formal briefing on aircraft landing zone safety and patient loading. Some of the key safety points to keep in mind are the following:

- Stay at least 50 to 100 feet away from a helicopter while it is landing or taking off. Consider shielding your eyes with goggles or a helmet shield because debris such as sand can be blown in a large perimeter.

- Do not approach the aircraft until the crew gives permission to do so or only when accompanied by a crew member.
- Watch flight crew for guidance and follow their instructions at all times.
- Approach the helicopter at a 30- to 45-degree angle from its front so that you can see the pilot and the pilot can see you.
- Never go to the rear of the helicopter.
- Do not place any part of your body higher than your body height (e.g., do not raise your arms above your head to elevate intravenous fluids).
- Secure all loose objects to protect them from rotor wash.

PREHOSPITAL TRAUMA RESUSCITATION

The goal of prehospital trauma resuscitation is to identify life-threatening injuries and to initiate therapy as soon as possible without delaying immediate transport to the trauma center. Because survival often is linked directly to the length of time from injury to trauma center care, prehospital care providers should strive to limit the time on scene by only addressing key tasks, such as airway control and immobilization of the spine. Some EMS services have a goal of no more than 10 minutes on scene (excluding time needed for extrication). All other assessments and interventions should be performed while en route to the trauma center. Physical assessment of the trauma patient at the scene often is hampered by poor access to the patient, lack of exposure, background noise, and other unfavorable conditions. The clinician therefore is challenged to develop assessment skills that overcome these evaluation obstacles. Field trauma resuscitation should follow the methodical but rapid Airway-Breathing-Circulation format for primary survey and intervention. Programs such as Prehospital Trauma Life Support and Basic Trauma Life Support are designed to facilitate an injury-guided assessment and treatment plan for prehospital care providers of all levels. These programs can be an excellent educational resource for managing trauma patients.

The prehospital trauma care provider should perform a systematic evaluation, with initial attention to the patient's level of consciousness and the patency of the airway. This assessment should be undertaken with simultaneous control of the cervical spine. These are the two most important field interventions for decreasing trauma morbidity and mortality. If a patient cannot maintain a patent airway, the airway must be secured at once. Endotracheal intubation is the most desirable method of securing the airway. This skill, however, can be difficult to perform in the field and should not be implemented without extensive provider training, strict protocols, and meticulous quality control. At all times, there must be a backup plan to manage the airway by reverting to basic maneuvers or by placing an alternative airway such as a laryngeal mask airway, Combitube, or surgical airway. The patency of the airway must be reensured at frequent intervals, especially when the patient is extricated or otherwise moved. This assessment should use clinical indicators, such as lung sounds and chest wall rise, and monitoring of end-tidal carbon dioxide and pulse oximetry.

Breathing should be assessed for rate, rhythm, and adequacy of air exchange. High-concentration supplemental oxygen should be administered. Ventilation should be assisted with a bag-valve ventilator whenever air exchange is inadequate. Prehospital care providers should be vigilant for signs and symptoms of a pneumothorax whenever providing positive-pressure ventilation. When caring for patients with brain injury, prehospital providers must maintain an awareness of the dangers of hypoxia, hypercapnia, and hypotension and must take measures to prevent or minimize these conditions as much as possible. Steps must be taken to avoid overaggressive ventilation, and ensure adequate oxygenation and blood pressure.

Circulation is assessed by checking for the presence of central pulses, such as the carotid or femoral pulse. Severe external hemorrhage is best managed with direct pressure to the wound. If bleeding is not controlled by this method, the prehospital care provider must resort systematically to the application of pressure to pressure points and, if necessary, tourniquet application. Large-bore intravenous access and infusion of fluids can be initiated while en route to the trauma center. The value of crystalloid administration remains controversial, but providers should follow local protocols, and enough volume should be provided to maintain adequate perfusion. Pneumatic antishock garments have not been proved to provide clinical benefit and are of limited utility in the management of trauma.

If at any time during the resuscitation, the prehospital provider is uncertain about how to proceed, or if there is an interruption in the plan of care, the provider should revert to fundamental assessments and interventions using the ABC format. Prehospital providers generally function under standing protocols for initial trauma care but should not hesitate to request medical direction for complicated cases.

COMMUNICATION AND DOCUMENTATION

Many of the communications that take place in the prehospital environment occur via radio systems that serve law enforcement, fire services, and EMS. When communicating by radio, remember to do the following:

- Speak clearly and briefly and directly into the microphone.
- Identify yourself by your service and unit number.
- Usual protocol is to say first who is being called and then who is calling. ("Beth Israel Deaconess Emergency, this is Boston MedFlight 1 with an entry notification for an adult trauma. Do you read?" "Boston MedFlight, this is Beth Israel Emergency, we read you loud and clear. Please go ahead with your transmission.")
- Protect patient confidentiality when conveying medical information. Remember that many persons, including citizens with radio scanners, are listening to these transmissions.
- Maintain professionalism; be patient when information or transmission is unclear. Never use profanity or jargon. Most systems tape all transmissions.
- Convey information in a systematic manner. Patient information should include age, gender, mechanism of injury, chief complaint, level of consciousness, including Glasgow Coma Scale score, brief description of suspected injuries, vital signs, interventions, and estimated time of arrival.
- At the completion of your transmission, ask if there are any questions. Answer the questions concisely, providing clarification when necessary. At the end of the transmission, advise that you have completed your transmission and are discontinuing radio contact.
- Sign off to indicate the end of your transmission.

Emergency department staff receiving the radio report should expect only a general understanding of the patient's condition. Nonessential questions should be held until the patient arrives to avoid tying up the radio channel or taking the EMS provider away from the patient.

On arrival at the trauma center, the patient report is given verbally to trauma team members. The report should include any changes that occurred during transport. Because the team simultaneously is assuming care of the patient, the prehospital provider should be prepared to repeat elements of the report. Written documentation of the prehospital care episode should be prepared and placed in the patient's medical record. The prehospital care report is important for patient care, quality improvement, research, and as a legal record. It must be accurate, legible, and complete.

TEAMWORK

Hospital-based trauma team members must encourage open communication with prehospital care providers, offer guidance and educational opportunities, and listen to concerns and suggestions. Inclusion of prehospital care providers in continuing education, case reviews, quality improvement programs, and research initiatives strengthens team relationships and improves patient care. Follow-up information given to prehospital providers on the trauma patient's injuries and outcome provides feedback and closure of the episode. Because of the stressful nature of prehospital care, there also should be opportunities for a team debriefing after difficult cases.

Nurses and physicians who work in emergency departments, critical care units, or trauma units are encouraged to ride as observers with EMS teams. This offers valuable insight into the early care of trauma patients, as well as improving the relationship between prehospital and hospital personnel.

Suggested Readings

Bledsoe B, Porter R, Cherry RA: *Essentials of paramedic care,* Upper Saddle River, NJ, 2002, Prentice-Hall.

Briggs S, Brinsfield K: *Advanced disaster medical response,* Boston, 2003, Harvard Medical International.

McSwain N Jr, Frame A, Salomone J, editors: *PHTLS basic and advanced prehospital trauma life support,* ed 5, St Louis, 2003, Mosby.

Moore E, Mattox K, Feliciano D: *Trauma manual,* ed 4, New York, 2002, McGraw-Hill.

CHAPTER 3

HOSPITAL SYSTEMS OF CARE

DIANNE M. DANIS

Trauma care optimally is provided within an inclusive regional system that encompasses prehospital, acute care, and rehabilitative components (see Chapter 1). Trauma centers are a key part of the system; in 2002, there were 1154 trauma centers in the United States.[1] This chapter discusses acute care facilities and the staff, equipment, and other resources necessary for trauma centers of any level, focusing primarily on the requirements related to emergency departments (EDs).

The concept of *commitment* to excellence in trauma care cannot be overemphasized. Within hospitals that aspire to be trauma centers, the commitment must be personal and institutional. Institutional commitment means that the hospital administration supports adequate personnel and resources on a 24-hour basis, along with priority access to these resources for major trauma patients. Institutional commitment also applies to providing continuing education for clinicians and to fulfilling a leadership and service role in the community in trauma care and injury prevention activities. Personal commitment demands that medical, nursing, and support personnel agree to provide dedicated and immediate availability 24 hours a day, as well as to participate in educational, performance improvement, injury prevention, and research activities.

TRAUMA CENTER CATEGORIZATION

The trauma care system has evolved to include different levels of trauma centers, based on need, geography, population density, and the capabilities and resources of each facility. Only 10% to 15% of all injured patients are estimated to require the resources of the highest-level trauma center, with the remainder of care being provided at other acute care facilities within the system.

The American College of Surgeons (ACS) has developed nationally recognized criteria and standards for level I to IV trauma centers. Many state, regional, or local systems apply the ACS criteria, modify the ACS criteria, or develop their own designation criteria. In the absence of a statewide system, some hospitals are simply self-designated or remain undesignated but still receive trauma patients.

Designation versus Verification

In formal trauma systems, each trauma care facility is officially *designated* by a regulatory body (frequently a state or regional emergency medical services agency) according to commitment, capabilities, and resources. Trauma center *designation,* a governmental process, differs from ACS *verification.* A verification survey may be part of a state or regional designation process but also may be voluntary on the part of a trauma center desiring to demonstrate excellence in trauma care.

The ACS verification process consists of the completion of an extensive presurvey questionnaire followed by a 2-day on-site survey. The survey, conducted by ACS surveyors, includes a dinner meeting, facility tour, multiple interviews with staff, review of program documents, and medical record review. Throughout the survey, emphasis is placed on evidence of institutional commitment, fulfillment of ACS standards, quality of care and patient outcomes, and the quality of the performance improvement program. The role of the individual trauma center within the regional or statewide system and community is examined as well. State or regional surveys have similar processes and components.

Trauma Center Levels

The following definitions of trauma center categories are excerpted from the ACS publication *Resources for Optimal Care of the Injured Patient: 2006.*[2] This document outlines essential and desirable criteria for trauma center organization, staff, facility resources and services, performance improvement, education, research, and injury prevention for all levels of trauma centers.

Level I

The level I trauma center is a regional resource trauma center and tertiary care facility central to the trauma care system. This facility must have the capability of providing leadership and total care for every aspect of injury, from prevention through rehabilitation. In addition to acute care responsibilities, level I trauma centers have the major responsibility of providing leadership in education, research, injury prevention, and system planning. This responsibility extends to all hospitals caring for injured patients in their regions.

Level II

The level II trauma center is a hospital that also is expected to provide initial definitive trauma care, regardless of the severity of injury. Depending on geographic location, patient volume, personnel, and resources, however, the level II trauma center may not be able to provide the same comprehensive care as a level I trauma center. Therefore, patients with more complex injuries may have to be transferred to a level I center. Level II trauma centers may be the most prevalent facility in a community, managing the majority of trauma patients.

Level III

The level III trauma center serves communities that do not have immediate access to a level I or II institution. Level III trauma centers can provide prompt assessment, resuscitation, emergency operations, and stabilization and also arrange for possible transfer to a facility that can provide definitive trauma care.

Level IV

Level IV trauma facilities provide advanced trauma life support before patient transfer in remote areas where no higher level of care is available. Such a facility may be a clinic rather than a hospital and may or may not have a physician available.

SPECIALTY TRAUMA CENTERS

Pediatric Trauma Care

Severely injured children require appropriate acute and rehabilitative care to improve survival and minimize long-term disability. The ACS verifies pediatric trauma centers—freestanding pediatric hospitals or hospitals providing care to adults and children—at levels I to IV, similar to adult trauma centers. However, trauma centers that make the commitment to care for injured children must have additional specialized resources available. Personnel requirements include a multidisciplinary team approach and staff with appropriate expertise in the care of injured children. Additionally, level I and II centers providing pediatric trauma care must have pediatric ED facilities (either a separate pediatric ED or a pediatric area within a combined ED), pediatric resuscitation equipment, a pediatric intensive care unit, and a pediatric-specific performance improvement program.[2]

Burn Centers

As in the larger trauma population, an inclusive system of care must provide for the entire spectrum of burn injury. Patients with major burn injuries require specialized acute and rehabilitative management in burn units. Burn units typically are located within level I or II trauma centers because of the resource intensity and specialized surgical critical care required. Burn centers are verified through a joint program of the ACS and the American Burn Association. Like trauma centers, burn units are expected to adhere to standards regarding specialized expertise, facility resources, performance improvement, education, research, injury prevention, and outreach responsibilities.[2]

TRAUMA RESUSCITATION TEAM

The trauma resuscitation team provides care to major trauma patients and is the core of a trauma care program. The team should operate according to the fundamental philosophy of a trauma resuscitation as a coordinated, standardized, multidisciplinary team process.

Trauma Team Members

Although the composition of the trauma team may vary among different institutions and trauma center levels, certain core personnel are necessary to provide appropriate evaluation and resuscitation. These personnel include the following:

- Trauma surgeon/team leader (attending surgeon or senior surgical resident)
- Additional physician assistance (surgery, emergency medicine, anesthesia, radiology)
- Primary registered nurse
- Additional nursing assistance (such as associate, circulating, and/or recording nurses)
- Radiology technician
- Respiratory therapist (as necessary)

A number of other disciplines and services may be part of the trauma team, some to respond as needed, others to be ready to provide services within their departments on demand. These include social services, pastoral care, computed tomography scan, the blood bank, operating room, intensive care unit, and laboratory.

The number of team members and the exact composition of the team should be determined by the needs of each facility. However, every team should have *one* clearly identified physician team leader who orchestrates a rapid, organized, and efficient resuscitation. Team members must be clear about their roles and responsibilities and perform them rapidly and simultaneously, with minimal direction and discussion.

Trauma Team Activation

Criteria for activating the trauma team and communication systems for notifying members of the trauma team to respond to the ED vary among different institutions and trauma center levels depending on capabilities and resources. Many trauma centers and regional trauma systems follow or modify ACS criteria as guidelines for determining when the trauma team needs to be activated (see Chapter 2).

Some trauma centers have refined their trauma team system further to incorporate a "tiered" response with the goals of more appropriately using resources, allocating staff, and reducing costs. In a nontiered response system, the full trauma team is activated for every trauma patient. In a tiered response, selected team members respond based on prehospital report of injuries and severity—the full team responds for patients with major trauma, and a smaller team for less severely injured patients. Box 3-1 lists typical criteria for a two-tiered trauma team. In some facilities, lower-level trauma resuscitations are conducted mainly by ED staff. Criteria for activating the trauma team should be defined collaboratively and clearly by a multidisciplinary trauma center administrative committee and must adhere to state and regional regulations, as well as ACS verification standards if applicable.

The system for activation of the trauma team usually includes a multiple-page beeper (voice or digital) system that announces the arrival or the estimated time of arrival of a trauma patient.

Box 3-1 **SAMPLE TWO-TIER CRITERIA FOR TRAUMA TEAM ACTIVATION**

Trauma Alpha: activate expanded trauma team

- Systolic blood pressure less than 90 mm Hg
- Respiratory rate less than 10 or greater than 29 breaths per minute
- Glasgow Coma Scale score less than 14
- Penetrating injuries to head, neck, or torso
- Flail chest
- Two or more proximal long-bone fractures
- Major pelvic fractures
- Paralysis
- Major burns

Trauma Beta: activate core trauma team

- High-speed auto crash, ejection, or rollover
- Motorcycle crash greater than 20 mph or with separation of rider from bike
- Bicycle versus auto with significant impact
- Auto-pedestrian injury with significant impact, or pedestrian thrown or run over
- Age younger than 5 or older than 55
- Pregnancy
- Serious preexisting medical disease

Early notification is important, so that the team can be prepared and assembled before the patient's arrival. However, the trauma team system also must be able to function efficiently in the absence of any advance warning.

Resuscitation Roles and Responsibilities

The first step in the evaluation and resuscitation of a trauma patient is for the team to receive a rapid and concise report from the prehospital provider. Reporting should occur while simultaneously moving the patient onto the hospital trauma stretcher, gaining exposure to the patient, and initiating the primary survey.

Trauma resuscitation evaluation and intervention traditionally follow the recommendations of the Advanced Trauma Life Support Course. The Trauma Nursing Core Course[3] (TNCC) teaches a similar approach. Both courses advocate a stepwise, standardized, and organized multidisciplinary team approach, prioritizing care by using "primary" (airway, breathing, circulation, and disability assessment, coupled with immediate intervention for life-threatening conditions) and "secondary" (head-to-toe identification of all other non–life-threatening injuries) surveys. This approach to evaluation and resuscitation enhances efficiency and minimizes delayed or missed diagnoses. Chapter 11 covers the specifics of the trauma evaluation and resuscitation.

Every trauma center should develop and define roles and responsibilities for each trauma team member, covering all the activities and tasks that need to be carried out during a resuscitation.

TRAUMA ROOM

The trauma resuscitation area should be designed to meet the needs of the major trauma patient by providing immediate access to all of the equipment necessary to perform a rapid and efficient resuscitation. The trauma resuscitation room or bay must be equipped and standing at the ready (or be *immediately* available) at all times to receive trauma victims (ideally two to three at once), with or without advance notice. A discrete, dedicated, and fully equipped resuscitation area for pediatric patients is also necessary, either contained within the larger trauma space or located in another part of the ED.

The space for trauma resuscitations must be able to accommodate the entire trauma team, as well as necessary equipment such as ventilators, x-ray machines, and ultrasound machines. Adequate lighting, the ability to warm the resuscitation area rapidly, telephone lines (including "hot lines" to blood bank, operating room, and trauma surgeons), computer terminals, an intercom system, and communication boards mounted in visible places (for communicating and documenting patient information, on-call schedules, standard drug doses and formulas, and other useful information) are important considerations. A sample trauma room layout is depicted in Figure 3-1.

The following equipment and procedure trays and sets should be marked clearly and placed strategically adjacent to the location where the procedure is likely to be performed:

- Airway management
- Phlebotomy/intravenous access
- Rapid infusor/warmer system
- Tube thoracostomy
- Urinary catheterization kit
- Gastric tube equipment
- Laceration stapling/suturing kits

Trauma Bay Setup

An example of a trauma resuscitation bay containing a single stretcher with strategically placed equipment.

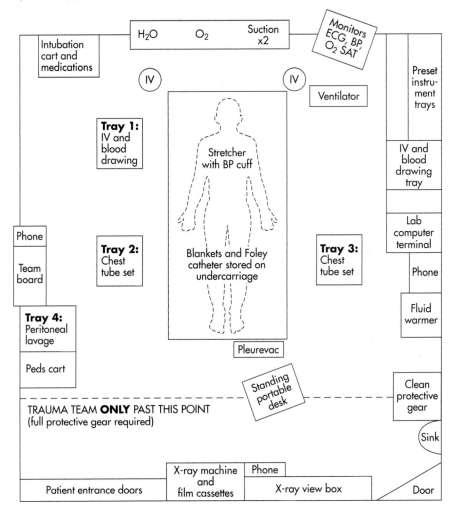

Figure 3–1. Trauma room layout. *(From Committee on Trauma, American College of Surgeons:* Resources for optimal care of the injured patient: 1999, *Chicago, 1999, American College of Surgeons.)*

- Diagnostic peritoneal lavage
- Open thoracotomy
- Pelvic fixators

Nurses and physicians awaiting a patient's arrival should always prepare the area further, being sure that equipment and supplies are ready for the specific type of patient expected. A convenient way to organize preparation is to use the ABCD mnemonic (airway, breathing, circulation, and disability assessment) and head-to-toe approach, the same as during patient assessment. Thus, airway and breathing equipment would be prepared first; then fluid resuscitation equipment; then equipment according to the reported or hypothesized injuries, starting with brain and spinal cord; and finally other injuries moving from head to toe. The resuscitation bay should be cleaned and restocked rapidly after every resuscitation and each shift.

Access to the resuscitation area should be limited strictly to those team members who will play an active role in the resuscitation. Many centers use some type of physical barrier to define clearly essential versus nonessential resuscitation personnel, for example, a yellow line on the floor. Anyone who crosses this line must have a legitimate reason for doing so and must don standard precautions garb (i.e., fluid-impervious gowns, gloves, and face protection). The importance of "crowd" and noise control cannot be overemphasized. Only the team leader should speak, directing the flow of the resuscitation, giving orders, and requesting information from team members. The primary nurse keeps the team leader apprised of the status of the patient and collaborates to implement the plan of care. Emergency nurses are in a good position to create the appropriate "culture" for resuscitations, one that encourages collaborative teamwork, is sensitive to and respects patients and families, and preserves confidentiality.

TRAUMA CARE DOCUMENTATION

The thorough, accurate, and legible documentation of all phases of the trauma patient's care is, of course, important for many reasons. In addition to allowing performance improvement activities, a good record also supplies data needed for the trauma registry, supports maximal financial reimbursement, and provides adequate legal justification for care that was (or was not) provided. Another important aspect of trauma documentation, but beyond the scope of this chapter, is the preservation of forensic evidence.

Designation of a separate flow sheet specifically for documenting trauma care is recommended to capture all necessary data for performance improvement and legal purposes. Reviewing examples from other institutions can be helpful. The flow sheet should be user-friendly to expedite and facilitate the capture of information. Even though it is recommended that there be a dedicated nurse recorder present during resuscitations, volume or staff limitations may not allow this at all times. A form that contains features such as checkoff lists, boxes, easily calculated scores (e.g., Glasgow Coma Scale score), anatomic diagrams to identify injury sites, and yes/no options makes documentation easier.

The emergent nature of trauma care certainly presents obstacles to documenting care at the time that it occurs, but nurses should not feel absolved from the responsibility of completing a sound record. Subsequent completion or amendment of records is acceptable as long as the appropriate notations are made to indicate when and by whom the additions were made.

Trauma documentation should include, at a minimum, the following:

- Time of arrival, procedures, significant events, and disposition to other diagnostic and/or definitive care areas; and, importantly, the notification and arrival times of the trauma team, trauma attending surgeon, and other subspecialists such as neurosurgeon or anesthesiologist.
- Key prehospital information: mechanism of injury, field interventions, patient responses
- Patient health history: medical history, medications, allergies
- Initial and frequent vital signs and Glasgow Coma Scale scores
- Results of the primary and secondary surveys with pertinent positive and negative findings
- All treatments, procedures, significant events, and patient responses
- All medications and fluids given before arrival and in the ED
- All laboratory study and x-ray results

- All team members present, family, and others
- Patient belongings and forensic evidence collected

Some trauma centers create separate physician and nursing forms, dividing up the data documentation burden. Any system that works well is acceptable. Also recommended is that trauma flow sheets be produced on multiple-copy paper to provide extra copies in the event of lost forms or for use by the trauma registry.

Regular performance improvement monitoring flow sheet documentation should be performed collaboratively by the trauma program manager and ED nursing staff to ensure compliance and to identify areas that require further education and/or counseling.

TRAUMA PERFORMANCE IMPROVEMENT

An effective performance improvement program for trauma care and trauma centers is essential (and is mandated by the ACS verification standards). The most common reason cited for the failure of an ACS verification review is the lack of an adequate performance improvement program. The trauma performance improvement program is multifaceted. The program incorporates peer review and credentialing, continuous and periodic monitoring of process and outcome indicators, mortality review, and other performance improvement activities. Although using ACS and other resources as a foundation,[2,4,5] the program should be designed carefully to address the unique aspects of the individual facility.

The goal of any performance improvement program is to improve patient outcome. In the same way that there must be institutional and personal commitment to being a trauma center, there must be mutual respect for and commitment to the performance improvement program by all who participate in the trauma care system. Nurses in all areas of the trauma center play a key role in defining a patient-focused performance improvement program, identifying deviations from standards, and monitoring compliance with protocol or policy changes. ED nurses have a critical role in effecting changes in practice to improve patient outcome. The trauma program manager will work closely with the ED nursing staff in this endeavor.

Performance Improvement Monitoring

Trauma centers are required to have an extensive performance improvement program, including systematic monitoring of quality indicators. Examples of indicators that apply specifically to the resuscitation phase of care include the following:

- All trauma deaths (including a determination of preventability, potential preventability, or nonpreventability of the death)
- Trauma team activation appropriateness (mistriage)
- Trauma surgeon response to trauma room
- Measurement of patient temperature in trauma room
- Hourly documentation of vital signs on trauma flow sheet
- Patients with a Glasgow Coma Scale score less than or equal to 8 who leave the ED without a definitive airway
- Patients with abdominal injuries and hypotension (systolic blood pressure less than 90 mm Hg) who do not undergo laparotomy within 1 hour of arrival
- Patients with an epidural or subdural hematoma who undergo craniotomy more than 4 hours after arrival
- Patients with an open tibial fracture, excluding a low-velocity gunshot wound, and an interval of longer than 8 hours between arrival and the initiation of débridement

Videotaping Trauma Resuscitations

The videotaping or digital recording of trauma resuscitations for performance improvement review and provider education is used in many trauma centers. Videotaping can be a valuable adjunct to the trauma performance improvement program. Watching and analyzing actual resuscitations are powerful learning experiences. Also, trauma videotapes allow the lessons learned during a trauma resuscitation to be disseminated among many clinicians.

The prospect of being videotaped can be intimidating and may lead to resistance among staff. How the program is presented is important in eliciting cooperation and willing participation. A nonthreatening, collaborative approach is essential.

Videotape reviews can improve resuscitations in the following areas:

- Prehospital report and patient entry
- Primary and secondary survey: performance and completeness
- Treatment priorities and decision making
- Procedures and techniques
- Standard precautions compliance
- System breakdowns: improving efficiency, eliminating delays
- Team leadership: organizational and communication skills
- Teamwork: improving communication and collaboration
- Clinical scenarios: correlating book learning with real life

The use of videotaping carries with it some significant concerns about peer review protection and patient confidentiality. The trauma center must approach this issue with careful planning after researching national, state, and hospital requirements concerning confidentiality and peer review protection. The Joint Commission on Accreditation of Healthcare Organizations has suggested that patient or family consent must be obtained prior to taping.[6] However, according to the ACS, "it has been recognized that this is impractical in most settings of trauma resuscitation and an institutional policy on videotaping dealing with confidentiality and subsequent tape destruction is used by many trauma centers to support this practice."[7]

A protocol for who will activate the camera, who will have access to tapes or digital recordings, and where and how long tapes will be stored must be defined clearly. The forums for review also should be defined clearly and covered under peer review laws, and access to these sessions should be appropriately limited as well.

QUALIFICATIONS OF NURSES CARING FOR TRAUMA PATIENTS

Nurses play a critical role in the assessment, management, ongoing monitoring, and planning of care for trauma patients. Expert care of trauma patients requires a combination of training and education, skill, and experience.

The *Resource Document for Nursing Care of the Trauma Patient*[8] makes recommendations concerning the trauma-related expectations of emergency nursing services. Emergency nursing services should provide a trauma-related component of orientation and an annual trauma skills validation. In collaboration with the trauma program, nurses should participate in the trauma performance improvement program and develop ED-specific trauma-related policies and procedures.

The ED should identify one or more trauma resource nurses. The trauma resource nurse may be a clinical nurse, clinical nurse specialist, nurse educator, or nurse manager. The trauma resource nurse possesses a special interest and expertise in trauma, serves as a consultant and role model, and works to develop the trauma skills of the rest of the staff.

The *Resource Document* recommends that at least 50% of the ED nursing staff be currently verified in TNCC, the Emergency Nursing Pediatric Course or Pediatric Advanced Life Support, and Advanced Cardiac Life Support. At least one nurse in every trauma resuscitation should be a TNCC provider.[8] State designation criteria also may have specific requirements for nursing qualifications.

Nurses who work in trauma center EDs will be expected to obtain trauma-related continuing education annually. Some of this education should be provided within the trauma center. In addition, there are many nationally accepted educational programs available to trauma nurses. These include TNCC, Course in Advanced Trauma Nursing, Advanced Trauma Care for Nurses, Advanced Trauma Life Support, Emergency Nursing Pediatric Course, Pediatric Advanced Life Support, and Advanced Burn Life Support. Other educational opportunities include regional, state, and national conferences.

BEYOND THE EMERGENCY DEPARTMENT

The evaluation and management of trauma patients is far from over when the patient leaves the ED. The continuum of care frequently extends from the ED to the operating room, intensive care unit, surgical floor, and on to the rehabilitation phase and may unfold over the next several weeks, months, or years. The care of trauma patients may require the services of every department in the hospital at one time or another, frequently as a top priority.

Trauma center expectations extend beyond the ED as well. A trauma center must have an organized trauma service, a trauma registry, a qualified surgeon trauma chief and surgical staff, and a trauma program manager (almost always a nurse). The areas that care for trauma patients, particularly the operating room and intensive care unit, are held to high expectations, similar to the ED, regarding personnel and resources. Additional standards apply to radiology and laboratory services and other services and departments throughout the hospital.

References

1. MacKenzie EJ, Hoyt DB, Sacra JC, Jurkovich GJ, Carlini AR, Teitelbaum SD, Teter H: National inventory of hospital trauma centers, *JAMA* 289:1515-1522, 2003.
2. Committee on Trauma, American College of Surgeons: *Resources for optimal care of the injured patient: 2006,* Chicago 2006, The College.
3. *Trauma Nursing Core Course,* ed 5, Des Plaines, Ill, 2000, Emergency Nurses Association.
4. Performance Improvement Subcommittee of the American College of Surgeons Committee on Trauma: *Trauma performance improvement,* Chicago, 2002, American College of Surgeons, available online at www.facs.org.
5. Fitzpatrick MK, Mattice C, Martin K: *Trauma outcomes & performance improvement course,* Sante Fe, NM, 2000, Society of Trauma Nurses.
6. Brown DM: Video recording of emergency department trauma resuscitations, *J Trauma Nurs* 10(3):79-81, 2003.
7. Performance Improvement Subcommittee of the American College of Surgeons Committee on Trauma: *Trauma performance improvement,* Chicago, 2002, American College of Surgeons, available online at www.facs.org, p. 16.
8. *Resource document for nursing care of the trauma patient,* ed 2, Des Plaines, Ill, 1997, Emergency Nurses Association.

CHAPTER 4

PATIENT TRANSFER

KAREN DRISCOLL

When the needs of a trauma patient exceed the capabilities of the facility caring for that patient, patient transfer is necessary. Positive patient outcomes depend on an efficient patient transfer process. The first step in this process is the development of a comprehensive transfer plan.

This chapter discusses interfacility transfers, but *intra*facility transfers (e.g., from the emergency department to the operating room, the intensive care unit, or the computed tomography scanner) also require planning and preparation. Appropriately trained staff and the proper equipment should accompany patients whenever they are in transit.

TRANSFER PLAN

Every institution should have a transfer plan that has been coordinated between transferring and receiving agencies before the need for actual patient transport. Agency policies and procedures should be consistent with local or regional policies, when they exist.

The transfer plan should include the following:

- Criteria defining types of patients to be transferred
- Criteria defining appropriate receiving facilities for each type of patient (trauma, burns, pediatric)
- Names and contact phone numbers of receiving facilities
- Guidelines for the selection of the appropriate transfer mode and accompanying personnel
- Names and contact phone numbers of ambulance and helicopter services
- Communications procedures with transport services and receiving facilities
- Requirements for stabilization before transfer
- Requirements and expectations of the receiving facility
- Forms for documentation before and during the transfer and documentation guidelines
- Lists of equipment and supplies (or prepackaged kits) to accompany patient, if hospital personnel conduct a transfer
- Guidelines for care en route
- Policy detailing who assumes financial responsibility for the transfer
- Provisions for families and friends of the patient

In addition, patient care plans should be developed for patients who have sustained multiple trauma, serious single-system injuries (such as head, cervical spine, chest, or abdomen), amputations, and burn injuries. Transfer care plans for infants, children, pregnant women, and elderly patients also should be in place.

LEGAL CONSIDERATIONS

Important legal considerations apply to transfer situations. The Consolidated Omnibus Budget Reconciliation Act (COBRA) is a federal law enacted in 1986. COBRA later was combined with the Emergency Medical Treatment and Active Labor Act (EMTALA). The most recent EMTALA regulations were published in 2003.[1] The overall purpose of COBRA and EMTALA is to provide guidelines for and to regulate the treatment and transfer of patients between hospitals. See Chapter 7 for more discussion of EMTALA.

The following are key points relevant to trauma patient transfers:

- Hospitals are obligated to provide *appropriate* medical screening examinations to all patients who arrive at their emergency department.
- The reason(s) for transfer and advantages of sending a patient to another facility must be documented clearly. Patients should be transferred only to a higher level of care (i.e., a level III trauma center should transfer to a level I trauma center) or to a lateral level of care (i.e., the patient is followed at a specific hospital that has at least the same capabilities as the sending facility).
- Ground and air ambulances must have appropriate personnel and equipment for the transfer. The level of care provided during interfacility transfers should not fall below the level of care provided within the referring hospital. Nursing organizations, such as the Emergency Nurses Association, have created specific position statements in regard to this issue. The Emergency Nurses Association recommends that if a patient requires specialized nursing care before transfer, the same expertise should be maintained during transfer.[2]
- All patients must be maximally stabilized, before transfer, within the capabilities of the sending facility.

Transfer documentation should include, when possible, permission to transfer the patient given by the patient or the patient's next of kin. The acceptance of the patient to be transferred at the receiving facility also should be documented along with the receiving physician's name.

PREPARATION FOR TRANSFER TO A TRAUMA CENTER

Decision to Transfer

Each institution should develop criteria for transfer based on the availability of specific personnel, skills, equipment, or technology. To be able to determine when a patient needs definitive care beyond the scope of what is available in the receiving initial hospital, community, or system is important. General guidelines concerning patients likely to require trauma center care are available from the American College of Surgeons (Box 4-1).

Modes of Transport

Clinical personnel should identify the various modes of transport available to the facility or community and should be familiar with the advantages and disadvantages of each so that an informed decision can be made as to the best means of transport for the patient requiring transfer. Personnel also should be familiar with the means to gain access to these transportation modes and know how to access regional resource centers. Having transport policies and plans in place before the need arises is wise. These policies and plans should be written with the mutual agreement of the referring and receiving facilities and the transporting agencies.

When determining the mode of transportation that would best serve the needs of the patient being transferred, clinical personnel should consider the urgency of the need for transfer; the

| Box 4-1 | CRITERIA FOR CONSIDERATION OF TRANSFER |

These guidelines are not intended to be hospital-specific.

A. Critical injuries to Level I or highest regional trauma center
 1. Carotid or vertebral arterial injury
 2. Torn thoracic aorta or great vessel
 3. Cardiac rupture
 4. Bilateral pulmonary contusion with Pao_2 to Fio_2 ratio less than 200
 5. Major abdominal vascular injury
 6. Grade IV or V liver injuries requiring >6 units red blood cell transfusion in 6 hours
 7. Unstable pelvic fracture requiring >6 units red blood cell transfusion in 6 hours
 8. Fracture or dislocation with loss of distal pulses

B. Life-threatening injuries to Level I or Level II trauma center
 1. Penetrating injury or open fracture of the skull
 2. Glasgow Coma Scale score <14 or lateralizing neurologic signs
 3. Spinal fracture or spinal cord deficit
 4. More than 2 unilateral rib fractures or bilateral rib fractures with pulmonary contusion
 5. Open long bone fracture
 6. Significant torso injury with advanced comorbid disease (such as coronary artery disease, chronic obstructive pulmonary disease, type 1 diabetes mellitus, or immunosuppression)

Note: It may be appropriate for an injured patient to undergo operative control of ongoing hemorrhage before transfer if a qualified surgeon and operating room resources are promptly available at the referring hospital.

(From Committee on Trauma, American College of Surgeons: *Resources for optimal care of the injured patient:* 2006, Chicago, 2006. The College.)

type and capabilities of the personnel involved in the transport; the type of equipment necessary to care for the patient during transport; the amount of patient care and work space required during transfer; and other limiting factors such as weather conditions, terrain, and transport distance.

Ground Ambulance

Advantages

- May be more readily available than airborne vehicles
- May be staffed by advanced life support (ALS) personnel with ALS equipment
- May be able to carry more than one patient or one patient plus large pieces of equipment
- Usually adequate space in which to provide patient care
- Can travel in most weather conditions

- Usually less noisy than aircraft
- Usually has space for additional personnel or family members

Disadvantages

- Increased transport times
- Possibility that ALS personnel and equipment are not available
- Possible need to travel on icy or muddy roads
- Limited access to certain terrain
- Sometimes bumpy or rough ride

Helicopter (Rotorcraft)

Advantages

- Relatively fast (twice as fast as ground travel for the same distances)
- Usually staffed by a combination of ALS and/or critical care personnel including nurses, physicians, respiratory therapists
- May be able to fly when road conditions are poor
- May be able to land on adverse terrain that is not prepared for fixed-wing aircraft or that cannot be reached by ground vehicle
- Can travel long distances
- Flight usually relatively smooth

Disadvantages

- Strict limits on number of crew and passengers it can carry
- May be limits on amount or size of equipment it can carry
- Very limited space in smaller models
- May be limited by adverse weather conditions
- Noisy
- Weight restrictions
- Usually most expensive mode of transportation

Airplane (Fixed-Wing Aircraft)

Advantages

- Usually holds more personnel and equipment than helicopter
- Usually has more patient-care space than helicopter
- Can sometimes fly *above* the weather
- Can travel long distances at high speeds
- Cabins usually can be pressurized

Disadvantages

- Not always on standby; therefore, may take longer to obtain service
- Has limited landing capabilities
- Noisy
- Low humidity

Physiologic Effects of Air Transport at High Altitudes

High altitudes can have the following physiological effects on patients transported by air:

- Possible hypoxia
- Acceleration or deceleration forces
- Gas expansion with altitude increase
- Motion sickness
- Dehydration
- Vibration or motion
- Increased noise
- Thermal changes (decreased ambient temperature at high altitudes)

Equipment Considerations for Transfer

Give consideration to the following equipment requirements for patient transfer:

- Oxygen and oxygen delivery mechanism (including ventilator)
- Airway adjuncts (including intubation equipment)
- Intravenous access supplies
- Intravenous fluids and infusion pumps
- Emergency medications
- Prescribed medications
- Monitor with electrocardiogram, noninvasive blood pressure device, pulse oximetry, and end-tidal carbon dioxide capabilities
- Defibrillator/pacemaker
- Suction equipment
- Stabilization devices (splints)
- Supplies for needle thoracostomy
- Heimlich valve with appropriate drainage or suction device
- Wound dressings
- Power source and backup power source (extra batteries) for all equipment

Information That Should Accompany the Patient

Information transmitted to receiving facilities by facsimile machine or electronic media before the patient's arrival assists the receiving team's preparation, but hard copies of this information should be sent along with the patient as well. This information includes the following:

- Patient's name and age
- Family status (whether or not members are en route and what information they have been given)
- Name, address, and phone number for next of kin
- Referring physician's name and phone number
- Receiving physician's name and phone number
- Name and phone number of contact person at referring facility
- Details of incident
- Patient assessment information
- Medical history, medications, allergies

- Flow sheet that includes the following:
  - Medications
  - Vital signs
  - Serial neurologic examinations
  - Any diagnostic and therapeutic interventions
  - Intake and output record
  - Laboratory results
  - Monitoring parameters
- Radiology (x-ray films, computed tomography scans) studies
- Pretransfer discharge note
- Time at which patient departed the referring facility
- Copies of patient's current and old medical records, if available
- Information about patient valuables (give to family when possible)

Stabilization of the Patient for Transport

An attempt to stabilize the patient before transport to another facility is essential. Clinical personnel should consider not only immediate needs but also those needs that may arise *during* transport. Anticipation of potential problems is the key to a safe and smooth transfer.

It is important to strive for the minimum amount of time possible in the referral facility by deferring all nonessential tests and interventions and by developing an efficient transfer process. Conducting a complete patient workup before transfer is not necessary. Once the need for transfer has been recognized, the patient should be stabilized and transferred as quickly as possible.

Airway

Clinical personnel should ensure that the patient has a patent airway. Endotracheal intubation should be considered if the patient has evidence of multisystem trauma with signs of hypoperfusion, anatomic disruption (e.g., burns or facial trauma), an altered level of consciousness, an increased risk of aspiration (e.g., difficulty handling secretions), or hypoxemia and hypoventilation (e.g., smoke inhalation or flail chest). If an airway adjunct is in place, personnel should be sure that it is secured for transport and that a spare is carried in the event of accidental removal.

Breathing

Patients should be placed on supplemental high-flow oxygen. The supply available should be sufficient to provide the patient with oxygen until arrival at the receiving facility. A full E-cylinder of oxygen lasts approximately 60 minutes at sea level if run at 15 L/min flow rate.

If the patient has sustained a pneumothorax, placement of a flutter valve or chest tube before transfer should be considered. Thoracostomy for pneumothorax is a clinical decision, and pneumothoraces generally do not require special or different treatment if patients are being transported by air. Once a chest tube is placed, it should be connected to a drainage system before patient transfer. If suction is required, personnel should include an additional suction device on the transport equipment list. A bulb syringe often can be used as an emergency backup suction device.

Equipment should be available to provide positive pressure assisted ventilation, if the need arises.

If the patient has an endotracheal tube in place or is at high risk for vomiting, an orogastric or nasogastric tube should be placed before transport to decompress the stomach and minimize the risk of aspiration, especially if the transport is over a long distance, over rough terrain, or by air when vibration and turbulence are anticipated.

Circulation

Appropriate therapeutic interventions should be performed with the goal of maintaining an adequate pulse and blood pressure and controlling external bleeding.

Clinical personnel should initiate and/or maintain two large-bore (14 gauge if possible) intravenous lines, and warmed crystalloid solutions (usually Ringer's lactate or normal saline) should be used to maintain the systolic blood pressure above 90 mm Hg. Plastic intravenous bags should be used to accommodate expansion and contraction of gases during high-altitude flights. Intravenous tubing should be minimized, and excess intravenous tubing should be coiled and taped to avoid inadvertent snagging and possible accidental removal.

An indwelling urinary catheter should be placed if the flight will take place over a long distance or if the patient requires it for comfort or monitoring.

Personnel should anticipate heat loss during transfer and promote normothermia with extra blankets and ambient heat.

Cervical Spine/Thoracic Spine

Clinical personnel should maintain alignment of the cervical and thoracic spine by providing stabilization with immobilization devices. Placement of the patient on a backboard minimizes patient movement during the transfer, decreases the likelihood of injury, and reduces the amount of pain the patient will experience. The patient should be secured adequately so that, if emesis occurs, the patient can be turned on his or her side without compromising spinal immobilization.

The need for restraints should be evaluated before departure from the referring facility. If restraints are not used at the outset, they should be within easy reach of the attendant during transfer in case the patient becomes agitated and creates a risk to treatment or his or her safety or that of the transfer crew. Physical or pharmacologic restraints may be needed.

Splints

All suspected or documented fractures, including pelvic fractures, and dislocations should be splinted appropriately. Air splints should not be used during air transport because expansion with altitude may cause tissue and circulatory compromise. A pneumatic antishock garment inflated to a splinting pressure or a linen sheet wrap may be used to splint pelvic fractures before transport. Personnel should check and document distal neurovascular status before and after splinting and after any movement of the patient. Traction splints may be used as appropriate.

Wound Care

External bleeding can be controlled by applying direct pressure. If pressure dressings have been applied, personnel should indicate this verbally and in writing in the patient's record.

Tetanus prophylaxis or tetanus immune globulin should be administered in accordance with standard guidelines. The appropriate antibiotics also should be administered.

Burn wounds should be covered with dry, sterile dressings. Clinical personnel should avoid wet dressings because they may cause the patient to develop severe hypothermia. The patient's level of pain should be assessed and treated with intravenous analgesia, such as fentanyl citrate (Sublimaze).

Radiology, Laboratory and Other Diagnostic Studies

After the decision to transfer the patient has been made, the emergency department physician may defer radiology, laboratory, or other diagnostic studies unless the benefit of completing these tests directly affects care during transfer and outweighs the risk of delaying transfer. The few truly necessary tests are listed next.

Radiographs

- Cross-table lateral cervical spine (Some tertiary referral centers recommend that cervical spine films *not* be taken before transfer if interventions performed before and/or during transport will not change regardless of findings on the cervical spine x-ray films.)
- Chest
- Pelvis

Laboratory Studies

- Blood glucose level
- Hematocrit and hemoglobin
- Human chorionic gonadotropin for female patients

Family Preparation

When family members are present at the sending facility, it is important to prepare them for what will happen to the patient during the transfer phase. Allowing family to see a patient at least briefly before the patient leaves the sending facility can be important, especially with patients who are critically ill or injured. When family will be traveling separately to the receiving facility, staff should ensure that a safe (emotionally stable) driver has been designated and should provide clear driving directions. Family should be directed not to leave the sending facility before the patient does in case the patient destination changes at the last minute and should be encouraged to drive at a safe speed because they will likely not be able to see the patient immediately after transfer.

CARE DURING TRANSFER

Ongoing, serial assessment of the patient must continue during the entire transfer. Assessment should include patency of airway, symmetric rise and fall of the chest, signs and symptoms of hemorrhage, vital signs including oxygen saturation and end-tidal carbon dioxide level (if available), neurologic status including Glasgow Coma Scale, temperature, and level of pain.

Humidified oxygen should be given throughout the transport. If the patient is receiving mechanical ventilation, settings should be monitored closely for any changes from air expansion and/or vibration. Expiratory tidal volumes should be monitored. If the ventilator does not have the capability to monitor expiratory volumes, an in-line manometer should be used for frequent tidal volume measurement, especially with air ambulances. The patient should be monitored for signs and symptoms of tension pneumothorax, and needle thoracostomy should be performed if necessary.

Intravenous fluids should be placed in pressure infuser devices for air transport to ensure a constant and regular rate of administration. All medications should be delivered through an infusion pump or flow regulating device. The patency of invasive monitoring lines, including arterial and pulmonary artery lines, should be maintained with a continuous flush device. In addition, arterial and pulmonary artery lines should be connected to a transducer to allow monitoring of the waveforms and to identify inadvertent dislodgment or malposition of the lines.

The transport team should be prepared to turn a patient quickly if emesis occurs, especially if the patient does not have an orogastric or a nasogastric tube in place. These tubes should be vented or attached to low suction. Analgesics and sedatives should be used judiciously, based on patient needs, neurologic status, and hemodynamic values. The patient and any passengers should be given safety briefings and should be provided with reassurance and support for the transport.

Communication

A brief, concise entry notification should be communicated to the receiving facility before arrival. This notification should include the patient's general condition, vital signs, any changes and interventions in transit, and the patient's response. An estimated time of arrival should be given, and any specific requests for equipment or personnel should be stated at this time.

On arrival, a brief verbal report is given. A written summary of events during transfer also should be given to the receiving facility. This summary should include any medications or intravenous fluids given and patient changes.

SUMMARY

The ultimate decision to treat the critically injured trauma patient in one's own facility or to transfer the patient to a regional referral center must be made by an objective appraisal of the level of care that can be delivered within a given facility. The trauma care team has an ethical and legal duty to transfer a patient to a facility where definitive care can be given whenever such a transfer is feasible and available.

References

1. Centers for Medicare and Medicaid Services: [Emergency Medical Treatment and Active Labor Act resources]. Retrieved March 16, 2005, from *www.cms.hhs.gov/providers/emtala*
2. Emergency Nurses Association: *Care of the critically ill or injured patient during interfacility transfer,* Park Ridge, Ill, 1999, The Association.

Suggested Readings

Air and Surface Transport Nurses Association: *Air and surface patient transport: principles and practice,* ed 5, St Louis, 2003, Mosby.

Committee on Trauma, American College of Surgeons: *Resources for optimal care of the injured patient: 2006,* Chicago, 2006, The College.

Emergency Nurses Association: *Care of the critically ill or injured patient during interfacility transfer,* Park Ridge, Ill, 1999, The Association.

Emergency Nurses Association: *Care of the pediatric patient during interfacility transfer,* Park Ridge, Ill, 2001, The Association.

Emergency Nurses Association: *Emergency nursing core curriculum,* ed 5, Philadelphia, 1999, Saunders.

Emergency Nurses Association: *Sheehy's emergency nursing: principles and practice,* ed 5, St Louis, 2003, Mosby.

Mass Casualty and Disaster Preparedness

Tener Goodwin Veenema

In no other situation do the concepts of interagency cooperation, communication, preplanning, and trauma team cohesion become more important than in the event of a mass casualty incident. On the local level, the principles of trauma team development, prehospital communication, and integration of community resources are truly put to the test. On a grander scale, regional, state, and federal agencies must be incorporated into the response system.

Disaster planning is only as good as the assumptions on which it is based. History suggests that, unfortunately, many of these assumptions have been false. Hospital planning efforts often are focused on what intuitively is expected to happen, which may not be at all what happens in actuality.

Defining Mass Casualty and Disasters

Disaster has many definitions. Disaster may be defined as any destructive event that disrupts the normal functioning of a community. Disaster has been defined as an ecologic disturbance or emergency of a severity and magnitude resulting in deaths, injuries, illness, and property damage that cannot be managed effectively by the application of routine procedures or resources and requires outside assistance. A more focused definition of a disaster for health care providers is when the number of patients presenting within a given period of time are such that the emergency department cannot provide care for them without external assistance.[1]

Disasters may be external or internal (Box 5-1). External events may be classified further into two broad categories: *natural* (those resulting from nature/environmental forces) or *man-made* (human-generated). Natural disasters include events such as tornadoes, hurricanes, earthquakes, floods, ice storms, and other geologic or meteorologic phenomena. Disasters or emergency situations caused by human beings are those in which the principal direct causes are identifiable human actions, deliberate or otherwise. Internal disasters, however, include events such as electric gas failure, water loss, medical gas failure, or elevator emergencies. Internal events refer to situations occurring within hospitals that disrupt the normal operations of patient care.

Mass casualty events or external disasters, whether natural or man-made, usually result in a sudden influx of injured or ill patients into the emergency department (ED). The size of the facility and its proximity to resources—such as transportation, additional personnel, and technical assistance on short notice—are factors that determine whether the situation is a disaster for the institution. Despite having different underlying causes, one type of disaster does not necessarily preclude the other, and an external and internal disaster may occur simultaneously as it did during the World Trade Center bombing in 2001 or Hurricane Katrina in 2005. During both of these events, a natural or man-made external event led to internal events in which staff were unable to reach the hospitals because of the devastation of the surrounding

| Box 5-1 | POTENTIAL CAUSES OF DISASTERS |

External events

Natural

Earthquake
Fire
Flood
Hurricane
Storm
Tornado

Man-made

Mass gathering: hysteria or unrest
Nuclear/biological/chemical materials incident: such as Chernobyl
Terrorism; such as the Oklahoma City or World Trade Center bombing incidents
Transportation related: such as airplane crash or railroad car derailment

Internal events

Bomb threat/explosion
Chemical or radiation release
Electric power failure: shutdown of medical equipment and electronic information
   systems
Elevator emergencies
Fire/explosion: potential situation for evacuation and victims
Flood
Inability of staff to reach hospital
Loss of medical gases: oxygen and air primarily for life support
Violence/hostage-taking
Water loss: heat, steam, and vacuum

environment. Regardless of the situation, safety and security of the patients and staff should remain a priority.

INSTITUTIONAL PLANNING FOR DISASTER

Disasters are not simply daily emergencies that are larger than usual. They often disrupt communication systems, interrupt transportation of patients and supplies, and constrain normal functioning. Disasters further overwhelm the monetary and personnel resources of local, state, and federal agencies in trying to manage the organizations, operations, and above all, the safety and health of all those involved. As a result, disasters can present complex and unique challenges for health care systems that mandate unique solutions. Planning for such an event thus becomes pivotal to anticipate what is likely to occur and to develop appropriate and cost-effective countermeasures in response. Response is the process of handling what actually happens whether the situation was anticipated or not. Effective planning ideally enhances response. As witnessed with Hurricane Katrina, the planning should be integrated at multiple levels of response, including municipal, state, and federal, with an established timeline for each.

A hospital-wide disaster committee should be created to develop the emergency operations plan (EOP) for the activation of resources in the event of an internal or external disaster. Representation from all departments in the institution, not only the ED, is essential to organize disaster response efficiently. The responsibilities of the hospital disaster committee include the following:

- Define what would be a disaster for the hospital.
- Review standards and guidelines developed by the Joint Commission on Accreditation of Healthcare Organizations and local regulators to address emergency preparedness.
- Create an EOP consistent with the incident command system (ICS), which would allow responders to manage the command, operations, planning, logistics, and finance and administration of an incident without being hindered by jurisdictional boundaries.
- Create, review, and update the hospital plan as the institution changes, regulations are amended, or a flaw in the plan is identified.
- Assist each department with clarifying the roles of responders and predetermining leadership within the department.
- Create a uniform format for each departmental plan; include external resources for personnel, equipment, and supplies.
- Create a concise notification system to contact on-duty and off-duty personnel.
- Integrate the local, regional, and state plans into the design of the hospital plan.
- Participate in the development of the local, regional, and state disaster plans.
- Orient, educate, and reeducate all personnel to disaster activation protocols.
- Conduct and evaluate drills testing the system; amend and improve the plan.
- Critique activations of the disaster plan within the institution and community.

The first step in effective disaster planning requires advance identification of potential problems for the institution involved. Although institutional, community, and regional uniqueness make the use of generic disaster plans impossible (Box 5-2), hospital EOPs should adopt the all-hazards approach. Hazard identification and mapping, vulnerability analysis, and risk assessment are the three cornerstone methods of data collection for disaster planning:

- Hazard identification is used to determine which events are most likely to affect a community or an institution. Hazard identification also is used to make decisions about who or what to protect based on established measures for prevention, mitigation (minimization of the effects of the event), and response.
- Vulnerability analysis is used to determine who is most likely to be affected, the property most likely to be damaged or destroyed, and the capacity of the community or institution to deal with the effects of the disaster.
- Risk assessment uses the results of the hazard identification and the vulnerability analysis to determine the probability of a specified outcome from a given hazard.

Even though a hospital has developed a written plan does not mean the hospital is prepared for a disaster or mass casualty event. Many hospital plans are so cumbersome that they cannot be implemented in practice and are thus likely to be ignored in an actual event. Successful hospital EOPs have the following characteristics:

- EOPs are based on valid assumptions of how individuals actually will behave in the event of a disaster and not how hospital administrators want them to behave.
- EOPs incorporate an interagency perspective and interface with other disaster plans.
- All personnel are aware of the EOP and receive regular training to support their role in the plan.
- EOPs are accompanied by the provision of adequate resources in terms of human capital, supplies, and equipment and funding.

Box 5-2	KEY ELEMENTS OF THE HOSPITAL DISASTER PLAN

1. Table of contents: for quick referencing
2. Definitions: to establish a frame of reference
3. Purpose and scope: to establish administrative authority
4. Plan activation: procedures for putting the plan into action
5. Notification and communication procedure: to ensure a smooth flow of information
6. Chain of command: to identify decision makers and authority figures
7. Command center: point of coordination and communication
8. Patient management plan: procedures for patient care functions
9. Patient staging area plan: readiness to receive victims, respond, and recover
   - Traffic flow: systematic entry into system to prevent confusion
   - Triage: classification of needs
   - Decontamination: if toxic agent suspected
   - Treatment areas: designated to maximize space use—critical, dead, minor, fractures, pregnant, unsalvageable, surgical, medical, psychiatric, discharges, uninjured
10. Specialized areas: to maintain control—family, media, employee volunteers, morgue
11. Individual departmental plans: to guide personnel
12. Internal disaster plans: individual procedures to respond to all categories of incidents
13. Evacuation plans: orderly routes to follow to secure patients and personnel
14. Interagency agreements: for specific resources, such as water suppliers or ambulances
15. Transfer criteria and agreements: for specialized treatment such as burns or pediatrics

- EOPs are acceptable to the end-users, which include the health care providers, hospital staff, and administrators at the local, state, and federal levels.
- The plans are tested at least once a year.

INCIDENT COMMAND SYSTEM AND HOSPITAL EMERGENCY INCIDENT COMMAND SYSTEM

In the event of a medically related disaster, the hospital and its staff widely experience confusion and chaos. Problems frequently seen in this type of event include the following:

- Too many persons reporting to one supervisor
- Different emergency response organizational structures
- Lack of reliable incident information
- Inadequate and incompatible communications
- Lack of structure for coordinated planning among agencies
- Unclear lines of authority
- Terminology differences among agencies
- Unclear or unspecified incident objectives

To address these problems, the ICS was developed to allow responders to manage the complexity and demands of an incident effectively in a structured fashion without being hindered by jurisdictional boundaries. To control the communication and planning of an emergency response, the ICS divided emergency response into five functions: command, operations, planning, logistics, and finance and administration.

In 1992 a generic disaster management plan, called the hospital emergency incident command system (HEICS), was created based on the ICS (Figure 5-1). HEICS was developed with the intent of minimizing the negative effects of a disaster by providing management with a structured and focused direction of activities. HEICS is an emergency management system that uses a logical management structure, defined responsibilities, clear reporting channels, and a common nomenclature to help unify hospitals with other emergency responders. HEICS has proved successful already in helping hospitals serve patients and communities in disaster situations, and it is quickly becoming the standard for emergency response. The HEICS plan offers several benefits:

- Predictable chain of management
- Flexible organizational chart allows flexible response to specific emergencies
- Prioritized response checklists
- Accountability of position function
- Improved documentation for improved accountability and cost recovery
- Common language to promote communication and facilitate outside assistance
- Cost-effective emergency planning within health care organizations

COMMUNITY PLANNING FOR DISASTER

Resources beyond local responders may be necessary for some mass casualty incidents. Team leadership, predetermined during community planning, directs and delegates which agencies or positions have responsibility during an incident for things such as triage, extrication, decontamination, and initial treatment at the disaster site. Determining the need for supplemental resources to assist with disaster site activities is a key element of the community plan, but these resources must be identified in advance and must be assimilated into the plan. The ED will continue resuscitation and will provide definitive care efficiently only if the staff members have understood and incorporated the initial community response into their disaster plan. At any time during the disaster or in the hours, days, or weeks following the disaster, victims may present to the ED without the benefit of emergency medical services involvement, or they may seek care at other locations in the community. The goal, therefore, should be to provide a coordinated, comprehensive response to patient care needs during all phases of the disaster continuum. The disaster continuum (or life cycle) is characterized by the phases of *preimpact* (before), *impact* (during), and *postimpact* (after).

This continuum provides a foundation for the disaster timeline. A community disaster management program has five basic phases: preparedness, mitigation, response, recovery, and evaluation.

- *Preparedness* refers to the proactive planning efforts designed to structure the response before its occurrence. Disaster planning encompasses the evaluation of all potential hazards, vulnerabilities, and risks, along with the probability that a disaster will occur.
- *Mitigation* includes all measures taken to reduce the harmful effects of the disaster by attempting to limit its impact on human health, community function, and economic infrastructure. Prevention measures include a broad range of activities, such as attempts to prevent a disaster from occurring and any actions taken to prevent further disease, disability or loss of life.
- *Response* refers to the actual implementation of the plan. Disaster response or emergency management is the organization of activities to address the event and focuses primarily on

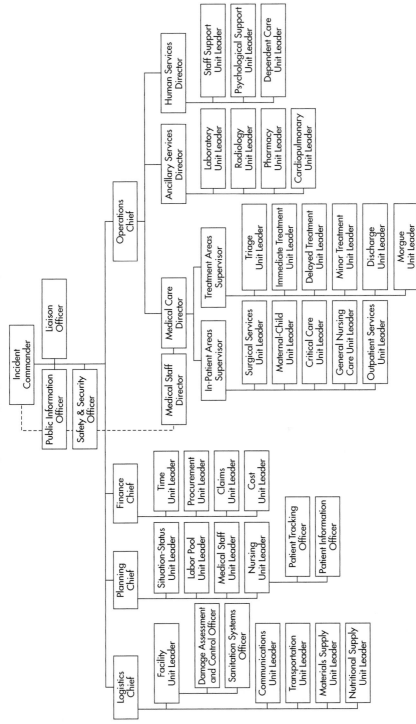

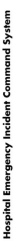

Figure 5-1. Hospital emergency incident command system. (*From Hospital Emergency Incident Command System Update Project: A project of the San Mateo County Emergency Medical Services Agency with support and funding from the California Emergency Medical Services Authority.*)

emergency relief: saving lives, providing first aid and medical care, and restoring damaged systems such as transportation and communication.

- *Recovery* actions focus on stabilizing and returning the community (or institution) to normal (preimpact phase). This can range from rebuilding damaged buildings or repairing infrastructure to relocating populations.
- *Evaluation* is the phase most often overlooked and underappreciated. After any disaster, it is essential that evaluations be conducted to determine what worked versus what did not work and to identify specific problems and challenges. Future disaster planning then should be based on empirical evidence derived from previous disasters.

Community disaster plans should accommodate needs specific to each phase of the disaster timeline. To provide a coordinated and comprehensive response, the community plan should incorporate the following essential points:

- Collaboration with all agencies that may be called on to respond in a disaster, including police, fire, emergency medical services, hospitals and urgent care centers, American Red Cross, utility companies, and the state/federal emergency management agency
- A clear understanding by all agencies of what communication system will be used and who will conduct the central communications
- A clear understanding by all agencies of the ICS and the leadership hierarchy
- Participation by all agencies in regular sessions to create a plan, simulate the plan, and revise the plan for the community or region
- A system for ongoing communication and reporting of activities in the aftermath of the disaster so that necessary services may be enhanced
- Compatibility with the National Response Plan and a clear interface with the National Incident Management System

Conducting a Disaster Drill

Annual evaluation of institutional response to disasters or emergencies is a requirement of Joint Commission on Accreditation of Healthcare Organizations. The management plan for the facility describes actions to be taken for external and internal disasters and outlines implementation of the educational component for personnel, as well as performance standards and evaluation criteria. The plan must be interpreted by the institution to fulfill Standard EC.1.6: A management plan addresses emergency preparedness. Disaster drills are executed by facilities to meet these requirements. The quality and effectiveness of the drill as an educational and evaluation tool is determined by the attitudes of the organizers and the participants. If all the stakeholders take the activity seriously, helpful information about emergency procedures can be shared, inconsistencies and inadequacies in the plan can be identified, and suggestions for improvement and revisions can be made. The following are several suggestions that may make the drill process more successful:

- Put the plan on paper first; be certain that all participating agencies have clearly defined roles and procedures to follow.
- Include all agencies in planning the disaster drill, from outcomes and goals for the exercise to choosing the scenario, site, date, and time of the drill.
- Conduct intradepartmental instruction for response so that each staff member has a clear understanding of his or her role in the drill; be certain to identify terminology that differentiates the drill from an actual event.
- Conduct an announced drill before an unannounced drill; although it may sound contradictory, actual events are infrequent, so having the opportunity to walk through the process is essential.

- In each department preassign an objective "observer," not involved with operational duties at the time of the drill, to collect data and provide feedback on the function of the department.
- Establish in advance measurable objective criteria for the evaluation of the drill.
- On completion, provide written evaluation for each department on its participation in the drill.
- Provide an opportunity for a representative from each department to participate in a hospital-wide evaluation of the drill as close to the conclusion of the drill as possible, and distribute a summary report internally of the evaluation results, identifying changes to incorporate into the disaster response procedure.
- Include all agencies in a discussion and critique of the drill, again as close to the end of the drill as feasible while impressions are fresh.
- Provide the community planning group with a summary report, including goals and outcomes met; make recommendations for amendments of the community drill process.
- Consider an unannounced community-wide disaster drill. Invite the press to cover the exercise, and use the opportunity to educate the community while working collaboratively with the media.

Much can be learned from the actual and simulated disaster experiences that have been published in nursing, emergency medicine, and hospital administration journals. A review of this literature would be of great assistance in establishing or revising a plan. The most important concept to consider is that every plan must be written to meet the specific needs of the institution and the community for which it is created. Collaborating with community members experienced in disaster response may prove to be the greatest asset in planning for the unexpected.

MASS CASUALTY EVENT MANAGEMENT

Mass trauma is defined by the Centers for Disease Control and Prevention as any multicasualty incident resulting from a large-scale natural disaster or from a conventional weapons (explosives, small arms, military munitions) terrorist attack that affects community health and access to vital services. Multicasualty incidents usually involve six or more casualties and directly or indirectly may result in injuries, deaths, disabilities, and emotional trauma. The most severe injuries in mass casualty events are fractures, burns, lacerations, and crush injuries; however, the most common injuries are eye injuries, sprains, strains, minor wounds, and ear damage.

In the event of an emergency, time is an important factor. The chances for recovery decrease the longer a seriously injured patient waits to receive care, and public health and medical care systems (including physical and mental health, public information, and social services) thus are encouraged to develop and review protocols that would allow them to respond quickly and efficiently to a mass casualty incident. In such an event, clinicians, hospitals, and public health agencies should be prepared to treat the negative health and behavioral effects that follow, and they also should be prepared to handle a large number of fatalities. They also are encouraged to develop and review hospital plans for dealing with surges in demand for emergency care because of complex injuries, psychosocial distress reactions, and the acute aggravation of chronic diseases that may be triggered by the psychological terror of such events. The nursing staff becomes a critical element in effectively handling a mass casualty incident, and during this disaster situation, the basic principles of nursing include the following:

- Rapid assessment of the situation and of nursing care needs
- Triage and initiation of lifesaving measures first
- The selected use of essential nursing interventions and the elimination of nonessential nursing activities
- Adaptation of necessary nursing skills to disaster and other emergency situations

PERSONAL PROTECTIVE EQUIPMENT

Disasters, whether natural or man-made, present a danger to the community and to those trying to help the victims. Health care providers, therefore, must protect themselves to avoid becoming victims of secondary contamination. Potential exposure to biologic or chemical agents occurs through several means:

- Direct contact with a hazardous substance
- Liquid (droplets or aerosols)
- Inhalation of vapors or aerosols
- Ingestion

Health care providers and other staff members can avoid exposure to hazardous agents by wearing personal protective equipment (PPE) when treating potentially infected patients. In the *Code of Federal Regulations,* Section 1910, the Occupational Safety and Health Administration defines the types of PPE and the situations in which employees are required to wear PPE. The different types of PPE offer different levels of protection and are designated A, B, C, and D.

Level A refers to a total encapsulating, chemical-resistant suit with a self-contained breathing apparatus, gloves, and boots. This suit provides complete protection from liquids and vapors.

Level B often is used when full respiratory protection is needed but the hazard from vapor is less. This form of PPE is not fully airtight, but it offers protection against liquids.

Level C uses a splash suit with a full-faced positive or negative breathing mask.

Level D consists of a work uniform using latex gloves and, if necessary, mouth and eye protection.

MASS CASUALTY INCIDENT RESOURCES

Information on injuries and stress related to mass casualty events can be found on the Centers for Disease Control and Prevention mass casualty event website at *www.jointcommission.org/ NR/rdonlyres/9C8DE572-4F28-AB84-3741EC82AF98/0/emergency_preparedness.pdf* (Reviewed November 6, 2006.) This site is designed to provide information and preparedness and response tools to help public health professionals and clinicians prepare for and respond to mass casualty events. The website also contains fact sheets in English and Spanish for the public. Box 5-3 contains a list of some of the available fact sheets. Additional information resources and descriptions of relevant research studies also can be found on the site.

Box 5-3	FACT SHEETS FOR PUBLIC HEALTH PROFESSIONALS AND CLINICIANS

Fact sheets for public health professionals and clinicians include the following:

- Brain Injuries and Mass Casualty Events: www.bt.cdc.gov/masscasualties/braininjuriespro.asp
- Lesiones cerebrales y sucesos traumáticos masivos:
- Coping with a Traumatic Event: www.bt.cdc.gov/masscasualties/copingpro.asp
- Cómo manejar un suceso traumático: www.bt.cdc.gov/masscasualties/es/copingpro.asp
- Injuries and Mass Casualty Events: www.bt.cdc.gov/masscasualties/braininjuriespro.asp

Preparedness tools for public health professionals and clinicians include the following:

- Explosions and Blast Injuries: A Primer for Clinicians—www.bt.cdc.gov/masscasualties/explosions.asp
- Mass Casualties Predictor: www.bt.cdc.gov/masscasualties/predictor.asp
- Predicting Casualty Severity and Hospital Capacity: www.bt.cdc.gov/masscasualties/capacity.asp

Response tools for public health professionals and clinicians include the following:

- Overview of Mental Health Survey Instrument: www.bt.cdc.gov/masscasualties/mhsurvey.asp
- Mass Casualty Event Preparedness and Response: www.bt.cdc.gov/masscasualties/index.asp

Resources for public health professionals and clinicians include the following:

- Glasgow Coma Scale: www.bt.cdc.gov/masscasualties/gscale.asp
- Disasters and Emergency Preparedness: www.nlm.nih.gov/medlineplus/disasterpreparationandrecovery.html
- Butler AS, Panser AM, Goldfrank LR, editors: *Preparing for the Psychological Consequences of Terrorism: A Public Health Strategy,* Washington, DC, 2003, National Academies Press. Available at http://search.nap.edu/books/0309089530/html/
- Information Networks and Other Information Sources, State and Local Health Departments: www.cdc.gov/doc.do/id/0900f3ec80226c7a

Suggested Readings

Hogan DE, Burstein JL: *Disaster medicine,* Philadelphia, 2002, Lippincott, Williams & Wilkins.

Joint Commission on Accreditation of Healthcare Organizations: *Health care at the crossroads: strategies for creating and sustaining community-wide emergency preparedness systems.* From www.jcaho.org/about+us/public+policy+initiatives/emergency+preparedness. pdf

Keyes DC, Burstein JL, Schwartz RB et al: *Medical response to terrorism: preparedness and clinical practice,* Philadelphia, 2004, Lippincott, Williams & Wilkins.

Landesman L: *Public health management of disasters: the practice guide,* ed 2, Washington, DC, 2005, American Public Health Association.

Langan JC, James DC: *Preparing nurses for disaster management,* Upper Saddle River, NJ, 2005, Pearson Education.

McGlown KJ: *Terrorism and disaster management: preparing healthcare leaders for the new reality,* Chicago, 2004, Health Administration Press.

Occupational Safety & Health Administration, US Department of Labor: *Incident command system etool.* From www.osha.gov/SLTC/etools/ics/

Veenema TG: *Disaster nursing and emergency preparedness for chemical, biological and radiological terrorism and other hazards,* New York, 2003, Springer.

TOPICS IN TRAUMA

INJURY PREVENTION

KAREN MACAULEY

The time has come to eradicate the word and concept of *accident* from our thought processes and vocabularies as trauma specialists. No longer do we believe that unintentional injury is related to factors beyond our control. Unintentional injury is predictable and preventable. Think of the many trauma patients you see, and take time to figure out whether you could have predicted their injury based on their risky behaviors, mechanism of injury, and/or lack of safety devices. Predictability and preventability are in no way an attempt to lay blame or make value judgments; this is simply science that allows us to predict what might happen and therefore to prevent the potential outcomes.

INCIDENCE

Unintentional injury is the leading cause of death for persons aged 1 to 44 years and in the top eight causes of death and disability for all persons. In 2002 the Centers for Disease Control and Prevention (CDC) reported 49,050 unintentional injury deaths in person aged 1 to 44 years and 97,835 unintentional injury deaths in all age groups.[1] The same year there were 161,269 deaths in all age groups from all causes, making unintentional injury responsible for 46.5% of all deaths in 2002. CDC data from 2003 show 27,127, 477 nonfatal injuries from unintentional injury.[2]

The leading causes of death from unintentional injury are falls in all age groups except 15 to 24 years. The other top causes of unintentional nonfatal injury are burn/fire, motor vehicle crash, struck pedestrian, and bicycle crashes. Each year unintentional injuries cost society more than $224 billion. Unintentional injuries are the leading cause of productive life lost, accounting for 18.6% of years lost.[2] Trauma never affects just an individual—families often are torn apart as a result of unintentional injury. The overall cost to society is astronomic.

TYPES OF INJURY PREVENTION

Injury prevention programs can address injuries at several places in the continuum of care. The American College of Surgeons recognizes several types of programs.[3] *Primary* prevention programs eliminate the actual traumatic event; *secondary* prevention programs reduce the severity of injury through the use of safety devices (helmets, seat belts); and *tertiary* prevention programs encompass all efforts following the trauma incident that optimize outcome, thereby preventing complications, long-term disability, or death. Comprehensive programs should look at potential interventions across this continuum: preventing the injury from happening (usually engineering), reducing injury (seat belts, helmets), and preventing mortalities and morbidities (trauma centers).

FOUR E'S OF INJURY PREVENTION

Enactment

It is important for trauma professionals to monitor safety laws closely, develop relationships with state legislators, and educate congressmen on trauma injury statistics, trauma center responsibilities, and injury prevention initiatives. Some of the most successful law changes have occurred from grassroots efforts initiated by trauma specialists.

Enforcement

No law can be effective without enforcement of the law. Behavior change usually does not occur without enforced consequences. Enforcement can be negative (punishment with non-compliance) or positive (reward with compliance). Bicycle helmet use often can be effective with positive enforcement, but seat belt use often requires negative enforcement for change to occur. Working closely with local law enforcement is a great tool to combine education, enactment, and enforcement together to accomplish injury prevention goals.

Engineering

Many specialists across the country and worldwide spend their entire professional life evaluating engineering changes to provide increased safety. Look at a car from 50 years ago and now look at today's cars. Cars today are full of collapsible compartments allowing the frame of the vehicle to absorb the crash forces instead of the occupant. All these changes occur because of research and engineering.

Education

Educational programs are often the easiest to implement but are most often not effective on their own. Take, for instance, bicycle crashes. Education of the rider about helmet use, rules of the road, and basic safety measures is important. However, a program would be more effective if it incorporated driver education as well because unsafe drivers often hit bicyclists.

Comprehensive programs that incorporate more than one E of injury prevention and are multidisciplinary are more effective than a one-sided strategy.

USING THE HADDON MATRIX FOR DEVELOPING PROGRAMS

Injury prevention is a science and thus requires scientific evaluation and implementation to show effectiveness. Using the Haddon matrix can assist you in developing a program that is well thought out and capable of being evaluated. Developed by Dr. William Haddon nearly 20 years ago, the Haddon matrix is a framework for understanding injuries.[4]

The Haddon matrix uses a systematic approach to establish potential causes of injury and intervention strategies. An example of its use is shown in Table 6-1. The first step is for you to determine what injury you want to evaluate. The matrix incorporates the host/agent/environment/setting of injury (human/vehicle-equipment/social environment/physical environment) against the preevent/event/postevent information. Each box of the matrix should be evaluated individually, listing all possible causes and potential interventions that could be done. A multidisciplinary collaborative approach works best to evaluate all potential solutions from many different angles to help determine that all program possibilities are evaluated.

T a b l e 6–1   Use of the Haddon Matrix in Motor Vehicle Collision

Phases	Human Factors	Agent or Vehicle	Physical Environment	Socioeconomic Environment
Preevent	Driver ability Driver distractions (cell phone use, children in the car)	Vehicle maintenance (brakes, tires) Vehicle inspection requirements	Weather conditions (rain, ice, snow, dry roads) Roadway factors (markings, surface)	Public attitude (drinking and driving, cell phone use while driving) Financial ability for individual purchase of car seats
Event	Seat belt use Use of car seats	Crashworthiness of vehicle Crushable vehicle frame	Breakaway off-road signage Side of roadway obstacles (trees, buildings)	Enforcement of laws (seat belt use laws, speed limit enforcement)
Postevent	Age Medical history	Gas tanks to prevent explosion	Emergency medical services response	Public attitude and support of trauma systems and community emergency medical services programs

Most injures are not a single event but part of a continuum of events. Therefore, potential solutions to the injury must cover all aspects of this continuum to determine the most effective overall strategy for prevention.

Once the potential intervention strategies have been identified, value ranking must be done to determine which intervention will be used. Values may include cost, feasibility, effectiveness, community preferences, or infringement of personal freedoms. Cost is often high on the list because prevention strategies most always cost money, and it is difficult to prove effectiveness (demonstrating the absence of an event/injury). Use epidemiology, data, research, and opinions as you make your intervention decisions.

Using the Haddon matrix to develop programs will be beneficial to guide the thought processes and keep program development systematic, comprehensive, and well thought out.

DATA SOURCES

Accurate data reporting lends credibility to program development. The CDC publishes mortality and injury statistics that can be focused to a specific city and state. Trauma registries have institution-specific injury and mortality data, and many states have state trauma registries that allow compilation of data from across the state. Other data sources include ambulance and police reports, detailed autopsy reports from the medical examiners, and the standardized emergency department discharge data set. Whenever possible, data must be community specific and applicable to the program catchment area. Data matching can be a useful tool when community-specific data are not available. Matching demographics closely is imperative, however, in order to extrapolate data from another community.

Relevant, accurate data also are important to have before any intervention to measure outcome after intervention. Proving efficacy of injury prevention programs is difficult, and working with an epidemiologist and statistician can be helpful.

SPECIFIC PREVENTION STRATEGIES

Child Passenger Safety

Despite many collaborative campaigns, 80% to 85% of all car seats continue to be used incorrectly. Misuses include not restraining the child, not installing the car seat properly in the car and positioning the seat improperly (rear facing car seats in the front seat). CDC data for 2003 report 7,713 nonfatal injuries from motor vehicle collisions (MVCs) in children less than 1 year, 43,495 in children aged 1 to 4 years, and 71,653 in children aged 5 to 9 years.[5]

Unrestrained children are at 3 times the risk for fatal injury in MVC. Most crashes continue to occur within 25 miles of home when many parents feel the safest allowing their children to ride unrestrained, and 14% of children under the age of 14 years continue to ride unrestrained. The cost of MVC for children under the age of 14 years is more than $25.8 billion, and each dollar spent on a car seat can save $32 in direct and indirect medical costs.[5]

Current recommendations from the American Academy of Pediatrics on car seat use are as follows[5]:

- Age less than 1 year AND less than 20 lb: rear-facing seat with a five-point harness in the back seat (NEVER in front of an airbag); current recommendations are to keep child rear facing as long as allowed by car seat–specified upper weight limit
- Age 1 year and older AND weight of 20 to 40 lb: forward facing in five-point harness, backseat is safest
- More than 40 lb until 80 lb (usually 8 years): booster seat (high or low back depending on presence of head rests) with three-point harness worn correctly (no shoulder harnesses behind back), back seat still safest
- After age 8/80 lb, all occupants should be belted with three-point harness.

Bicycle Safety

In 2002, there were 113,513 injuries from bicycle crashes in riders aged 5 to 9 years and another 141,252 injuries in riders aged 10 to 14 years. Seventy percent of children aged 5 to 14 years ride bicycles, and these children account for 21% of all bicycle injuries. Head injury is the leading cause of death from bicycle crashes, yet only 15% to 25% of riders wear helmets. A nonhelmeted rider is 14 times more likely to die, and it is felt that bicycle helmets could prevent 75% of head injury deaths and decrease head injury by up to 85%. The cost of bicycle injuries exceeds $2.2 billion per year, and for each dollar spent on a bicycle helmet, a $30 decrease in direct medical costs would result.[5] Comprehensive bicycle injury programs must incorporate enactment (bicycle helmet laws), enforcement, and education. Education must include rider and driver education. Engineering also should be considered to get riders off the main roads to prevent car collisions. Media events can include share-the-road campaigns.

Pedestrian Safety

Children under the age of 10 years do not possess the cognitive and developmental ability to cross streets alone and therefore require close supervision when out and about. Each year children are killed in their own driveways when parents and visitors do not see them and run over them.

The National Safe Kids Campaign, now Safe Kids Worldwide, did an observational study of driver behaviors (1999) and found the following: 45% of drivers violate stop signs by not coming to a complete stop—37% rolled through the stop sign, 7% did not even slow down, 32% violated the stop sign with children present, and 24% did not stop completely even with pedestrians crossing the intersection.[5]

Programs need to address not only pedestrian educational programs but also driver education. Developing safe playgrounds for kids also can have a huge impact on pedestrian injuries, as shown by Barbara Barlow in Harlem.[6] Children who have safe and supervised play areas away from traffic are less likely to be injured.

Violence

Violent injuries continue to increase in the United States each year. The CDC reports approximately 14,500 deaths from homicide, with another 30,600 deaths from suicide in 1998.[7] Homicide is a complex social disease, and prevention programs must encompass many diverse social programs, as well as education, enactment (gun control), and enforcement. Engineering specialists also are working on developing trigger locks controlled by fingerprint that do not allow a gun to fire unless fingerprints match in an attempt to decrease accidental home shootings from children playing with parent's firearms.

Alcohol/Substance Abuse and Trauma

Alcohol is one of the leading factors in MVCs, and driving impaired after drinking is thought to be one of the most frequently committed violent crimes in the United States. Every 15 to 33 minutes someone in the United States is killed in an alcohol-related crash, and every 2 minutes someone is injured in an alcohol-related crash. Twenty-two percent of injuries in children in MVCs can be attributed to driver alcohol use. Alcohol-related crashes cost society more than $100 billion each year. Alcohol and other drugs are a factor in 45% to 65% of all fatal MVCs and 20% of nonfatal crashes.[8] Studies show that up to 69% of trauma patients meet diagnostic criteria for substance abuse or dependence.

Mandatory substance abuse screenings and intervention protocols are useful tools to evaluate substance abuse in the trauma population. School programs addressing substance abuse are a worthwhile endeavor. Enactment has played an important part in alcohol-related crashes, with all states adopting a legal age of 21 years for alcohol consumption and many states adopting 0.08 blood alcohol content for legal intoxication. Sobriety checkpoints and enforcement also contribute significantly to the solution of substance abuse, and engineering will continue to play a role as development of breathalyzers in vehicles continues and they become readily available.

INJURY RISK FACTORS

The risk for injury changes based on environment, development, and social factors. Toddlers are high risk for injury related to their curious nature and their inability to understand risk and consequences. Adolescents are at high risk for injury related to their risky behaviors—substance use, speeding, feelings of invincibility—and to their inexperience as drivers and emotional lability. Older Americans are at risk from their underlying medical conditions and decreasing cognitive abilities.

Young children, males, and poor children suffer trauma in a disproportionate share. Children in rural areas are at greater risk for unintentional death than their urban counterparts. Poverty can be a primary predictor for injury and is more relevant than ethnicity in most cases related to resources available and hazardous environments.

YOUR ROLE IN INJURY PREVENTION

First, and foremost, be a role model for safety. Wear a bicycle helmet; wear a seat belt; do not drink and drive. The community looks to trauma specialists to set the safety standard for the community.

Work with local legislators to change and develop injury prevention laws. Grassroots efforts are effective in making stronger laws related to injury prevention strategies. Invite legislators to visit trauma centers and emergency departments. Educate them about trauma and prevention.

Develop programs. Identify an injury that is severe, common, or easily preventable. Collaborate with other disciplines and colleagues to develop a prevention program. Be persistent. Carefully evaluate the program: first attempts are rarely as successful as initially hoped, but persistence and evaluation will work together to make a strong program. Consult injury prevention experts from across the country, and ask them what worked for them and what did

---

Box 6-1   INJURY PREVENTION RESOURCES

American Trauma Society
www.amtrauma.org
Center for Disease Control and Prevention
www.cdc.gov
WISQARS (Web-Based Injury Statistics Query and Reporting System)
www.cdc.gov/ncipc/wisqars
National Center for Injury Prevention and Control
www.cdc.gov/ncipc
Emergency Nurses Association—EN CARE
www.ena.org
Injury Free Coalition for Kids
www.injuryfree.org
National Highway Traffic Safety Administration
www.nhtsa.dot.gov
Crash Injury Research and Engineering Network
www-nrd.nhtsa.dot.gov/departments/nrd-50/ciren/CIREN.html
Safe Kids Worldwide
www.safekids.org
ThinkFirst National Injury Prevention Foundation
www.thinkfirst.org
Society of Trauma Nurses
www.traumanursesoc.org
Trauma Nurses Talk Tough
www.traumarn.com/page6.html

not. Learn from other's less successful programs and from their successful programs. Box 6-1 lists resources for injury prevention.

Each and every one of us makes a difference in injury prevention activities.

References

1. *Injury Fact Book (2001-2002),* Atlanta, Ga, 2002, National Center for Injury Prevention and Control, Centers for Disease Control and Prevention.
2. National Center for Injury Prevention and Control. CDC fact sheets: *www.cdc.gov/ncipc/ factsheets/children.htm* Reviewed November 6, 2006.
3. Committee on Trauma, American College of Surgeons: *Resources for optimal care of the injured patient: 1999,* Chicago, 1999, The College.
4. Christoffel T, Gallagher S: *Injury prevention and public health,* Sudbury, Mass, 2006, Jones and Bartlett.
5. National Safe Kids Campaign: *Promoting child safety to prevent unintentional injury. www.usa.safekids.org/content_documents/Ped_pdf* Reviewed November 6, 2006.
6. Injury Free Coalition: www.injuryfree.org
7. Injury and violence prevention. In *Healthy people 2010,* vol 2, Washington, DC, 2002, US Department of Health and Human Services.
8. Shankar U: *Pedestrian roadway fatalities,* Washington, DC, 2003, National Center for Statistics and Analysis Advanced Research and Analysis.

CHAPTER 7

LEGAL AND FORENSIC CONCERNS IN TRAUMA

SANDRA A. JUTRAS

This chapter focuses on several areas in which the trauma nurse may experience legal challenges or concerns, including potential malpractice and risk management, ensuring patient safety, and adhering to state and national laws and regulations. The chapter also reviews the trauma nurse's responsibilities in the area of potential criminal or civil cases and how to handle forensic evidence correctly.

Trauma nurses not only perform an important role in the initial care and stabilization of victims of violence and trauma but also assist in the investigation of crime and the legal process for victims living and deceased. For example, questions related to trauma that may be of later relevance in a court of law may remain unanswered because of a trauma nurse's lack of awareness of forensic issues. Frequently, cases are won or lost based on the methods of handling evidence.

A major concern is protecting the trauma nurse from potential legal claims of malpractice. The following section provides basic definitions of the components of malpractice and other legal terms.

DEFINITIONS OF MALPRACTICE TERMS

Nursing malpractice or negligence contains *four key elements.* All four elements must be present for medical or nursing malpractice to exist:

1. *Duty:* A relationship must be established between the patient and the health care provider. This occurs when the health care provider accepts responsibility for the care and treatment of the patient.
2. *Breach of duty:* This concept is related to the standard of care ("duty") applicable to the professional. The standard of care for the specific specialty and treatment involved must be determined to see whether an act of omission or commission has caused damage to the patient.
3. *Damages/injury:* This area must include one or more of these factors:
   - Physical and mental pain
   - Medical expenses
   - Lost wages
   - Loss of earning capacity
   - Loss of companionship, society, affection, and sexual relationship (loss of consortium)
   - Hedonistic damages: damages that attempt to compensate for the loss of the pleasure of being alive
   - Punitive or exemplary damages, which are awarded in addition to actual damages
   - Acts of recklessness, malice, or deceit
4. *Causation:* A *direct* causal relationship between the act of negligence and the resulting injury must be established. This is the most difficult aspect to prove in a court of law.

Other Legal Definitions

Other legal definitions the trauma nurse needs to know are these:

Negligence: The failure to exercise the standard of care that a reasonably prudent person would have exercised in a similar situation; any conduct that falls below the legal standard established to protect others against unreasonable risk of harm, except for conduct that is intentionally, wantonly, or willfully disregardful of others' rights[1]

Gross negligence: Reckless disregard of a legal duty; requires willful, wanton, and reckless misconduct[1]

Vicarious liability: Liability that a supervisory party (such as an employer) bears for the actionable conduct of a subordinate (such as an employee)

Respondeat superior ("let the superior make the answer"): The doctrine holding an employer or principal liable for the employee's or agent's wrongful acts committed within the scope of employment or agency

RISKS FACED BY TRAUMA NURSES IN THE FIRST HOUR

The major risks that involve nurses during the first hour of acute trauma care can be subdivided into two major categories: patient safety and documentation. Related to all these issues is the importance of timely, complete, and accurate communication. Collaborative communication between medical, nursing, and allied health providers and the patient not only is vital to provide the optimum level of trauma care but also reduces the medical-legal risk.

Patient Safety Issues

Patient safety has become an area of increased emphasis in the health care arena. This includes issues such as patient identification, verbal orders, management of high-alert medications, use of the universal protocol, handoff communications, and use of restraints.

Patient Identification

Correct identification of the patient is absolutely essential. Standards set by the Joint Commission on Accreditation of Healthcare Organizations[2] (JCAHO) require that patients be identified by two separate identifiers whenever medications, treatments, or procedures are administered or when specimens of any type are acquired. If a patient is able to volunteer his or her name correctly when asked, this can serve as one identifier. Hospital number is the most common second identifier; others are the individual's telephone number, photograph, or other person-specific identifier. Room number cannot be used as an identifier; this is particularly important in the emergency department (ED) when patients are being moved around constantly. In the event that an accurate identification cannot be made and the patient's name is unknown, additional bar codes or other identifiers must be matched. Additionally, one should use special care when two or more patients in the ED have the same last names or multiple family members are involved in a trauma.

Verbal Orders in the Emergency Department

The taking of verbal orders should be avoided to the extent possible. At times this is difficult in the midst of an active trauma resuscitation. When a verbal order must be taken, the preferred procedure is for the recipient to write it down and then read back what has been written.

However, according to safety recommendations from JCAHO, during a "code" situation, it is sufficient if the physician calls out a medication order and the nurse repeats it back before administration. In this instance, a "repeat back" rather than "read back" verification is acceptable. Also acceptable is for a different person to record or document the medication.[2]

High-Alert Medications

The Institute for Safe Medication Practices[3] has a list of high-alert medications that have a significant risk of causing serious patient harm if errors are made during administration. For these medications, special safeguards should be in place to reduce errors. The institute recommends risk reduction strategies such as limiting access; using auxiliary labels and automated alerts; standardizing ordering, preparation, and administration; and use of double-checks. Box 7-1 lists some of the drug classes and specific medications most relevant to trauma care.

Box 7-1   HIGH-ALERT MEDICATION CATEGORIES AND SPECIFIC MEDICATIONS RELEVANT TO TRAUMA CARE

High-alert medication categories

- Adrenergic agonists, IV (e.g., epinephrine)
- Adrenergic antagonists, IV (e.g., propranolol)
- Anesthetic agents, general, inhaled and IV (e.g., propofol)
- Inotropic medications, IV (e.g., digoxin and milrinone)
- Moderate sedation agents, IV (e.g., midazolam)
- Moderate sedation agents, oral, for children (e.g., chloral hydrate)
- Narcotics/opiates, IV and oral (including liquid concentrates and immediate- and sustained-release)
- Neuromuscular blocking agents (e.g., succinylcholine)
- Radiocontrast agents, IV
- Thrombolytics/fibrinolytics, IV (e.g., tenecteplase)

High-alert medications

- Heparin, low molecular weight, injection
- Heparin, unfractionated, IV
- Insulin, subcutaneous and IV
- Lidocaine, IV
- Nitroprusside sodium, for injection
- Sodium chloride injection, hypertonic, more than 0.9% concentration
- Warfarin

(Modified from *ISMP's list of high-alert medications*, Huntingdon Valley, Pa, 2005, Institute for Safe Medication Practices. Retrieved March 7, 2006, from www.ismp.org/Tools/highalertmedications.pdf)

Universal Protocol

The JCAHO has developed the *Universal Protocol for Preventing Wrong Site, Wrong Procedure, Wrong Person Surgery.*[4] The protocol includes preoperative verification, site marking, and a procedural pause or time-out immediately before the initiation of any invasive procedure. During the time-out, the team verifies that the *correct procedure* will be performed on the *correct patient* at the *correct site* and that all necessary documents are available. The entire team participates in the time-out, and the communication should be active (spoken verification, not just the absence of objection). The pause is applicable to a number of trauma procedures, such as chest tube placement and central line insertions. However, JCAHO standards advise that these precautions should not delay urgent care required during an emergency situation and that the time-out procedure *does not* apply if it is too risky to pause. The pause does not need to be used before minor procedures such as venipuncture, peripheral intravenous insertion, nasogastric tube placement, or urinary catheter insertion.

For any procedures which involve laterality (right side versus left side), multiple structures (fingers), or multiple levels (vertebrae), the JCAHO mandates marking of the correct site on the skin before the procedure. The marking should be done directly on the skin at the site where the procedure is to be done using a hospital-approved mark. If the patient is alert, he or she should be asked to confirm that the correct site has been marked. If the procedure is to be done in a procedure room, the site should be marked before the patient is moved to the room. Again, site marking can be deferred if the patient is too unstable to delay the procedure. Another exception is when the provider who will be performing the procedure is with the patient continuously from preprocedure preparation until the start of the procedure. Site marking is not necessary for procedures to be performed on obvious wounds.

Handoffs

The JCAHO added a new patient safety goal related to handoff communications[2] in 2006. A handoff is any transfer of responsibility for a patient from one clinician to another. The safety implications of incompletely or inaccurately transmitting information about a critical trauma patient are obvious. Many handoffs occur during trauma care, including first responders to prehospital personnel; prehospital to ED or flight crew; referral hospital to receiving trauma center; and ED to operating room, intensive care unit, or floor staff. The JCAHO requires that institutions adopt a standardized approach for handoffs. The opportunity for verbal interaction and the opportunity to ask and answer questions must be provided. All handoffs should include information about a patient's care, treatment, status, and recent/anticipated changes. Verbal report often is reinforced with a standardized guide to the handoff components or with a written form.

Use of Restraints

Trauma patients may need to have physical restraints applied for protective purposes, that is, to preserve the safety of the patient and of the staff. Restraints may be necessary to prevent removal of endotracheal tubes, central and peripheral intravenous lines, monitors, or catheters. The rationale for restraints and the trial of less intrusive measures (when feasible) should be documented in the medical record. Restraints must be applied safely, observed frequently per protocol, and documented in timely fashion. Failure to reflect close observation and documentation leaves the nurse vulnerable should an adverse event occur.

Documentation

Documentation must be clear and must include a description of injuries, vital signs and other assessment data trends, diagnostic tests performed and available results, and medical interventions. All procedures must be documented in their order of occurrence. Initials next to procedures must be legible with full name and professional status indicated within the document. Flow sheets with checklists facilitate the ease of documentation. If times are recorded in a format other than the 24-hour military clock (preferred), AM and PM must be clearly indicated with the date. Each page must contain the patient identification information. Pages are photocopied for legal/insurance reasons and may not be admissible if identification information is missing from the record.

Trauma flow sheets must include details, starting with the patient's arrival, that document the entire ED stay. Where possible, one nurse should be assigned to document during a trauma resuscitation. Documentation must be written in real time, rather than from memory when the event is over. Interventions such as endotracheal intubation, chest tube insertion, IV insertion and fluid administration, medication administration, and portable x-ray films and other diagnostic tests should appear in chronologic order.

Abbreviations

Abbreviations that may lead to patient error must be avoided. The JCAHO has compiled a list of common abbreviations that have led to nursing/medical errors (Table 7-1).

Medication Administration

Medications need to be documented thoroughly, including the following:

1. Full name of medication
2. Dose or strength
3. Route
4. Sites of injections for agents such as tetanus toxoid and immune globulin
5. Infusion rate
6. Patient response

Proper Use of Medical Equipment

Proper use of medical equipment includes the following:

1. The time of application and discontinuance of equipment should be documented, including warming of equipment used for hypothermia or autotransfusion equipment, along with any equipment settings or other procedure details.
2. For patients requiring defibrillation, the documentation should include the number, time, and strength of defibrillator charges delivered.

NURSING LIABILITY DURING TRAUMA

The nurse, as part of the trauma team, may be held liable for actions committed or omitted during care of the patient. Most commonly, the hospital as the employer also will be named under the theory of *respondeat superior.* If the nurse departs from acceptable standards of

Table 7–1   Dangerous Abbreviations

Abbreviations to be Avoided and Intended Meaning	Potential Problem	Recommended Terms
U (unit)	Mistaken as zero, four, or cc	unit
IU (international unit)	Mistaken as IV (intravenous) or 10 (ten)	international unit
Q.D. Q.O.D. (once daily and every other day)	Mistaken for each other. The period after the Q can be mistaken for an "I," and the "O" can be mistaken for "I."	daily every other day
X.0 mg (use of trailing zero) [Note: Prohibited only for medication-related notations]	Decimal point is missed	X mg (never write a zero by itself after a decimal point)
.X mg (lack of leading zero)	Decimal point is missed	0.X mg (always use a zero before a decimal point)
MS MSO₄ MgSO₄	Confused for one another Can mean morphine sulfate or magnesium sulfate	morphine sulfate *or* magnesium sulfate
µg (microgram)	Mistaken for mg (milligrams) resulting in one thousandfold dosing overdose	mcg
H.S. (half-strength or Latin abbreviation for bedtime)	Mistaken for half-strength or hour of sleep (at bedtime). q.H.S. mistaken for every hour. All can result in a dosing error	half-strength *or* at bedtime
T.I.W. (3 times a week)	Mistaken for 3 times a day or twice weekly, resulting in an overdose or underdose	3 times weekly *or* three times weekly
D/C (discharge)	Interpreted as discontinue whatever medications follow (typically discharge meds)	discharge
c.c. (cubic centimeter)	Mistaken for U (units) when poorly written	mL (milliliters)
A.S., A.D., A.U. (Latin abbreviations for *left ear, right ear,* and *both ears*)	Mistaken for OS, OD, or OU (*left eye, right eye,* or *both eyes*)	left ear, right ear, *or* both ears

Modified from *FAQs about the 2004 National Patient Safety Goals, Questions about Goal #2 (Communication),* Oakbrook Terrace, Ill, 2003, Joint Commission for the Accreditation of Health Care Organizations. From www.jcaho.org/accredited+organizations/patient+safety/04+npsg/04_faqs.htm
Note: These preferred practices apply to all documentation—including orders, progress notes, consultation reports, and operative notes—and to written, preprinted, and electronic formats.

care or does not follow the policies and procedures outlined by the employer, the hospital or institution may not stand behind the nurse's actions. For this reason, some professionals elect to carry individual malpractice insurance policies rather than rely solely on employee coverage. The potential for malpractice exists in the areas of communications, treatment issues, monitoring issues, medications, supervision, and the chain of command[5]:

- Regarding verbal or written *communications*, the nurse should take care to communicate all pertinent information as completely, accurately, quickly, and frequently as is dictated by institutional policy and the patient's clinical condition.
- When performing or assisting with a *treatment or procedure*, the nurse is expected to provide the correct treatment and provide it correctly and to initiate the procedure in an appropriate time frame.
- When *monitoring* a patient, the nurse needs to monitor the appropriate parameters in the appropriate frequency according to institutional policy and the patient's clinical condition. Monitor alarms must be active. Nursing actions in response to any deterioration in a patient's condition need to be prompt, appropriate, and documented.
- When administering *medications*, the nurse should always keep in mind the "Five Rights":
  - Right medication
  - Right dose
  - Right time
  - Right route
  - Right patient

Orders need to be clarified if there is any question about their content or correctness. After administration, the patient needs to be assessed for the effect of the drug and for possible adverse reactions, side effects, or toxicity.

- *Supervision* issues are related to expectations that nurses will supervise and delegate to assistive staff appropriately, following institutional policy and adhering to statutory/regulatory requirements.
- Last, the nurse must follow the *chain of command* when indicated. In the event that the trauma nurse feels that the treatment plan is incorrect or may cause potential and/or unnecessary harm to a patient, the nurse should activate the chain of command in the nursing and/or physician structure. The charge nurse, supervisor, or attending physician must be made aware of the nurse's concerns.

LAW RELEVANT TO TRAUMA NURSES

Nurse Practice Act

Every state has its own nurse practice act. Every nurse is expected to be familiar with nursing practice legislation and regulations promulgated within their practice arena.

Good Samaritan Law

A Good Samaritan law is a statute that exempts from liability a person, such as an off-duty physician or nurse, who voluntarily renders aid to another in imminent danger but negligently causes injury while rendering aid. Some form of coverage is offered in all 50 states and in the District of Columbia. According to Heilig, "The trauma nurse who becomes involved in the care of a victim of a car crash or of a violent crime during off-duty hours is not liable for negligent acts. When an off-duty nurse happens to be at an incident scene, there is an ethical, moral, if not legal, duty to stop and render assistance."[6]

Consent Issues

Consent issues are encountered commonly during trauma care.

Types of Consent

Blanket Consent for Treatment. The blanket consent usually is obtained when a patient enters the ED and refers to general measures such as medications, diagnostic tests such as laboratory tests, and noninvasive radiologic studies.

Informed Consent. The term *informed consent* signifies that the patient has full understanding of the risks and benefits and possible undesirable effects or risks of a procedure. To give informed consent, the patient must be competent and not under the influence of any drugs or other agents that could impair judgment. The patient also must have the legal right to give consent.

Implied Consent. Implied consent is activated when the patient is not in a condition to give consent and when no next-of-kin is present. Implied consent should be used only when danger to life and/or limb exists and it is regarded that the patient would have preferred care to no care in this situation. This is an exception to informed consent and should be used judiciously.

Consent for an unconscious, mentally impaired, incoherent, or combative patient should include all efforts to reach responsible parties, family members, or institution administrators if the patient is in the custody of a state or federal facility. Treatment under implied consent can be used only if there is a life-threatening emergency. Careful documentation of all efforts and responses to attempts to obtain consent must be documented clearly.

Minors

The status of minority is defined by state law. With minors, consent must be sought from parents or legal guardians before care and invasive procedures whenever possible. In the event of urgent and emergent care, the potential hazard of waiting for consent must be weighed against the need to initiate lifesaving interventions. Documentation within the ED records should reflect efforts and results in attempts to locate family members. At times, the hospital may involve a judge or court to issue an order to implement treatment, such as the situation when a parent refuses treatment for a minor child.

Prisoners

Prisoners are in the custody of federal, state, local, or immigration authorities. Their individual rights may be diminished because of their legal status. Hospital administration should be notified if legal counsel needs to become involved regarding treatment or consent. Staff cannot be compelled by authorities to provide evidence obtained from the patient, such as drug-filled condoms expelled after the use of laxatives or obtained through a cavity search of the patient. This violates the patient's fourth amendment constitutional right of unlawful search and seizure.

Religious Considerations and Consent

Certain religions prohibit organ and tissue transplantation, blood transfusions, or autopsies. The ED staff should be familiar with common considerations of various religions because they have a duty to honor and respect the wishes of the patient and family, even when they conflict with the personal beliefs of the caregiver.

Refusal of Treatment

Competent patients have the right to refuse any form of treatment. The ED staff has the responsibility to ensure that the patient and family are educated about the need for procedures. If the patient has been given appropriate information and understands the implications of not receiving treatment, then the refusal is within the rights of the patient. If the treatment or procedure is forced on the patient, then charges of assault and battery may be made against the staff.

Signing out Against Medical Advice. At times, patients elect to sign out against medical advice. It is imperative that the patient be mentally competent to make this informed decision and that he or she has been told the risks of leaving without treatment. If the ED staff believes that the patient is incompetent, then obtaining a signature on an against-medical-advice form may be considered legally invalid.

Elopement. Some patients "elope," or just leave the ED without notice. Documentation of this must be included in the ED records, including the time the elopement was detected by the staff.

Court Orders for Treatment. Hospital administrators may ask for a court order to deliver medical treatments when refusal by family or a patient may compromise a patient's life. For example, a court order may need to be obtained for a child who needs a blood transfusion but whose parents refuse because of religious beliefs.

Mandated Reporting

Mandatory reporting to appropriate agencies or authorities in certain situations is the responsibility of trauma care providers. The physician, administrator, or nurse may be the one to inform authorities. Each hospital should maintain policies and procedures for conditions that must be reported. Situations commonly reported include the following:

- Animal bites
- Burns
- Gunshot wounds
- Poisonings
- Sexual assault
- Stabbings
- Suspected abuse of a child, elder, or dependent adult
- Suspicious deaths

Child abuse, infanticide, partner abuse, elder abuse, and abuse of disabled, custodial, and institutionalized patients are mandated-reporting events. This topic is covered in Chapter 23, where detailed information can be found on interpersonal violence. The potential ramifications of mandatory reporting often worry nurses who interact with the patient. It may be reassuring to keep in mind that nurses or physicians cannot be held liable if the suspect signs of abuse ultimately are determined to be unfounded.

Emergency Medical Treatment and Active Labor Act

The Emergency Medical Treatment and Active Labor Act (EMTALA), a federal statute passed in 1986, was designed to stop "patient dumping" of uninsured and poor patients to other facilities. EMTALA and its accompanying regulations and guidelines cover many facets of antidumping; only trauma-related aspects are reviewed in this section[7,8]:

- All individuals who arrive at the ED are entitled to an appropriate medical screening to determine whether an emergency medical condition exists.
- An assessment must be completed to ascertain the clinical situation. This may be done at triage and within the ED.
- Patients with emergency medical conditions must be stabilized.
- Patients may be transferred for provision of care beyond the capability or capacity of a hospital.
- Patient transfer according to regional protocol within the context of a trauma system is acceptable.
- Patients must be stabilized to the extent possible before any transfer; the goal is to "ensure, within reasonable medical probability, that no material deterioration is likely to result from or occur during the transfer."[6] However, it is recognized that the inability to stabilize a patient completely may in itself be an indication for transfer.
- Four requirements for appropriate transfer are the following:
  1. The transferring facility provides medical treatment within its capacity.
  2. The receiving agency agrees to accept the patient and has available space and qualified personnel.
  3. The transferring hospital sends all relevant medical records to the receiving facility.
  4. Patients are transported in an appropriately equipped vehicle with qualified personnel. The level of care and skill previously provided must be maintained during transfer. For additional information about patient transfer, see Chapter 4.
- Referral centers such as trauma centers and burn units are obligated to accept all appropriate transfers of patients if they have the capacity to treat the individual.

Health Insurance Portability and Accountability Act

The Health Insurance Portability and Accountability Act of 1996 imposed a number of requirements on hospitals in the areas of patient privacy and confidentiality. The law and accompanying regulations are extensive. Only key points relevant to trauma care are outlined next[9-11]:

- Providers must protect what is known as personal health information (PHI). This includes information related to a patient's health status or health care.
- PHI may be disclosed for the purposes of treatment or health care operations. Health care operations include quality assessment/improvement and education activities. Providing follow-up to referral agencies is acceptable.
- PHI may be disclosed for 12 national priority purposes, among which are mandated reporting, law enforcement, disclosures to coroners or medical examiners, organ donation, and worker's compensation claims.

■ With appropriate permission, PHI may be disclosed to family members or significant others. Verification of identification before disclosing PHI is expected.

FORENSIC CONSIDERATIONS IN TRAUMA CARE

Trauma nurses perform an important role in the investigation of crimes and the legal process related to victims of violence. In particular, cases may be won or lost based on the handling of evidence. The emergency nurse is often the first to assess and observe the initial arrival of the trauma patient. Nurses working with trauma patients should have the knowledge and ability to describe various types of crime-related injuries. Inaccurate descriptions can result in confusion and lead to the legal case against the perpetrator being weakened or dismissed. Documentation should include the location and dimensions of all injuries. Diagrams, body maps, or photography help to reconstruct injury patterns.

Many EDs are building a cadre of forensic nurse experts. In the trauma room the forensic nurse is responsible for preserving evidence, interviewing the witnesses, collecting evidence, and managing forensic issues until the case is turned over to the proper authority. Forensic nurses are skilled in forensic technique and appropriate medical-legal procedures.[12]

Evidence

Emergency nurses become involved in evidence collection when a patient is admitted for trauma care from suspicious injuries that may be crime-related or self-inflicted. Hospital EDs are regularly in contact with essential evidence in criminal cases. Clinicians should keep in mind that it is not always possible to predict whether a trauma incident will result in future criminal or civil action. Therefore, ED staff should approach most trauma cases as potentially litigious and should consider evidence collection wherever possible.

Forensic evidence may be lost by the ED staff when crime victims are treated if the staff are not aware of its presence or potential value. The most common types of evidence include clothing, bullets, bloodstains, hairs, fibers, and small pieces of material such as fragments of metal, glass, paint, and wood. Also, any personal property may constitute forensic evidence and should never be released to the family without the permission of the police. However, information regarding a blood alcohol level or toxicology screens cannot be released to the police without the patient's consent. If necessary, lawyers can request a subpoena later to obtain such material. Documentation must reflect the accurate identification, description, and security of medical-legal evidence.

Preserving Clothing Evidence

It is imperative that nurses in the clinical environment recognize and preserve vital fragments of trace evidence by careful handling of the patient's clothing and personal property. This is one of the most important actions by nurses that can aid the investigation process. Clothing worn at the time of the incident may contain trace evidence useful in linking the victim with the assailant or crime scene.

Careful examination of defects in clothes can be compared to the wounds of the victim, and often clothes provide insight into the type of weapon or wounding instrument used. Clothing from automobile or pedestrian incidents may display tire impressions or conceal trace evidence, such as paint chips or broken glass, that could identify the vehicle that struck the victim. Gunshot residues surrounding bullet holes in the clothes may determine the distance of the firearm from the victim at the time of firing (range of fire).

Documentation of the condition of the patient's clothing should be noted carefully, including the color, type, unusual markings, and tears or other damages.

Processing Clothing. Clothing should be removed carefully to protect any foreign fragments adhering to them:

1. Clothing should not be shaken.
2. Clothing frequently is cut away during resuscitation. The ED staff should avoid cutting through tears, rips, and holes that may have resulted from the weapon or the assault.
3. Clothing should never be discarded or thrown on the floor because this can result in cross-contamination of trace evidence with debris from the treatment environment.
4. A clean, white sheet can be placed on an empty trauma table, equipment stand, or on the floor in the corner of the room to receive clothing until time permits appropriate packaging.
5. Clean white paper should be placed over stains to avoid cross-contamination with other articles.
6. If a victim can remove his or her clothes, this should be done standing on a clean sheet or a large sheet of paper. This will collect any microscopic evidence that may become dislodged during removal.
7. The collection sheet must be placed in a separate paper bag and labeled for transfer to the crime laboratory.

Preservation. Use the following guidelines for preserving forensic evidence:

1. If possible, moist clothing should be hung up to dry in a secure area.
2. Police should be told whether clothing they are to retrieve is in a damp condition.
3. Each item of clothing should be stored in separate paper, *not plastic,* bags. Plastic bags are inappropriate because there is a tendency for condensation to accumulate, resulting in degradation of the integrity of the evidence.
4. Each bag should be sealed and clearly marked with the date, time, and signature or initials of the individual doing the sealing.

Wound Characteristics

Wound characteristics constitute evidence that may be obscured by emergency trauma care. The nurse's initial documentation should include the location of injuries and their approximate measurements. This includes sharp, blunt, and fast-force injuries, such as contusions, cuts, lacerations, stab wounds, and bullet wounds, as well as uniquely patterned injuries such as bite marks. Diagrams, body maps, or photography are helpful in reconstructing injury patterns in subsequent investigations or at autopsy. For patients who survive, or whose wound is excised or extended surgically, later reconstruction of the injury is impossible. Also, treatment procedures and the natural healing process may alter the condition of the wound.

Nurses should be knowledgeable about the types of injuries generally resulting in medical-legal cases and should be familiar with the appropriate terminology. In general, however, rather than labeling injuries in terms such as entrance or exit wound, defense wounds, or hesitation wounds, it is far better simply to describe and/or photograph or diagram the wound.

Any bullet or bullet fragments recovered during treatment should be packaged properly and turned over to the crime scene officer in an unaltered condition.

Chain of Custody

The evidence chain of custody begins with the person who collects the evidence. Items placed in bags should be labeled with the patient's name, date, time of placement, and full signature of the person collecting the evidence. The items must remain in view or under lock and key until the police investigator or coroner sign as having received them. Each individual must maintain the chain of custody to ensure it can be used as evidence. Rules of evidence require a chain of custody for each item recovered from the patient. This includes trace and physical evidence, laboratory specimens of blood and body fluids, clothing, and personal articles. The integrity of every specimen or piece of evidence seized must be ensured to protect its admissibility in a court of law. Failure to maintain the chain of custody renders potentially important evidence worthless if lost, damaged, or unaccountable from the hands of the nurse to the police officer.

SUDDEN AND UNEXPECTED DEATHS

Sudden and violent deaths most frequently represent the initial interface between the hospital staff and police in the ED. Considering the number of sudden and unexpected trauma deaths that occur in the clinical setting, nurses have a critical role to play in providing answers in questionable death situations. Deaths that occur because of trauma or unknown causes require investigation. Generally, any death that occurs during the first 24 hours after admission is reportable to the medical examiner/coroner system regardless of the history, and the medical examiner's office may take custody of the body at its discretion. The medical examiner legally may overrule the wishes of a family. Suspicious or unexpected deaths may warrant an autopsy in spite of family objections.

If a death occurs in the trauma room, the room immediately becomes a scene of legal inquiry and is listed as the place of death on the death certificate regardless of where the initial incident occurred. The death scene must be protected until the body and evidence have been removed at the completion of any medical-legal investigation.

Maintaining an index of suspicion is essential for the ED staff when considering criminal activity as a cause of sudden and unexpected death. Preservation of evidence and careful documentation of the circumstances surrounding the death and the decedent's social and medical history may form the basis for deducing the cause of death when it is not obvious. Nurses are among the first to come in contact with the patient, interview family members, and handle the patient's property and laboratory specimens. They serve as a vital link among the victim, police, and medical examiner or coroner.

Advance Directives

In 1991, hospitals began to implement the Patient Self-Determination Act by asking all patients admitted to the hospital about their individual wishes in the event of a life-threatening situation. Several types of advance directives are in use in the United States today. Advance directives often are not applicable during an initial trauma resuscitation, but they are important components of the total plan of care. Advance directives include the following:

- Living will: This document outlines exactly what treatment measures should and should not be used in the event of a critical situation in which resuscitation may be necessary. The living will is intended to be prepared by the patient during a nonurgent time and shared with family members.
- Health care proxy (also called durable power of attorney for health care): Some states do not recognize living wills but use health care proxies instead. A health care proxy is a written document that takes effect when a patient is unable to speak for himself or herself and names a proxy who will pass on the wishes of the patient. It is understood that a discussion of the patient's wishes has taken place with the proxy before it is implemented. The health care proxy is not valid if the patient can communicate with mental clarity.

- DNR orders: A "do not resuscitate" decision may be made by the patient or, if the patient is incapable, the family, if they know the patient's wishes. In the event of an unexpected emergency, family members are called on to make these decisions and rely greatly on the medical and nursing personnel to understand the current diagnosis and prognosis. Family conversations should be documented carefully and completely.
- Uniform Anatomical Gift Act (1987): The option of organ and tissue donation should be offered when it is anticipated that a trauma patient might die in the ED or need to be kept on pharmacotherapy to allow perfusion of organs with the potential for donation. The hospital organ donation coordinator should be notified and will work with the trauma team and family in educating them about possible options for donation of tissue or organs. See Chapter 9 for more details on organ and tissue donation.

PRODUCT LIABILITY

Another area of legal concern is that of product liability. This area has ramifications for patients and clinicians and includes the following:

- Competency with equipment use: For all medical equipment used during trauma care, the trauma nurse is accountable for being oriented to its use and competent in its use. Competency usually is established during orientation to the ED and periodically is refreshed or renewed as needed. The professional nurse is responsible to know how to operate equipment correctly and safely or to ensure another person will do this if there is a knowledge deficit.
- Malfunctioning medical equipment: If a piece of medical equipment malfunctions, the trauma nurse is responsible for ensuring that the equipment is replaced or fixed immediately. A record of such malfunction must be reported through the chain of command. This includes electronic, battery, computer, and manual equipment. It becomes a safety issue if the item simply is marked "broken" and is not replaced or repaired.
- Malfunctioning industrial equipment: If a trauma patient's injury is a result of a faulty piece of industrial equipment, the notation should be made in the medical record that the injury was reported as resulting from a malfunctioning piece of equipment or machine. This notation should be made in the patient's own words and placed in quotation marks. This piece of information is necessary for investigations by the Occupational Safety and Health Administration and any legal proceedings evolving from the incident.
- Industrial accident cases: A notation should be included in the trauma record that the injuries occurred at work. Worker's compensation may be awarded (or denied) based on the documentation within medical records.
- Motor vehicle malfunctions: If a faulty motor vehicle is thought to be the cause of injury, then descriptions from witnesses, driver, or passengers should be documented using quotation marks.

SUMMARY

The trauma nurse faces areas of potential interaction with legal issues many times during the initial hour of care. Issues of privacy, consent, forensic concerns around documentation and evidence collection, and risk management in avoiding hospital-based errors during care abound. Nevertheless, staying on top of the basic legal principles covered in this chapter can protect not only the trauma victim but also the trauma team.

References

1. Garner B, editor: *Black's law dictionary,* ed 7, St Paul, Minn, 1999, West Group.
2. *Joint Commission 2006 National Patient Safety Goals: implementation expectations,* Oakbrook Terrace, Ill, 2006, Joint Commission on Accreditation of Healthcare Organizations. Retrieved March 7, 2006, from www.jointcommission.org/NR/rdonlyres/DDE15942-8A19-4674-9F3B-C6AE2477072A/0/06_NPSG_IE.pdf
3. *ISMP's list of high-alert medications,* Huntingdon Valley, Pa, 2005, Institute for Safe Medication Practices. Retrieved March 7, 2006, from www.ismp.org/Tools/highalertmedications.pdf
4. *Universal protocol for preventing wrong site, wrong procedure, wrong person surgery,* Oakbrook Terrace, Ill, 2003, Joint Commission on Accreditation of Healthcare Organizations. Retrieved March 7, 2006, from www.jointcommission.org/NR/rdonlyres/E3C600EB-043B-4E86-B04E-CA4A89AD5433/0/universal_protocol.pdf
5. Bogart JB, editor: *Legal nurse consulting: principles and practice,* Boca Raton, Fla, 1998, CRC Press.
6. Heilig RW: Legal concerns in trauma nursing. In McQuillan KA, Von Ruden KT, Hartsock RL, et al, editors: *Trauma nursing from resuscitation through rehabilitation,* ed 3, Philadelphia, 2002, Saunders.
7. US Department of Health and Human Services, Centers for Medicare and Medicaid Services: *State operations manual: appendix V—interpretive guidelines—responsibilities of Medicare participating hospitals in emergency cases,* Baltimore, Md, 2004, The Centers. Retrieved October 25, 2006, from www.cms.hhs.gov/manuals/Downloads/som107ap_v_emerg.pdf
8. Brown LC, Cochran RG: CMS issues much-anticipated EMTALA guidelines, *J Trauma Nurs* 11(3):107-110, 2004.
9. Office for Civil Rights, US Department of Health and Human Services: *Summary of the HIPAA privacy rule,* Washington, DC, 2003, The Department. Retrieved October 25, 2006, from www.hhs.gov/ocr/privacysummary.pdf
10. Moscop JC, Marco CA, Larkin GL, et al: From Hippocrates to HIPAA: privacy and confidentiality in emergency medicine. Part I: conceptual, moral, and legal foundations, *Ann Emerg Med* 45:53-59, 2005.
11. Moscop JC, Marco CA, Larkin GL, et al: From Hippocrates to HIPAA: privacy and confidentiality in emergency medicine. Part II: challenges in the emergency department, *Ann Emerg Med* 45:60-67, 2005.
12. Lynch VA, Duval JB, editors: *Forensic nursing,* St Louis, 2005, Mosby.

CHAPTER 8

CRISIS INTERVENTION IN TRAUMA

PATRICIA MIAN

A crisis is an acutely time-limited state of disequilibrium resulting from situational, developmental or societal sources of stress. A person in this state is temporarily unable to cope with or adapt to the stressor by using previous methods of problem solving.[1]

Death, grief, loss of a body part, disfigurement, concerns about the cost of care, loss of property, and family relationships are issues than can factor into crises experienced by the trauma patient and family.

Whatever the cause, a crisis can threaten to overwhelm a person's emotional resources.

Traumatic injury is a situational crisis that is unexpected and is defined by the following:

1. The event is sudden, without warning, and there is not adequate preparation time to handle the event.
2. The event is perceived as a threat to life and bodily integrity, whether realistic or not.
3. A sense of displacement and detachment from familiar surroundings and persons occurs.
4. A loss or threat of loss of person, health, or hope occurs.

STAGES IN CRISIS

Crisis and response are considered in four generally accepted stages.

Stage One: Impact/Shock

The initial response to shock occurs on physical, cognitive, and emotional levels:

Physical

- Arousal triggered by the fight-or-flight response
- Increased epinephrine output and sensory input with increased anxiety and tension
- Physical distress such as nausea, dizziness, and difficulty breathing

Cognitive

- Denial of the trauma
- An attempt by the mind to try to reframe the information into an unthreatening interpretation

Emotional

- Disbelief
- A sense of unreality as if the world were in slow motion

Stage Two: Confusion and Disorganization

Confusion and disorganization give way to a multitude of emotions including feelings of helplessness and inability to cope.

Stage Three: Problem Solving and Reorganization

The third stage involves problem solving and reorganization:

- Attempting to problem solve as the reality of the situation is faced
- Use of new and different ways to cope

Stage Four: Resolution

- In the last stage the trauma patient comes to resolution concerning the crisis:
- Work toward resolution and resumption of normal life
- Hope is that positive growth will occur as a result of the crisis

GOALS OF CRISIS INTERVENTION

In crisis intervention, it is important to define the crisis as the individual sees it, not as the health care provider perceives it. Some may manage a seemingly overwhelming event, whereas others can be overwhelmed by lesser stress. Concurrent stressors in the individual's life also can affect how the crisis is handled. The goals of crisis intervention include the following:

1. To decrease the emotional distress to tolerable limits
2. To mobilize internal and external resources
3. To return to the precrisis level of functioning and gain positive benefit from coping with the crisis

BALANCING FACTORS

Aguilera[2] defines three balancing factors that determine how the individual will experience the crisis:

1. Perception of the event: The cognitive or subjective meaning of the event to the individual
   One's perception of the event rather than the actual event determines how the situation is perceived. What is the meaning of the event to the person?
2. Situational supports: The person's significant relationships and who the individuals are on whom the person can count for help
   This can include family, friends, co-workers, or spiritual supporters. The lack of a support network can lead to increased isolation and vulnerability.
3. Coping capacities: The individual's internal strengths
   How does this person cope with stress and what has worked for that person in the past? Individuals have different vulnerabilities to stress and different coping strategies.

STEPS IN CRISIS INTERVENTION

Most crises resolve on their own, and the changes experienced become integrated into a person's life over time. However, early intervention helps prevent long-term negative effects. Be proactive and reach out to those in crisis by using the following guidelines:

ASSESSMENT

- Establish rapport and use language that is appropriate to the person's level of understanding.
- Identify the degree of distress defined by the behaviors exhibited, emotions expressed, and cognition of the response.

PLAN INTERVENTIONS

- Acknowledge the problem, and move toward resolution.
- Encourage the individual and family to problem solve and generate new solutions.
- Draw on resources to develop small, manageable goals.
- Help individuals maintain self-esteem and portray an individual's attempt to cope in a positive light.

ANTICIPATORY PLANNING

- Continually reassess the situation and the individual's response.
- Assist the patient in moving toward independence and formulating realistic plans for the future.

IDENTIFICATION OF MALADAPTIVE COPING

When a person is not coping well, it is important to recognize the signs and to help redirect the process. The following are some possible signs of maladaptive coping:

- Excessive denial or withdrawal. The individual uses fantasy to replace or merge with reality. For example, a mother who continually tells her child to wake up when the child is dead.
- Impulsive behavior and scapegoats used to vent rage. For example, an individual who continually lashes out at staff members and has no insight into the behavior.
- Denial of feelings—overcontrol of emotions. An overly stoic individual who insists that he or she is fine in the face of devastating circumstances.
- Too much dependence or too much independence. The individual cannot make any decision on his or her own or cannot accept help from staff members.
- Inability to ask for or use help when it is offered or needed.
- Ritualistic behavior. An attempt to control anxiety and fears related to impending danger or loss. For example, the patient constantly may check the medical equipment, straighten out the sheets, or wash hands.

STAGES OF CRISIS IN THE TRAUMA PATIENT

Trauma patients are confronted with their own vulnerability and an overwhelming threat to their life. Morse and O'Brien[3] describe the four stages of crisis for the trauma patient. The degree of stress is determined by the patient's physiologic state and perceptions, coping styles, and support system.

Step One: Vigilance

Initially, there is a heightened sense of awareness of the event and an attempt to control or direct activities. Time slows down. Internally, the patient feels calm and detached, although the visual imagery is frightening. Once the medical system intervenes, the patient surrenders control to it.

Interventions are as follows:

- Provide patient with information.
- Make environment safe and private.
- Explain all procedures.

Step Two: Disruption

Patients in the critical stage of disruption experience great fear and confusion. The focus shifts from surviving to the reality of the trauma and the losses associated with it. These losses include body alteration, inability to communicate, and loss of emotional autonomy. The patient feels powerless, and the environment may be perceived as hostile and threatening.

Interventions are as follows:

- Ensure that family members are present.
- Keep communication open, provide specific information, and answer patient's and family members' questions.
- Develop effective means of communication; for example, for an intubated patient, ask questions that require a "yes" or "no" answer.
- Reorient the patient to time, place, and person.
- Provide medication or other forms of relief from pain and anxiety.

Step Three: Regrouping

Regrouping is the beginning to adjust to the implications of the injury and learning to live with setbacks and disappointments. The patient accepts dependence on others for care.

Interventions are as follows:

- Begin exploring circumstances of injury with patient.
- Empower the patient by giving positive feedback.
- Provide realistic hope.

Step Four: Striving to Regain Self

The final stage is integrating the old self with the new self, including acceptance of the traumatic injury and reintegration into society.

Interventions are as follows:

- Help the patient integrate details of the trauma event. The patient reviews trauma as it becomes part of his or her life story.
- Assess the patient for risk of psychological complications.

TRAUMA AND THE FAMILY

During the resuscitative stage and initial stage of treatment, families of trauma patients are in a crisis state. Fear and uncertainty about the patient's condition and lack of information increases the stress. Because trauma is such an unexpected event, there has been no preparation or "worry" time. Along with the abrupt separation from the patient, families feel they have no control over the events that are happening. They are coping with a traumatic event in an unknown environment with strangers. During a crisis, individuals are impressionable and there is a heightened awareness of their surroundings.

During the first two stages of crisis, families generally experience the following:

Anxiety: The family member experiences pacing, hyperventilation, and a feeling of "jumping out of one's skin."

Denial: The family member cannot process what has happened. This helps the individual buy psychological time to adjust. "He'll be fine."

Anger: Helplessness and feelings of powerlessness about the trauma may be expressed in anger, which may be misdirected to others, such as staff members. Anger can delay the feelings of grief and sadness, which may be too painful to tolerate.

Remorse and guilt: The patient may have feelings that he or she should have been able to prevent what happened and could have done more. The family member says many "if only" statements. If the relationship with the patient is complicated or conflicted, family members may experience even more guilt.

Sadness and grief: This is an expression of pain as the reality of the trauma or loss is experienced. Crying, a longing for the patient, and sharing of the patient's life as the family begins to understand the magnitude of the event.

INTERVENTIONS FOR FAMILIES

A critical and significant therapeutic way of helping families of trauma patients is simply "being with them" at this difficult time. This is the ability of the staff member to bear witness to another's grief and to let the family know they are not alone and will be helped through the crisis. Simply sitting with the family or listening quietly can be a powerful intervention. A calm presence in the middle of chaos is reassuring and comforting for the family.

Communication

Communication with the family should include the following:

- Use the patient's name: This makes the crisis more real and shows respect for the patient. It helps staff members develop alliance.
- Short, simple sentences: The family is too disorganized to take in a great deal of information. You may need to use nonmedical terminology.
- Repetition: Review and repeat medical information. This helps the family process the event and stay focused on the topic.
- Feedback: Have the family repeat back what they have heard. This makes the situation more real and helps family members to assess their perceptions of the event.
- Clarification: Clarify and correct distortions so that the family has a realistic perception of the situation. "I know you wish everything would be fine."

Safety and Structure

To provide safety and structure for the family, do the following:

- Ensure privacy. Families should be brought to a private room when they arrive and should be protected from others (such as well-meaning friends and reporters).
- Provide medical information as soon as possible.

- Meet basic comfort needs. Offer water, coffee, juice, and blankets.
- Provide orientation. Families need to be oriented to the structure of the trauma center and the expectations of staff and family. Give time frames because time is distorted during a crisis.

Information and Validation

Provide the following information and validation for the family:

- Medical information: Staff members should inform family members of the severity and critical nature of the trauma as quickly as possible. The information should be clear, concise, and factual. This helps give families "worry time" and helps break down denial.
- The event: Obtain as much information about the circumstances of the trauma as possible. Rescuers, if available, should talk to family. Even seemingly unimportant information can be helpful. The family may need to repeat what happened numerous times to make sense of it and make it real.
- Acknowledge reactions and feelings: Listen and support family members' expressions of feelings.
- Normalize feelings: Explain the wide and unexpected range of emotions in crisis. Help legitimize feelings, such as guilt, in sudden and unexpected trauma. However, do not rationalize away feelings, but put them in the context of reality.

Mobilize the Support System

Ensure that the family has a strong support system:

- Have the family identify and contact significant support persons.
- Help mobilize internal resources: "Have you been in this situation before?"
- Offer spiritual resources.
- Identify cultural resources or concerns.

FAMILY PRESENCE

Current research has demonstrated the benefits to families of being present during resuscitation and invasive procedures. Organizations such as the American Heart Association and the Emergency Nurses Association have endorsed this practice. Family presence has become a more accepted practice in medical resuscitations and treatment, less so in trauma situations. The importance of having the family be with the patient, even briefly, cannot be underestimated. Families report that family presence helped them know that everything possible was done to save the patient, provided relief from wondering what was happening, and allowed them to say good-bye and feel that they provided comfort to the patient. The majority of families also felt that being present facilitated their grieving process and adjustment to the death.[4] The following guidelines are useful when offering the family the option of being present:

- Designate a family facilitator not involved with patient care.
- Assess the family for desire/appropriateness to see patient.
- Ensure that the resuscitation team is agreeable to having family with the patient.
- Clarify the structure for family members, such as number of family members and amount of time, stressing the importance of patient care. Prepare family members for what they will see, hear, and smell.

- Have the family facilitator stay with the family during the visit and explain interventions. Encourage family members to talk and touch the patient if desired.
- After the visit, the family facilitator stays with the family members to assess their needs, concerns, or questions.

DEATH OF THE PATIENT

If the patient dies during the resuscitation or before the family arrives, the family obviously will experience extreme distress and much difficulty comprehending the sudden loss.

When the family members arrive, do the following:

- The family members should be told in an empathic way by using the term *death* rather than *passed on* or other more abstract terms. This information may need to be repeated until the family can understand the reality of the death.
- The family should be offered the opportunity to see the patient and should be given time to make the decision. Research has demonstrated that families that decide not to see the patient may later regret the decision, so it is important to keep that option available. However, support the ultimate decision of the family.
- The family should determine the amount of time that they need with the patient.
- Because of the abrupt separation, mementos from the patient may ease the transition. Cutting a lock of hair has been helpful to families of adult patients and of children.
- Because of the unexpected nature of trauma and the psychological reaction, many families may have questions later about the care in the emergency department, such as whether the patient was in pain or "shocked." It is helpful for families to have the opportunity to follow-up because these lingering questions may impede the grieving process. Either the names of the primary clinicians caring for the patient/family and their hospital telephone numbers should be given to the family, or staff members should provide telephone follow-up to the family, usually within a few weeks.

References

1. Kneis LC, Riley E: *Psychiatric nursing,* ed 5, Menlo Park, Calif, 1996, Addison-Wesley.
2. Aguilera D: *Crisis intervention: theory and methodology,* ed 8, St Louis, 1998, Mosby.
3. Morse JM, O'Brien B: Preserving self: from victim to patient, to patient, to disabled person, *J Adv Nurs* 21:886-896, 1995.
4. Meyers TA, Eichhorn DJ, Guzzetta CE et al: Family presence during invasive procedures and resuscitation, *Am J Nurs* 100(2):32-43, 2000.

Suggested Readings

Burgess A: *Advanced practice psychiatric nursing,* Stamford, Conn, 1998, Appleton & Lange.

Hoff LA: *People in crisis: clinical and public health perspectives,* ed 5, San Francisco, 2001, Jossey-Bass.

Lindemann E: Symptomatology: management of acute grief, *Am J Psychiatry* 101:101-148, 1944.

O'Connor S, Gervasini A: Trauma death of a 28-year old: two clinicians help a family to view the body and keep a lock of hair, *J Emerg Nurs* 27(2):159-161, 2001.

CHAPTER 9

ORGAN AND TISSUE DONATION

ROBIN L. OHKAGAWA

In the United States alone, more than 93,000 persons are on a waiting list for the "gift of life"—organ transplant. Although there were almost 7,600 deceased organ donors in 2005, there are still more than 10,000 persons waiting for a suitable organ to become available.[1] Trauma professionals have important roles to play in identifying potential donors and working with an organ procurement organization (OPO) during the donation process in order to maximize transplant success.

SUCCESS OF TRANSPLANTATION AND NEED FOR DONORS

The first successful organ transplant occurred in 1954 when doctors at Peter Bent Brigham Hospital in Boston performed a kidney transplant on identical twins. In 1967, the world was astonished when Christian Barnard of South Africa completed the world's first heart transplant. Since then, thousands of successful transplants have been performed, giving recipients a chance to live longer and fuller lives. During 2003, 25,451 transplants were performed in the United States.[3] In addition to organs, donors can provide valuable tissues that can be used in a myriad of ways to enhance recipients' health and well-being.

Up to 100 persons can benefit from a single donor. The organs that can be recovered for transplantation are the heart, lungs, liver, kidneys, pancreas, and small bowel. Some of the tissues that are transplanted include corneas, heart valves, skin, bone, and vessels.

As the frequency of organ donation and transplantation grew, the need for regulation and coordination increased. In 1986 the Department of Health and Human Services established a single network to act as a clearinghouse for the identification and distribution of organs and tissues to be transplanted. A private agency, the United Network for Organ Sharing (UNOS), was contracted to carry out this task.

All clinical transplant centers, OPOs, and tissue typing labs are members of UNOS. Membership criteria include education, training, and experience of medical personnel. UNOS maintains the national waiting list of all patients in the United States waiting for a solid organ transplant. UNOS performs organ-recipient matching and operates the organ placement center. It also tracks organ recipients throughout their lives.[3]

In addition to UNOS at the national level, there are 59 OPOs across the United States. Each of these OPOs has been federally designated to serve one of 11 regions. Every hospital in the United States has been assigned an OPO. OPOs are not-for-profit organizations, are members of UNOS, and work in accordance with allocation policies governed by UNOS. OPOs work collaboratively with hospitals through the entire donation process, including the evaluation, consent, management of the donor, and coordination of the recovery of the organs. OPOs provide education regarding the identification of potential donors and the donation process. They also provide data to assist hospitals in improving their referral rates and therefore compliance with the Centers for Medicare and Medicaid Services (CMS) regulations, which are monitored routinely by the Joint Commission on Accreditation of Healthcare Organizations.

OPO personnel are trained to work with donor families, presenting the option of donation, educating family members about donation choices, understanding possible cultural and religious differences, and documenting consent. They often maintain contact with donor families in the weeks and months after the donations and transplants have been completed.

The waiting list for organs has doubled in the last 10 years.[4] Because of this need, a number of government regulations have been enacted. In 1998, the CMS (formerly the Health Care Financing Administration) declared that in order for hospitals to receive Medicare funding, all patient deaths and impending deaths must be referred to the local OPO. In 2003, Health and Human Services Secretary Tommy Thompson initiated a national collaboration of OPOs and hospitals to meet the challenges of increasing the number of organs available for transplantation and ensuring that all families have the opportunity to choose donation when appropriate.

ORGAN DONATION PROCESS

Identification

The organ donation process starts with the identification of a potential organ donor. Because most trauma patients enter the hospital system though the emergency department, emergency staff members often have the vital role of initiating this process. For example, a trauma patient who has a significant head injury and has a Glasgow Coma Scale score of 5 or less may become a possible donor and should be referred to the local OPO.

When a referral is made, it does *not* mean that the hospital staff has given up on treating the patient. A number of referrals to the OPO do not result in donation because patients survive their injuries. Although a patient may have incurred multiple trauma, it does not mean that donation is not an option. For example, a patient who has suffered a closed head injury as a result of a motor vehicle collision and other injuries such as rib fractures, heart and lung contusions, and a liver laceration still has the potential to donate. A liver laceration does not preclude transplantation, and in the foregoing example, the kidneys, pancreas, and small bowel may be unaffected completely by the trauma so that the donor may save the lives of five persons.

Trauma patients are not the only patients who have the potential to become organ donors. Nontraumatic neurologic events, such as cerebral vascular accidents, aneurysm ruptures, or anoxic insults, can result in a devastating condition with a poor prognosis, and patients with these conditions also should be referred to the OPO. It should be noted that patients with a medical and social history that includes hypertension, coronary artery disease, diabetes mellitus, and alcohol abuse also have the opportunity to provide the gift of life.

Referral

Once a potential organ donor has been identified, it is up to the hospital employee to make a referral to the local OPO. At this point, ongoing collaboration between the hospital and the OPO begins. The hospital employee must share with the OPO coordinator detailed information regarding the potential donor, such as medical and social history, patient status, family understanding and acceptance of the gravity of the situation, and plan of care. This information allows the OPO to evaluate the medical suitability of the potential donor. Timely and detailed referrals best prepare hospital staff and the OPO coordinator to offer the patient's family the option of donation, if appropriate.

During the evaluation period, it is important that organ perfusion and oxygenation be maintained. If they are compromised, the option of donation may no longer be available to a family. By maintaining an adequate perfusion pressure (usually a mean arterial pressure greater than 60 mm Hg) with intravenous fluids and vasopressors as needed, partial pressure of oxygen in arterial blood of 100 mm Hg on the lowest fraction of inspired oxygen required, and a urine output of approximately 100 mL/hr, the organs will be appropriately perfused and oxygenated. A study done at a California hospital demonstrated that use of resuscitative and maintenance protocols developed for patients declared dead by neurologic criteria resulted in more organs being recovered during the 3 years after the initiation of the protocols than in the 3 years before the interventions.[5]

Declaration of Death

In the late 1970s the determination of death by neurologic or brain criteria ("brain death") was increasingly recognized. The 1980 Uniform Determination of Death Act legalized this brain-based definition of death.[6] This legislation was a breakthrough for organ donation because it now allowed medical personnel to maintain clinically dead patients with mechanical support (thus keeping the organs perfused and oxygenated) and minimize ischemic injury and allow for a better outcome of the subsequent transplant. Although patients can be maintained on mechanical support, the effects of brain death begin to manifest themselves fairly soon; therefore, for the best outcome, the donation process needs to proceed quickly.

For a patient to be declared clinically dead by neurologic criteria, one must be able to prove the sustained absence of cerebral and brainstem function. The clinical exam includes checking for the pupillary, corneal, cough, and gag reflexes. The exam also requires the absence of movement to noxious stimuli, the presence of posturing, and a negative response to cold caloric irrigation and doll's eye reflex testing. To determine whether the patient has an intact brainstem, apnea testing must be performed. The absence of respiratory effort despite a partial pressure of carbon dioxide in arterial blood of 60 mm Hg or greater indicates that apnea is present, that is, the patient is apneic and therefore does not have a respiratory drive. Commonly, two clinical exams are performed, which are separated by a minimum of 6 hours, in order to prove that the findings on the initial negative clinical exam are not reversible, for example, because of hypothermia at the time of the first exam. A confirmatory test often is used to shorten the waiting period or in addition to the clinical exam. The most common confirmatory test used is the measure of brain flow scan or four-vessel cerebral angiogram. Every hospital should have a written policy that establishes death determination using brain death criteria. This policy should outline clearly the expectations and specifically list the step-by-step process. The policy should identify who or what physician specialty is credentialed to make the determination of brain death, and the policy should be clear for adult and pediatric patients.

Once the tests are complete and the results are confirmed, the patient is pronounced dead. The heart is still beating because the patient is maintained on mechanical support, but the brain has died; that is the time of death recorded on the death certificate. At this point the medical examiner may need to be notified to give permission for donation. This sign-off is particularly relevant in deaths involving accidents and suspected homicide and suicide and those occurring within less than 24 hours after hospital admission. These days, organ donation rarely is restricted by the medical examiner, and frequently a forensic photographer accompanies the procurement team during the operative course.

Donation after Cardiac Death

Donation after cardiac death–that is, irreversible cessation of cardiac and pulmonary function—has resurfaced recently as a way for families whose loved ones do not meet the requirements for death by neurologic criteria to donate organs. Once a family has consented to a do not resuscitate order and comfort measures only and therefore withdrawal of treatment, the family may have the option of donation after cardiac death. The Institute of Medicine Committee on Non-Heart-Beating Transplantation II practices and protocols recommended that OPOs should pursue donation after cardiac death because it is a medically and ethically appropriate source of organs.[7] Kidneys transplanted from donation after cardiac death donors have a successful 1 year postgraft survival rate similar to those kidneys transplanted from patients dead by neurologic criteria. At 10 years posttransplantation, there is a 78.7% graft survival rate in recipients transplanted with a donation after cardiac death kidney versus 76.7% from donors dead by neurologic criteria.[8] The liver, pancreas, and (in some institutions) lungs also can be recovered through donation after cardiac death. For donation after cardiac death to occur, there must be an organized extubation: the operating room must be available and set up, and the transplant staff must be in-house and available. It should be noted that the longer it takes for the patient to become asystolic, the greater the chance that hypoxic and ischemic injuries to the organs can affect the transplant outcome.

Option of Donation

The benefit of organ donation to the recipient is obvious. The benefit to the donor family is not as readily apparent. Organ and tissue donation can help the grieving process. Donation may give families comfort through knowing that the tragic death of their loved one will provide continued life to others. Fulfilling a family member's documented request for his or her organs to be donated may make relatives feel that they can do something to assist their loved one, even at a time when events make them feel helpless.

Offering the family the option of donation is a collaborative process involving the hospital and the OPO. Unless the family raises the subject, donation should not be discussed with a family until it is determined that the family has accepted and acknowledged the death.[9] Once a family has consented to withdrawal of treatment, it is appropriate to provide families with information about their donation options.

Research has shown that requestors specializing in organ and tissue donation have a higher consent rate.[10] Partly because of this, the CMS regulations state that OPO staff or others trained by OPO staff are the only ones who should discuss donation with a potential donor family. The accuracy of the information exchanged with the family is imperative. Because the OPO staff is ultimately responsible for the recovery of organs and tissues, there must be a fully informed consent.

The timing of offering families information regarding their option to donate is critical. Families need to have understood the gravity of their loved one's prognosis and/or death. Premature conversations almost always result in lack of consent and mistrust of the hospital staff with fear that they are not taking adequate care of their loved one. The environment in which the conversations occur also can have an impact on families. The family needs to be escorted to a quiet and private room; these conversations should never take place in the patient's room or in the hallways.[11] Hospital staff plays a vital role in supporting families through the hospital course and in ultimately preparing a family for the donation discussion. Social workers, chaplains, and other support personnel are vital to families experiencing a crisis. Often a cup of water, assistance with hotel accommodations, or a familiar face in the confusion of the event can give families comfort, resulting in a positive experience. Also important is that hospital staff continues to update families on their loved one's condition and plan of care, and this starts in the emergency room.

The option of donation should never be withheld from a family. Often hospital staff feels uncomfortable with approaching families about donation. A clear separation between the hospital staff members who are treating the patient and the OPO staff can assist families in separating the two. Donation provides families great comfort, and "protecting" families from this option is a disservice to families and their loved ones. Donation should be considered one of the end-of-life options for families whose loved ones face a nonsurvivable injury and whenever possible should be a family-centered event.

First Person Consent

Several states have moved forward to enforce "donor rights," that is, respecting the patient's decision before his or her death to be a donor. Similar to a living will, the patient's documented decision to donate, indicated on a donor card or driver's license, now is respected. The 1968 Uniform Anatomical Gift Act states that a legal adult can make the decision to donate any part of his or her body in the event of death.[6] Most persons are surprised to learn that this is not the practice everywhere and that despite their written designation that their organs and tissues be used, donation only occurs with the written consent of the patient's family. If the would-be-donor resides in a state that does not enforce first person consent, it is important that the donor make his or her wishes clear to the family. OPO and hospital personnel are required to obtain consent in accordance with state laws in effect.

Allocation and Procurement

The donor blood type, tissue typing, height and weight are entered into the UNOS national computerized network of wait-listed potential recipients. Based on the donor information entered and the recipient's degree of illness, time listed on the waiting list, and location, a list of potential recipients is generated for each organ. The OPO coordinator uses this list and works with the transplant surgeons identified for each recipient to locate the most appropriate recipient. Once the organs have been "placed" with potential recipients, the recovery process begins. The transplant surgeons for the accepted organ come to the donor hospital to procure the organ. The organ then is sent to the transplant center where the recipient is being prepared for transplantation. Often teams travel great distances to perform organ retrieval. The donor continues to be hemodynamically maintained while in the operating room. The heart and lungs must be transplanted within 6 hours of removal, in contrast to the kidneys, which when on a pulsatile pump, can be transplanted up to 72 hours after recovery, although most are transplanted within 12 to 24 hours.

TISSUE DONATION

Hundreds of persons can benefit from the gifts of a single tissue donor. Several types of tissue can be donated; for example, corneas, heart valves, bone, vessels, and skin. Box 9-1 lists the different tissues and their uses. In general, anyone from newborn to the age of 80 can donate some form of tissue. Hospitals are required by CMS regulations to notify the local OPO in the event of a death. When this referral is received, a preliminary screening process is done. If a patient is a candidate for tissue donation, the local OPO contacts the patient's family and offers the family the option. Hospital staff should refrain from mentioning donation to families without OPO collaboration because the criteria frequently change and not every person is a candidate for tissue donation.

SUMMARY

Trauma professionals have an important role in initiating the donation process. The Society for Critical Care Medicine endorses this important role, stating, "If, in the process of delivering

Box 9-1	SUMMARY OF TISSUES THAT CAN BE TRANSPLANTED				
Bone	**Ear**	**Eye**	**Heart**	**Other**
Femur	Incus	Cornea	Heart valves	Cartilage
Fibula	Ligaments			Dura mater
Humerus	Malleus			Fascia lata
Ilium	Stapes			Skin
Mandible	Tendons			
Radius	Tympanic membrane			
Ribs				
Tibia				
Ulna				

(Adapted from Phipps WJ, Monahan FD, Sands JK, et al: Medical-surgical nursing: health and illness perspectives, *ed 7, St Louis, 2003, Mosby. Data from United Network for Organ Sharing, www.unos.org)*

high-quality end-of-life care, organ donation is possible, then critical care professionals should help enable that outcome."[12] By the identification of potential donors, making a referral to the local OPO and working collaboratively with the OPO coordinators on site, health care professionals act as advocates to ensure that each family that has the option of donation is given that choice appropriately. A trauma professional's goal is to save lives. Through facilitation of organ and tissue donation, even when a patient dies, a trauma professional can help to save and improve the lives of many others and provide lasting solace to the donor's family.

References

1. United Network for Organ Sharing: National Data Statistics. Retrieved November 6, 2006, from www.unos.org
2. Organ Procurement and Transplantation Network: April 6, 2004
3. United Network for Organ Sharing: Who Are We, History. Retrieved November 6, 2006, from www.unos.org/WhoAreWe
4. Organ Procurement and Transplantation Network: *Data resources.* Retrieved November 6, 2006, from www.optn.org/data/data_resources.asp
5. Roth BJ, Sher L, Murray JA et al: Cadaveric organ donor recruitment at a Los Angeles County Hospital: improvement after formation of a structured clinical, educational and administrative service, *Clin Transplant* 17(suppl 9):52-57, 2003.
6. Uniform Law Commissioners: The National Conference of Commissioners Uniform State Laws, Final Acts, Official Site http://people.bu.edu/wwildman/WeirdWildWeb/courses/thth/projects/thth_projects 2003_lewis/udda.pdf Reviewed November 6, 2006.
7. Committee on Non-Heart-Beating Transplantation II: the Scientific and Ethical Basis for Practice and Protocols, Division of Health Care Services, Institute of Medicine: *Non-heart-beating organ transplantation: practice and protocols,* Washington, DC, 2000, National Academies Press.
8. Weber W, Dindo D, Demartines N et al: Kidney tranplantation from donors without a heartbeat, *N Engl J Med* 347(4):248-255, 2002.

9. Rocheleau CA: Increasing family consent for organ donation: findings and challenges, *Prog Transplant* 11(3):194-200, 2001.
10. Beasley CL, Capossela CL, Brigham LE et al: The impact of a comprehensive, hospital-focused intervention to increase organ donation, *J Transpl Coord* 7:6-13, 1997.
11. Ehrle RN, Shafer TJ, Nelson KR: Referral, request, and consent for organ donation: best practice—a blueprint for success, *Crit Care Nurse* 19(2):21-33, 1999.
12. Society for Critical Care Medicine, Mission Statement. Retrieved 2004, *www.sccm.org*

III

CLINICAL CONCEPTS

CHAPTER 10

MECHANISM OF INJURY

JOSEPH S. BLANSFIELD

The optimal care of a trauma patient combines a careful history with a physical assessment. Identifying and understanding the mechanism of how a patient was injured can be useful in early management of the patient. We know that certain patterns of injury may heighten the "index of suspicion" for the trauma team. Additionally, certain "triggers" or markers for significant injury could alert the clinician for specific injury or severity of injury. The trauma team can use the history to anticipate the patient's needs and to plan care before arrival. Certain diagnostic studies and interventions can be anticipated and performed in a timelier manner for those that may require them. This allows the trauma team to be proactive instead of reactive.

HISTORY

Important information about the mechanism of injury begins with the prehospital providers. They become the eyes and ears for the trauma team, relaying pertinent details about the scene that otherwise would not be available (Figure 10-1). Concerted efforts should be made to collect this "perishable" data and incorporate it into the medical record because once the emergency medical services personnel leave, that data may become lost or difficult to collect after the fact.

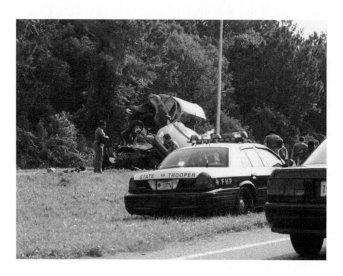

Figure 10-1. Prehospital scene information.

Motor Vehicle Collision

Important details relevant to a motor vehicle collision include the following:

- Speed of vehicles involved
- Size of vehicles involved
- Type of impact (frontal, lateral, off-center, rear, sideswipe, or rollover; Figure 10-2).
- Occupant position relative to vehicle before and after the collision
- Pedestrian involvement
- Safety devices (lap belt, shoulder belt; air bag, child car seat) and if properly applied
- Vehicle deformity and/or magnitude of intrusion
- Possible interior structures of contact with occupant (windshield, mirror, steering wheel)
- Smoke, fumes, or potential hazardous materials in the injury environment
- Other occupants' conditions and injuries or deaths.

Penetrating Injuries

Important details relevant to penetrating injuries include the following:

- Number and type of wounds
- Size of wounding instrument (weapon caliber, missile velocity, distance traveled, length of knife or impaled object)
- Direction of wounding tract (if possible)

One must take care not to destroy potential forensic evidence that may be useful in determining injury or for medical-legal cases. Do not cut through holes in clothing that may have resulted

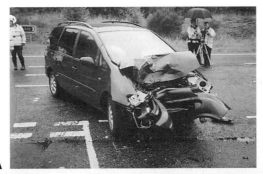

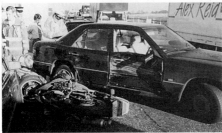
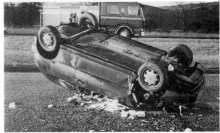

Figure 10-2. Types of impact. **A,** Frontal impact. **B,** Side/lateral impact. **C,** Rollover. (Courtesy trauma.org)

from penetration. Use paper bags for clothing collection because they are breathable. Avoid using plastic clothing bags for storage because it may hasten deterioration of evidence.

Falls and Jumps

Important details relevant to falls and jumps include the following:

- Distance of fall or jump
- Landing surface of victim (to estimate force absorption)
- Body part making initial contact (feet, head, back, buttocks)
- Victim activity before fall or jump (falls are often unintentional and unplanned, whereas jumps may be intentional or planned events and have the potential follow-on considerations of caring for a patient who may have tried to harm himself or herself or may have been in the act of fleeing from authorities).

Fires

Important details to collect for fires include the following:

- Thermal or chemical injury to body structures (e.g., approximate body surface area and depth of burn and smoke or heat inhalation)
- Field therapy for surface injury
- Environment (e.g., closed space or open area with ventilation)
- Explosive forces involved (e.g., if protected from or exposed directly to blast wave, additional injury by flying debris, collapsing structures, and onto what surface victim was thrown)
- Potential for secondary injuries from chemicals, toxic gases, burning products, victim's attempt to escape (e.g., jumping from building)

A common pitfall in dealing with burn injuries is initially to overestimate the body surface area burned and underestimate the wound depth. Percentages and amounts of tissue damage should be reassessed, and this is often a progression of the burn injury process.

Occupational Injuries Related to Machines

Important details to collect for injuries related to machines include the following:

- Length of time since injury and extrication
- Function of machine (e.g., grinding, chopping, rotary, or high-energy source)
- Potential contaminants (e.g., bacterial, animal manure, pesticides, herbicides, lubricants, or fuel)

Environmental and Substance Considerations

It is helpful to remember that the term *injury* also includes physiologic damage caused by extremes of temperature or absence of life-sustaining substances, such as oxygen; therefore, it is also important to relate the conditions of the scene. Extreme cold or heat, wet conditions, and smoke can create additional injuries that may not be as visible as other injuries.

Medical conditions and the consumption of alcohol or other drugs can alter a patient's response to injury significantly. Especially helpful is if field personnel survey the scene for evidence of the victim using medications, beverages, or illicit substances.

FORCE OF INJURY

Tissues are injured when exposed to excessive amounts of mechanical, electrical, thermal, or chemical energy and/or are deprived of heat and oxygen. The injury can be a structural or physiologic disruption. Because most cases of trauma involve mechanical energy, a brief overview of several key points is provided.

Kinetic energy

The wounding potential of an event is affected greatly by the amount of kinetic energy (energy in motion) that is transferred to the victim. Kinetic energy *(KE)* is determined by the mass of the object in motion and its velocity, or amount of acceleration. The following formula demonstrates the relationship:

$$KE = {}^{1}/_{2} \text{ Mass} \times \text{Velocity}^2$$

By this formula one can note that kinetic energy can be increased in two ways; doubling the mass results in doubling the kinetic energy; however, doubling the velocity results in quadrupling the kinetic energy.

Laws of Motion

Newton's first law of motion holds that when an object is set in motion, it tends to remain in motion until acted on by an outside force. A person riding in a vehicle, thrown, falling, or suddenly struck by an object will remain or be set into motion and remain at that rate of acceleration until another force inhibits that motion (i.e., causes deceleration): the vehicle crashes or the person contacts a surface. Deceleration forces cause deformation of tissues referred to as *strains,* which are classified as *tensile* (stretching), *shear* (opposing forces across an object), or *compressive* (crushing). When the deforming force exceeds the ability of the tissue to regain its original shape *(elasticity)* or its ability to resist a change in shape during motion *(viscosity),* the tissue will be injured, resulting in lacerations, contusions, fractures, ruptures, and other types of injuries.[1]

The patterns of injuries noted with deceleration can be attributed to multiple factors, which include point of impact and rate of deceleration. During a motor vehicle collision (MVC), the vehicle travels at a set speed until stopped. An occupant continues to travel at that speed until an outside force or object (safety belt, air bag, or striking the vehicle interior) causes him or her to stop. We know certain organs and anatomic structures within the body are not "fixed" in position and are able to shift position during rapid deceleration. As a result, these organs continue in motion until they strain flexible points of attachment. This often is referred to as the *crash within a crash within a crash.* For example, the first impact is the car to tree, the second impact is driver to steering wheel, and the third impact is heart to sternum. External injuries are related directly to the force or objects that strike the body in a sudden deceleration. Internal injuries are related to deceleration, which causes deforming forces to underlying structures and organs that are not "fixed" and therefore are able to shift and/or rupture from points of attachment (e.g., brain, heart and great vessels, spleen, and kidney).

TYPES OF INJURY MECHANISMS

In describing the types of injury mechanisms, a distinction is made between penetrating and blunt forces.

Penetrating forces involve direct contact with an instrument that pierces the skin, require less energy to injure, and result in fewer body structures harmed. Penetrating injuries are the result of stabbings, bullet or missile fragmentation wounds, impaled foreign objects, or high-pressure injections.

Blunt forces involve compression, deformation, or sudden change in atmospheric pressure. They usually result in more injuries, involve more severity and more body systems, and can include contusions, lacerations, fractures, or ruptures of solid tissue masses. Injuries sustained from a blunt force tend to be more difficult to manage because more structures can be affected, the lack of external signs with occult injuries may delay diagnosis, and the patient may experience more complications as a result of the injuries.

PATTERNS OF INJURY ASSOCIATED WITH VARIOUS INJURY MECHANISMS

Motor Vehicle Collision

Patients who are injured as a result of an MVC can have patterns of injury that vary according to their position in the vehicle and the use of safety restraints.

Position in the Vehicle

The driver is at risk for hitting the steering column, dashboard, gearshift handle, rearview mirror, windshield, a pillar (between windshield and door), and the door. The reported patterns of injury correspond with the body parts most likely to hit these structures:

- Facial lacerations, facial bone fractures
- Scalp lacerations, skull fractures, intracranial injuries
- Spinal injuries
- Chest wall lacerations, contusions; rib, clavicle, and sternal fractures, pulmonary contusions, or lacerations with corresponding pneumohemothorax
- Thoracic aorta laceration at area of attachment (i.e., superior to left subclavian artery)
- Abdominal wall lacerations, contusions; rupture or avulsion of liver, spleen, kidney, pancreas, bowel, or bladder
- Fractured pelvis; posterior hip dislocation; fractured femur, tibia, fibula, ankle, or foot; ligamentous injury to knee
- Several common patterns of skeletal injury in an MVC involve the knees: striking the instrumental panel (causing a patellar fracture and ligamentous disruption in the knee joint), the force transmitted along the axis of the femur (producing a posterior hip dislocation and femoral shaft fracture), or the feet becoming entangled in the floor pedals and causing fractures or strain on joints

Front-seat passengers are not exposed to the same number and type of internal vehicle structures and have a different pattern of injuries. Although they have a higher incidence of head, abdominal, and upper torso fractures, they have fewer thoracic injuries and lower torso fractures.[1]

Rear-seat passengers' incidence of severe injury can be as high as front seat occupants if they are not restrained.

Use of Safety Restraints

Shoulder and lap restraints reduce the incidence and severity of injury by reducing the force with which a person strikes a surface, preventing the victim from striking multiple surfaces or preventing ejection from the vehicle. Consequently, restrained occupants have fewer or less severe head, facial, and thoracic injuries or upper and lower torso fractures. In a crash with substantial forces or cases in which the restraints are used improperly, the restraint can produce injuries to the following structures:

- Chest (fractured ribs, lung or blunt cardiac injury)
- Abdomen (tear or rupture of liver, spleen, kidney, pancreas, bowel, or iliac artery or aorta)
- Cervical spine (fracture, dislocation of spine, blunt injury to cervical blood vessels) or lumbar spine (disrupted ligaments, vertebral fractures)

Air bags installed in vehicles are part of the supplemental restraint system in frontal crashes. They work with the windshield to provide protection. Automobile manufacturers now also have included side air bags for lateral impacts. Air bags have been associated with a reduction in the severity of brain injury and incidence of facial fractures and lacerations and lower extremity fractures.[2]

As with other types of safety restraints, air bags also can pose a risk for injury for certain high-risk individuals. Occupants who are out of position (leaning forward, riding with seat close to air bag, or unrestrained) or infants and children in car seats can be struck by the air bag or module cover. The air bag can produce *direct contact injuries* (contusions, abrasions, lacerations, fractures), trauma to internal organs (eye, heart, intraabdominal organs), and severe head and neck injuries in children.[3]

Pedestrian Struck by a Motor Vehicle

A moving vehicle strikes a pedestrian with its bumper and hood, causing the individual to lose balance or become airborne and finally land on a surface, which provides a third area of impact. The areas of impact can vary depending on the victim's height and the size of the vehicle. Typical injuries occur in a triad pattern:

- Hood strikes an adult on lower abdomen, hip, or upper femur region; a child in the head, chest, or abdominal region
- Bumper strikes adult on lower leg; child in femur or tibia/fibula region
- Victim lands on hood or ground (producing head, chest, and/or abdominal injuries)

Pedestrians who have received a side impact may have sustained a fracture of a femur or tibia/ fibula on the "affected" side, which may be obvious during the physical assessment. However, ligamentous injury to the knee on the "unaffected" side also may occur and may not be obvious until later. This has implications for the patient's ambulatory status if this injury is missed.

If a patient has injuries that correspond to one or two of the aforementioned regions, the provider should be alert to the possibility of additional injuries that fit this pattern.

Cyclists

The patterns of injuries can vary between riders of motorcycles and bicycles. Motorcycles tend to be heavier and tip sideways, entrapping lower extremities and producing lateral injuries and pelvic fractures. Bicycles are lighter than motorcycles. The front tire catches or becomes destabilized, causing forward-leaning cyclists to be propelled forward, striking their face, head, shoulders, chest, or upper extremities.

Falls or Jumps

Whereas an MVC represents a form of horizontal deceleration, a jump or fall creates a vertical deceleration if the person lands on the feet, buttocks, or top of the skull. The mobile internal structures move up and down, stressing different points of attachment than if the motion were anterior or posterior. This is known as axial loading. The patterns and severity of the victim's injuries depend on the following:

- Distance traveled
- Impact surface (i.e., absorbing or rigid)
- Body area(s) making initial contact on impact

If the victim lands on his or her feet, buttocks, or top of the head, the impacting force is transmitted along the axis of the skeleton causing the following injuries:

- Compression fractures of the calcaneus, long bones of the lower torso, pelvis, and lumbar spine, and if the person is propelled forward and stretches out his or her arms to brace for fall, bilateral distal radius (Colles') fractures
- Pelvic vascular injuries
- Descending aortic disruption at area of attachment (i.e., above diaphragm)
- Separation of the heart from the aortic valve
- Pulling away of the kidney from the renal artery

Penetrating Wounds

Objects that penetrate the skin can produce a wide variety of injury patterns depending on the degree of penetration, the ability to release kinetic energy, and the untoward effects that the missile produces. Objects with low kinetic energy (i.e., low velocity), such as knives, produce *stab wounds* that are limited to the length of the penetrating object, direction or trajectory of the stabbing motion, and the structures that are in line with the wounding tract produced. An impaled object should be left in place whenever possible to aid in the diagnosis of the injury and to help tamponade any possible bleeding surfaces. Objects that appear to be close to a bone should be evaluated to determine whether the wound constitutes a compound fracture and requires surgical débridement and infection prophylaxis.

Objects that enter the body as missiles can be classified as *gunshot wounds, fragmentation wounds,* or *impaled foreign objects.* Bullets produce a wide range of injuries, and wound ballistics (i.e., the study of how a missile interacts with target tissue) depend on characteristics of the missile, weapon, and body part(s) struck.[4]

When assessing the severity of a gunshot wound, obtain the following information whenever possible:

- Caliber (size or diameter of missile)
- Type of missile (potential to deform or fragment)
- Type of gun (handgun, high velocity; rifle, very high velocity)
- Trajectory of missile in body (structures involved)
- Range (distance between victim and weapon)

Missiles produce tissue injury by two methods: *direct* (laceration, heat) or *indirect* mechanisms (cavitation, shock wave). Prediction of the exact internal injuries associated with a gunshot wound is difficult because kinetic energy and the tissue response vary. A low-velocity missile, which cuts or lacerates tissue, can be fatal if it strikes a highly vascular structure, such as the aorta, or inconsequential if it strikes a less vital structure. This type of missile produces little cavitation and does not exceed the elasticity of the tissue.

Temporary cavitation is more of an issue with high-velocity missiles. A high-powered missile can be discharged at close range and pass through an extremity, creating just a laceration because of the high elasticity of the muscle. However, if the kinetic energy is transmitted to less-elastic tissue, that same extremity may need to be amputated because the bones are shattered and neurovascular structures are destroyed beyond repair. Cavitation is most destructive in nonelastic tissue, such as bone, liver, spleen, and brain.[1]

Fragmentation wounds are caused by devices that break apart when detonated and explode, sending multiple pieces of shrapnel in all directions. These shrapnel fragments are hot, jagged pieces of metal that tear into the body with high velocity, often leaving large soft tissue defects and burns.

Other types of impaled objects are dangerous because the initial appearance of the wound may not look serious. *High-pressure injection wounds* come from the inadvertent introduction of a liquid into tissue, such as in the hand. Initially, the wound appears to be a minor puncture site, painless and nonedematous. Within hours, the injected foreign substance (water, cleanser, paint) begins an inflammatory response that leads to infection and potentially compartment syndrome. Patients with injection wounds need to be evaluated immediately and considered for surgical exploration and débridement.

PATTERNS OF INJURY ASSOCIATED WITH KNOWN INJURIES

Patterns of injuries also can be predicted according to the anatomic area involved. When certain body areas are subjected to a sudden deceleration or compressive force, the rigid bony skeleton and mobile tissue mass can produce underlying contusions or rupture.

Scalp

Scalp tissue is vascular and does not readily vasoconstrict; therefore, direct pressure and possibly surgical closure (sutures or staples) is required to control blood loss. Large, bulky dressings cannot generate the point-specific pressure required.

Skull

A linear fracture over the temporal region could be associated with injury to the underlying middle meningeal artery and subsequent epidural hematoma. A depressed skull fracture requires substantial force, therefore underlying intracranial soft tissue and dural layers also may be contused, lacerated, or contaminated.

Brain

The brain is mobile within the rigid skull and, if set into motion (acceleration or deceleration forces), can strike multiple surfaces within the skull and cause multisite contusions (i.e., coup-contrecoup mechanism). The mobile brain strains at the points of attachment, which are the bridging veins beneath the dura (creating a subdural hematoma), brainstem, and cranial nerves. When these points of attachment are severed, bleeding and injury occur.

Eye

The eye is a liquid-filled globe generally protected by the bony rim created by the facial bones. Eye trauma is the result of an object smaller that the circumference of the rim (e.g., golf club, fist, steering wheel) coming in direct contact with the eye and causing an increase in intraorbital pressure. Any pressure applied to a fluid in a container is transmitted undiminished in all directions throughout the fluid (Pascal's principle), resulting in stretching of ocular structures (e.g., retina, iris, choroids, and ciliary body) and blowout fractures of the weaker medial orbital floor. Clinically, backward displacement of the eye into the orbit causes a blowout fracture of the inferior orbital floor, and possibly hypoesthesia (decreased feeling) below the eye may result.

Facial Bones

The bones in the face fracture from direct impact and involve multiple sites. Fracture may be suspected clinically when facial structures are edematous and asymmetric and eye movement is limited, specifically upward gaze. The patient's airway can be compromised easily by hemorrhage or edema. Direct trauma to the face may involve concomitant intracranial and/or cervical spine injuries.

Neck

Penetrating injury of the soft tissues near the thoracic outlet (base of neck) should be assessed carefully for possible involvement of underlying structures, including apices of the lung, major vascular structures, esophagus, trachea, or cervical spine; penetrating injury of the esophagus can produce sepsis from bacterial contamination of surrounding tissue. Cervical spine injury should be suspected with blunt forces to the neck. Children can be more difficult to assess because of a syndrome called SCIWORA—spinal cord injury without radiologic abnormality. This occurs when ligaments are stretched beyond their elastic limits and the spinal cord becomes injured, but on radiologic exam the anatomy appears normal.

Chest

Deceleration forces cause the heart, aorta, and bronchus distal to the carina (point of bifurcation into left and right bronchi) to tear from points of attachment. Compressive forces can cause fractures of relatively strong skeletal structures, and underlying organ damage should be suspected when fractures are found (e.g., ribs, [pulmonary contusion, injury to proximal artery, lacerated liver or spleen, ruptured diaphragm], scapula [pulmonary contusion, brachial plexus disruption], or sternum [blunt cardiac injury, lacerated liver]). Ecchymosis or abrasion in areas consistent with the safety belt should alert clinical personnel to the potential for pulmonary and/or blunt cardiac injury or rib fracture with or without flail segment.

Abdomen

Compressive forces cause solid organs to rupture and hemorrhage if pressure is great enough; hollow organs, such as the bowel and bladder, can rupture and spill their contents at the time of injury; fractures of lower ribs may lacerate abdominal structures; ecchymosis of abrasion in areas consistent with the safety belt should alert clinical personnel to the potential for small bowel, pancreatic, and lumbar spine injury (Chance fracture).

Deceleration forces can tear the bowel at points of attachment, including the retroperitoneal duodenum and intraperitoneal small bowel. Penetrating objects may produce wounds that involve the chest wall, pleura, diaphragm, and/or multiple sites in the bowel (because of the proximity of bowel loops); they may produce eventual sepsis if the bowel is penetrated.

Pelvis

The pelvis is made up of multiple durable and injury-resistant bones that protect the lower abdomen and major blood vessels. The bones and soft tissues are highly vascular and can produce a substantial blood loss if disrupted. The pelvic bones form a ring, which usually disrupts in more than one area. A fractured pelvis should be considered a sign that the victim has sustained a major force, likely has substantial intraabdominal and bladder injuries, and has a high potential for major blood loss. Males may experience urethral disruption if a pelvic fracture causes strain in rigid soft tissues that anchor the urethra on the inferior surface of the prostate gland.

Extremities

Compressive strain on the skeleton causes forces to be transmitted along the axis of the bone to weaker, less elastic structures (joints). Fractures may appear alone or in association with ligamentous injuries in distal joints. Because many nerves and blood vessels are close to bones, the possibility of neurovascular compromise should be considered. Wounds on an extremity with a known or suspected fracture should be considered a possible open fracture (if examined closely, clinical personnel may note golden globules, evidence of bone marrow in a wound, in serous drainage).

Compartment syndrome should be suspected in blunt or penetrating injury when the pain is out of proportion to the apparent injury. If bleeding is occurring in the muscle such that it prevents adequate arterial inflow and venous outflow, tissue can become ischemic and potentially necrotic. This is a surgical emergency and may require urgent fasciotomy.

References

1. Hunt JP, Weintraub SL, Wang YZ, Buechter KJ: Kinematics. In Moore EE, Feliciano DV, Mattox KL, editors: *Trauma,* ed 5, New York, 2004, McGraw-Hill.
2. Marx JA, editor: *Rosen's emergency medicine: concepts and clinical practice,* ed 5, St Louis, 2002, Mosby.
3. National Highway Traffic Safety Administration: Air bag related injuries, *Ann Emerg Med* 42:285-286, 2003.
4. Department of Defense: *Emergency war surgery,* Third United States Revision, Washington, DC, 2004, US Government Printing Office.

INITIAL ASSESSMENT OF THE TRAUMA PATIENT

MARY M. CUSHMAN

The initial assessment of the trauma patient plays a pivotal role in establishing the priorities of patient care, and it defines the "road map" by which the trauma team will achieve the treatment goals of a critically injured patient. A trauma patient who presents to the resuscitation bay will be managed more efficiently by an orderly, comprehensive, and consistent assessment process. The intent of an initial assessment is to identify life-threatening injuries and intervene with appropriate maneuvers. Once the primary survey and initial resuscitation are complete, adjuncts to the primary survey are implemented, and a secondary survey is done. The secondary survey is a head-to-toe evaluation, history, and physical examination. The adjuncts to the secondary survey then are implemented and reevaluated. This latter action assures the clinician that injuries are not missed. Any intervention that has been done during the patient's resuscitation, including diagnostic tests and patient disposition, are defined at the end of the initial assessment. This chapter outlines the essential components of the initial assessment of a patient with multiple injuries.

PLANNING AND PREPARATION

A multidisciplinary team approach is essential for comprehensive care of the trauma patient. Patient interventions often are initiated at the scene of injury by prehospital providers through the use of protocols, preestablished management plans, medical control directives, and regional practices. Our complex health care system extends beyond the walls of the hospital and coexists with many agencies; a coordinated and inclusive system of patient care is crucial for optimal patient outcome. Strong communication systems within the region, appropriate medical facilities, broad-based commitment to a trauma system, competent health care practitioners, performance management initiatives, and adequate resources are valuable aspects that must be established before trauma patients are introduced into the system. Established trauma systems standardize patient care, increase professionalism among the providers, and optimize patient outcomes. A regional trauma system must be established and periodically reviewed and revised to ensure competency. Planning and preparation within a trauma system optimizes patient care and maintains cost efficiencies in a complex health care system.

PRIMARY SURVEY

The primary survey identifies the life-threatening injuries and interventions that are necessary to prevent subsequent morbidity and/or mortality in the trauma patient. This process is intended to be efficient, sequential, and timely. The key aspects of the primary survey are summarized by the mnemonic *ABCDE*. *A* symbolizes airway control with cervical spine protection, *B* identifies breathing and ventilation aspects, *C* is circulation with hemorrhage control, *D* is disability (neurologic assessment), and *E* is for exposure or environment control. Resuscitation of the trauma patient occurs simultaneously with the primary survey, and reassessment is a dynamic process. The primary survey may be repeated multiple times until the team is assured that no additional life-threatening injuries exist. As with all patient care, personal protection against the transmission of infectious diseases is a high priority for all team members who come in contact with the patient.

Airway Management with Cervical Spine Protection

Airway management and cervical spine protection are the first priorities in care of the trauma patient. All multiple-trauma patients should receive supplemental oxygen until it is proved that they can maintain their airway, they are breathing well, oxygen is perfusing their brain adequately, and that no neurologic deficit exists. If the initial survey of the patient reveals a patient who is alert, talking, moving all extremities, and oriented, you may assume that the airway is patent. If the patient is agitated or combative, it may be indicative of hypoxia or an inadequate airway. A chin lift–jaw thrust or nasopharyngeal/oropharyngeal airway may be useful to support or maintain the patency of a patient's airway. Head, facial, neck, and inhalation injuries pose potential airway disruptions and should have early and aggressive airway control. Obstructed airways initially may present as noisy respirations, and any patient with a Glasgow Coma Scale score of 8 or less may need an intervention to support the airway. If the mechanism of injury suggests that the patient may have a laryngeal injury, the patient may exhibit hoarse or weakened phonation. These patients may need the controlled environment of an operating room and specialized equipment to intubate.

Consider the following:

- Clinical personnel must assume that the patient has a cervical spine injury until it can be ruled out by x-ray films or computed tomography scan and clinical evaluation. All trauma patients should have a cervical collar and full immobilization in place to maintain the neck in a neutral, immobilized position until injury can be ruled out. Head position is essential in preventing or causing additional cervical spine injury.
- Semirigid cervical collars, long boards with appropriate padding, or logroll precautions should be used for the patient until the stability of the cervical spine is clarified by diagnostic tests or clinical exams.
- Manual immobilization of the patient's neck during movement of the patient is important to avoid additional injury to the spinal cord/vertebral column.
- Patients with an altered level of consciousness resulting from a head injury, drugs, or alcohol must have vigilant protection of their spinal column by the health care team.
- The very young and the elderly are at high risk of exhibiting spinal cord injuries without any radiographic abnormalities. The clinical exam of these patients must be conducted carefully.
- Any life-threatening issues that are identified during this phase of the assessment must be corrected before advancing in the primary survey. Examples of these conditions include partial or complete obstruction of the airway from foreign bodies, debris, or the patient's tongue. The airway itself may be disrupted by a penetrating injury or the larynx and/or other airway structures may be injured by blunt forces.

Airway Adjuncts

The use of airway adjuncts may be essential to the management of the patient's airway. Familiarity with the various types of adjuncts available, including their indications and contraindications, is essential. A variety of techniques may be used to open or clear an obstructed airway. The jaw thrust or chin lift may reposition the tongue and open the airway, whereas suctioning may remove any debris that has accumulated in the oral cavity (blood, vomitus, secretions, teeth). Suctioning must not be aggressive because this may stimulate the gag reflex and subsequent vomiting and/or aspiration. The cervical spine must be maintained in the neutral position, without any hyperflexion, hyperextension, or rotation.

Oropharyngeal Airway. The oropharyngeal airway should be used only in *patients who are unconscious and without a gag reflex.* Even if the patient is intubated endotracheally, the oropharyngeal airway may be used as a bite block to prevent the patient from biting the endotracheal tube.

Nasopharyngeal Airway. The nasopharyngeal airway may be used on patients *who are conscious and have an intact gag reflex.* This airway is contraindicated in patients with severe facial fractures. The airway is better tolerated by the responsive patient and is less likely to induce vomiting.

Laryngeal Mask Airway. The laryngeal mask airway is used as an alternative to mask ventilation or as a temporizing measure until an endotracheal tube can be secured.[1] The laryngeal mask airway has an advantage in trauma patients who are unable to maintain a seal with mask ventilation. The laryngeal mask airway does not protect against aspiration and therefore is not a definitive airway for trauma patients.

Endotracheal Tube. An endotracheal tube should be considered when total airway management is essential. In the trauma patient, absolute care must be taken to avoid hyperextension of the neck before diagnostic studies to rule out a cervical spine injury. The patient must be well ventilated with a bag-valve-mask device before instituting an endotracheal intubation, and an assessment of the patient's neurologic status should be obtained before the administration of sedatives, narcotics, or paralytic agents. The endotracheal tube may be inserted orally or nasally. Nasotracheal intubation is not used commonly in the trauma patient and is contraindicated in those patients with severe midface fractures or basilar skull fractures or with patients without respiratory effort.

Correct tube placement must be confirmed by auscultation and subsequent chest x-ray film. Stabilization of the tube is an important consideration before transportation of the patient. Frequent reassessments ensure that proper placement is maintained. Inadvertent extubation during movement or transport should be anticipated and corrected as indicated.

Cricothyroidotomy. Cricothyroidotomy is a procedure that should be used only when airway management by another means cannot be accomplished. This technique provides oxygen to a patient in an emergent situation, but it is considered to be a temporary airway until a definitive one can be established (Figure 11-1). Cricothyroidotomy may be carried out by the following procedures:

- *Needle placement and transtracheal jet insufflation.* Carbon dioxide rapidly accumulates with this method (usually within 30 minutes), so a definitive airway must be established quickly.

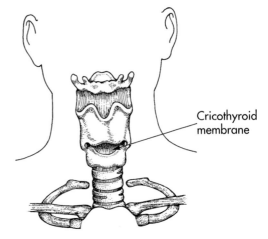

Figure II–I. Cricothyroidotomy.

Cricothyroid membrane

- *Surgical incision and tracheal tube placement.* A surgical cricothyroidotomy should be converted to a formal tracheostomy as soon as the patient's clinical condition allows. Open cricothyroidotomy is generally *not* indicated in pediatric patients.

End-Tidal Carbon Dioxide Detector. An end-tidal carbon dioxide detector confirms placement of the endotracheal tube by indicating the presence of carbon dioxide in the exhaled gases.

Pulse Oximeter. A pulse oximeter is a noninvasive method to measure oxygen saturation of arterial blood continuously.

Breathing and Ventilation

The function of breathing and ventilation is for gas exchange at the respiratory membrane. Adequate oxygenation must be maintained. If oxygenation is not being accomplished adequately by the patient, staff must provide assistance to optimize oxygenation and gas diffusion. The effectiveness and adequacy of ventilation can be evaluated by arterial blood gas measurement.

Life-threatening clinical findings that impair ventilation include tension pneumothorax, tension hemothorax, flail segment with pulmonary contusion, open pneumothorax, and cardiac tamponade. These conditions are diagnosed by clinical exam rather than diagnostic tests and, if found, must be corrected or addressed immediately. These injuries should be identified in the primary survey. Simple pneumothorax or hemothorax, fractured ribs, and pulmonary contusion may interfere with ventilation but usually are addressed in the secondary survey. See Chapter 18 for management of chest injuries.

Assessment of breathing effectiveness may be measured by the patient's facial expression (distress, anxiety, or agitated), quality of respirations (shallow or labored), skin color (pallor, cyanosis), or use of accessory muscles (chest wall, neck, and abdomen).

Assess the trachea for its position (midline versus shifted to the left or right) and whether crepitus exists, indicating a disruption in the system. Evaluate neck veins for whether they are flat or distended, and assess breath sounds for whether they are present, diminished, or absent. Evaluate the chest wall for its integrity (flail segment, splinting, open wounds) and symmetry during expansion. Evaluate the respiratory rate for its quality (rate, depth). Central cyanosis would indicate ineffective gas exchange. Pulse oximetry and end-tidal carbon dioxide monitors are helpful pieces of equipment to have in your resuscitation bay.

Circulation and Hemorrhage Control

Assessment of the trauma patient's circulatory status during the primary survey can be accomplished rapidly by evaluating the patient's level of consciousness, skin color, and pulse. The patient's level of consciousness may be impaired when there is a decrease in the circulating blood volume, thereby causing diminished cerebral perfusion. The patient possibly may have had a significant blood loss and still be conscious. The patient's skin may be indicative of inadequate organ perfusion if it is pale, cool, and/or diaphoretic and the nail beds have delayed capillary refill (>2 seconds). Central pulses (femoral or carotid artery) are best evaluated bilaterally. Tachycardia is the most common sign of hemorrhagic shock. The peripheral pulse rate that is full, slow, and regular usually represents normovolemia, but this will not be the case in a patient who takes beta-adrenergic blocking medications. A rapid, thready pulse usually represents hypovolemia, but there may be other influencing factors. An irregular pulse usually signifies a potential cardiac dysfunction. If pulses are not present, or if they are ineffective, an emergent resuscitation is necessary to replenish blood volume and cardiac output. Any external hemorrhage must be identified and controlled during the primary survey. Direct manual pressure is the best method to control external hemorrhage, and elevation of the extremity and application of pressure to arterial pressure points also may help to control bleeding. Tourniquets and other pneumatic splinting devices are not recommended because they may cause tissue damage and ischemia. Under extenuating circumstances, tourniquets may have a limited role.

The primary goal of hemorrhage management is to identify the source of bleeding and control it. Arterial bleeding in open wounds can be ligated by the physician, and scalp lacerations may be closed with staples to control the bleeding. If there is an open book pelvic fracture or a vertical sheer injury, a bed sheet that is tied around the pelvis may be a good temporizing measure until definitive repair can be accomplished.

A number of other circumstances may influence your ability to assess the volume status of your patient accurately, and they include the elderly, children, athletes, and those individuals with chronic medical conditions. Geriatric patients may have a limited physiologic ability to compensate for blood loss, so they may not exhibit tachycardia, an early sign of volume depletion. Children often are able to compensate for hypovolemia through an extensive physiologic reserve, and their deterioration is often sudden and catastrophic. Athletes have a similar capacity to compensate, typically with bradycardia, so an early sign of blood loss or hypovolemia often can be undetected. Comorbid medical conditions and their medication regimen may mask, or exacerbate, the patient's true physiologic status.

Hypovolemic shock is the most common type of shock that occurs in the trauma patient. It results from a decrease in the amount of circulating blood volume, with a subsequent decrease in venous return, causing a decreased stroke volume, decreased cardiac output, and impaired tissue perfusion because of diminished oxygen availability at the cellular level. Two large-bore intravenous lines should be initiated, if not already in place, and 2 L of Ringer's lactate solution or normal saline should be infused rapidly in the adult patient. In children, a crystalloid fluid bolus of 20 mL/kg should be infused rapidly when you suspect hypovolemia. If the patient's hemodynamic status does not stabilize after the bolus, administration of blood products should be considered. Type-specific blood is preferred, but if the patient is unstable, uncrossmatched blood can be used until definitive interventions are implemented. For those patients who respond initially to the infusions but subsequently deteriorate, ongoing blood loss must be considered. If the patient does not have a pulse, immediate cardiopulmonary resuscitation and advanced life support measures must be initiated. An emergent thoracotomy or transportation to the operating room may be indicated. Ongoing, frequent reassessments are critical for identifying any trends in the patient's hemodynamic parameters. Any life-threatening conditions that interfere with circulation and are identified during the primary survey must be addressed as they are found.

Hemorrhagic shock is classified into four different categories, based on the amount of blood loss, as shown in Table 11-1.

Patients experiencing hypovolemic shock will be restless and anxious, and their skin will be cool, diaphoretic, and pale. Their distal extremities will be cool, and their capillary refill will be delayed (>2 seconds). Their pulse will be weak and at a rate that is greater than 100 beats/min. Their blood pressure will be less than 90 mm Hg systolic, and their respirations will be shallow and rapid (>29 per minute) or depressed (< 10 per minute). Their Glasgow Coma Scale score will be less than 13, and they will have a decreased level of consciousness. If they are conscious, they may complain of being cold and/or thirsty.

Other considerations at this point in the initial assessment include preventing hypothermia in the patient with multiple injuries. Controlling any hemorrhage, applying warm blankets,

Table II-I Classification of Hemorrhagic Shock

	Class I	Class II	Class III	Class IV
Blood loss (mL)	<750	750-1500	1500-2000	>2000
Blood loss (% blood volume)	Up to 15%	30%	30%-40%	>40%
Pulse rate	<100	>100	>120	>140
Blood pressure	Normal	Normal	Decreased	Decreased
Pulse pressure	Normal or increased	Decreased	Decreased	Decreased
Respiratory rate	14-20	20-30	30-40	>40
Urine output (mL/hr)	>30	20-30	5-15	Neglible
Central nervous system/mental status	Slightly anxious	Mildly anxious	Anxious and confused	Confused and lethargic
Fluid replacement	Crystalloid	Crystalloid	Crystalloid and blood	Crystalloid and blood

Reproduced with permission from American College of Surgeons' Committee on Trauma, *Advanced trauma life support (R) for doctors (ATLS[R]) Student Manual, 7th edition,* Chicago, American Surgeons, 2004.

increasing the ambient air temperature, administering warmed fluids, and removing saturated dressings can help to minimize and/or prevent hypothermia. All clothing and wet dressings should be removed as soon as possible. All patients should be monitored continuously to assess for dysrhythmias, pulseless electrical activity, or other cardiac rhythm or rate disturbances.

Assessment of Patient's Neurologic Disability

Once the life-threatening injuries have been identified and the essential interventions have been done, a brief neurologic examination should be completed to establish a baseline for subsequent evaluations. A more in-depth exam can be done once the patient is hemo-dynamically stable. An abbreviated neurologic exam should include the Glasgow Coma Scale (Table 11-2) because this scoring system evaluates the patient's eye opening, verbal response, and best motor response. The sum of these scores provides the clinician with a simple and efficient method to predict the patient's outcome, as well as a way to quantify the patient's neurologic status. Sequential assessments of the Glasgow Coma Scale will identify changes in the patient's neurologic status.

The Glasgow Coma Scale reflects the function of the patient's central nervous system, its degree of integration, and brainstem function. The scores can range from 3 to 15 and increase as the patient's level of consciousness and integration skills improve. A score of 8 indicates coma. A patient who is intubated or paralyzed by pharmaceutical agents for airway control will have a prognosis different from a patient who has a head injury. Both will have a Glasgow Coma Scale score of 3, but they may have very different outcomes. The patient's motor function

Table 11-2 Glasgow Coma Scale

Eye Opening	
Spontaneous	4
To voice	3
To pain	2
None	1
Best Verbal Response	
Oriented	5
Confused (imprecise)	4
Inappropriate words	3
Incomprehensible words	2
None	1
Best Motor Response	
Obeys simple commands	6
Localizes noxious stimulus	5
Withdraws (pain)	4
Flexion (pain)	3
Extension (pain)	2
No motor response	1

From Teasdale G, Jennett B: *Lancet* 2:81-84, 1974.

should be assessed carefully and documented before the administration of any pharmacologic agents.

Exposure and Environmental Considerations

Patients must be exposed completely to have their injuries assessed thoroughly. Warm blankets, warm intravenous infusions, elevated room temperature, and warmed, inspired air encourage normothermia. Monitoring the patient's temperature early in the resuscitation is important, and subsequent evaluations will identify any trends toward impending hypothermia. If the patient has ongoing hemorrhage, the patient will be more susceptible to hypothermia, so the primary goal in this circumstance is to stop the bleeding.

Adjuncts to the Primary Survey

Once the primary survey is complete and all life-threatening injuries have been addressed appropriately, the following adjuncts, if not already implemented, should be considered before initiating the secondary survey.

A cardiac monitor, pulse oximeter, and an end-tidal carbon dioxide monitor should be placed on the patient on arrival into the trauma resuscitation area. The patient's vital signs—to include a pulse, arterial blood pressure, respiratory rate, and temperature—should be measured and trended. Arterial blood gas, nasogastric or orogastric tubes, intravenous catheters and fluids, and a Foley catheter should be implemented at the earliest opportunity (if not contraindicated). These interventions should not interfere with the team leader's resuscitative efforts (airway, breathing, circulation, or neurologic evaluation). Two large-bore (14- or 16-gauge) peripheral intravenous lines should be placed—and if this is not possible, consider a large-bore central line—administering warmed Ringer's lactate solution or normal saline. Blood samples should be drawn when the intravenous lines are placed. If the patient continues to be hemodynamically unstable after a 2-L infusion of intravenous fluids, consider administration of blood products.

Limited radiographic studies may be done at this time, leaving additional studies to be completed during the secondary survey, but x-ray films should not delay the patient's resuscitation. The anterior/posterior chest x-ray film and an anterior/posterior pelvic x-ray film can identify potentially life-threatening injuries in patients who have sustained blunt trauma. A lateral cervical spine x-ray film may identify an injury that is critical during the initial resuscitation, but an inadequate film does not exclude such an injury, so protection of the cervical column is essential until more thorough radiologic studies can be completed during the secondary survey.

SECONDARY SURVEY

After the primary survey has been completed and appropriate therapeutic interventions have been accomplished, clinical personnel should continue to the secondary survey, examining the patient carefully and methodically from head to toe, checking for obvious injuries, deformities, impaled objects, bruises, bleeding, and complaints of pain. Ongoing monitoring of vital signs is imperative.

To perform an adequate assessment, the patient should be undressed. The patient should be kept warm with blankets, a heat shield or other heating device during the physical assessment and therapeutic/diagnostic interventions. A complete neurologic evaluation (including Glasgow Coma Scale) should be performed.

Perform the following tasks for each part of the secondary survey.

Patient History

- Obtain a prehospital history of the scene, events, conditions, mechanism of injury, field physical assessment, and clinical data.
- Obtain a list of prehospital treatments and interventions.
- Obtain a medical history, surgical history, comorbidities, medications, allergies and transfusion history.

Head

- Observe the head for bruises, lacerations, and deformities.
- Palpate the head for deformities.

Face

- Observe the face for bruises, lacerations, deformities, and asymmetry.
- Palpate the face for deformities and step-offs.

Eyes

- Observe the eyes for injuries, foreign bodies, periorbital ecchymosis, hemorrhage, contact lenses, enucleation, and extraocular movement.
- Check pupil size and reaction to light.
- Check visual acuity, if appropriate.
- Palpate the orbital rims.

Nose

- Observe the nose for injuries, foreign bodies, epistaxis, and cerebrospinal fluid rhinorrhea.
- Palpate the nose for deformities.

Mouth

- Observe the mouth for injuries, foreign bodies, hemorrhage, missing or broken teeth, and malocclusion of teeth.
- Palpate the mouth for foreign bodies and malocclusion of teeth.

Ears

- Observe the ears for injuries, foreign bodies, cerebrospinal fluid otorrhea, Battle's sign, and hemotympanum.

Neck

- Observe the neck for penetrating or soft tissue injuries, ecchymoses, distended jugular veins, and deviated trachea.
- Palpate the neck for deviated trachea, subcutaneous emphysema, cervical vertebrae deformity, and pain response.
- Auscultate the neck for bruits.

Chest

- Observe the chest for injuries, impaled objects, ecchymoses, chest wall bruising, chest expansion, respiratory rate, rhythm and depth, use of accessory muscles of respiration and work of breathing.
- Palpate the chest for pain response, subcutaneous emphysema, and deformities (sternum, clavicles, ribs).
- Auscultate the chest for breath sounds and heart sounds.

Abdomen

- Observe the abdomen for injuries, impaled objects, ecchymoses, evisceration, distention, and scars.
- Auscultate the abdomen for bowel sounds.
- Palpate the abdomen for pain response, guarding, and rigidity.

Pelvis and Genitalia

- Observe the pelvic area for injuries, bleeding, and priapism.
- Palpate for pelvic instability.
- Check rectal sphincter tone.
- Note pain and/or urge to void but inability to urinate.

Lower Extremities

- Observe the lower extremities for injuries, open wounds, deformities, edema, and angulation.
- Palpate the lower extremities for crepitus, pain response, deformities, discolorations, pulses distal to injury, skin temperature, motor and sensory function, and capillary refill.

Upper Extremities

- Observe the upper extremities for injuries, open wounds, deformities, edema, and angulation.
- Palpate the upper extremities for crepitus, pain response, deformities, discolorations, pulses distal to injury, skin temperature, motor and sensory function, and capillary refill.

Posterior

- Inspect the patient's back; patient should be logrolled, maintaining spinal alignment.
- Observe the patient's back, thorax, buttocks, and posterior legs for injuries, bruises, deformities, impaled objects, and bleeding.
- Palpate the back for pain response and deformities.

Assessment and reassessment of the parameters of the primary survey is important throughout the secondary survey. After a secondary survey has been completed, calculate the trauma score (Table 11-3) and document all findings. The nursing diagnosis box contains a list of nursing diagnoses frequently used for trauma patients.

Table II–3   Trauma Score

	Points
Respiratory Rate	
10-24 breaths/min	4
25-35 breaths/min	3
36 breaths/min or greater	2
1-9 breaths/min	1
0	0
Respiratory Effort	
Normal	1
Shallow, retracted, none	0
Blood Pressure (Systolic)	
≥90 mm Hg	4
70-89 mm Hg	3
50-69 mm Hg	2
1-49 mm Hg	1
0	0
Capillary Refill	
<2 sec Normal	2
Delayed	1
None	0
Glasgow Coma Scale (Score)	
14-15	5
11-13	4
8-10	3
5-7	2
3-4	1
Total =	———

From Champion HR, Sacco WJ, Copes WS et al: *J Trauma* 29:623-629, 1989.

HIGH-FREQUENCY NURSING DIAGNOSES FOR PATIENTS WITH TRAUMA

- Ineffective airway clearance
- Risk for aspiration
- Ineffective breathing pattern
- Impaired gas exchange
- Fluid volume deficit
- Decreased cardiac output
- Ineffective tissue perfusion: cerebral, cardiopulmonary, renal, gastrointestinal, and/or peripheral
- Hypothermia
- Impaired skin integrity
- Impaired tissue integrity
- Risk for peripheral neurovascular dysfunction
- Impaired physical mobility
- Acute pain
- Fear
- Anxiety
- Knowledge deficit: aftercare for injury
- Risk for infection
- Risk for injury
- Risk for trauma
- *Nursing diagnoses specific to injury or unique patient population*

From NANDA International: *NANDA nursing diagnoses: definitions & classification, 2005-2006,* Philadelphia, The Association.

Reference

1. Sheridan RL, editor: *The trauma handbook of the Massachusetts General Hospital,* Philadelphia, 2004, Lippincott, Williams & Wilkins.

Suggested Readings

Champion HR, Sacco WJ, Copes WS et al: A revision of the trauma score, *J Trauma* 29:623-629, 1989.

Committee on Trauma, American College of Surgeons: *Advanced trauma life support instructor manual,* Chicago, 1993, The College.

Teasdale G, Jennett B: Assessment of coma and impaired consciousness, *Lancet* 2:81-84, 1974.

CHAPTER 12

SHOCK AND FLUID REPLACEMENT IN TRAUMA

MAUREEN A. HARRAHILL

Shock is an abnormality of the circulatory system that results in inadequate organ perfusion and tissue oxygenation.[1] Shock can be initiated by a number of different mechanisms, including inability of the heart to pump adequately (cardiogenic and obstructive), the loss of vascular tone (neurogenic and inflammatory), and the loss of circulating fluid (hypovolemic and hemorrhagic). Some authors describe an additional category of "traumatic shock." As conceptualized, this form of shock represents the result of a series of insults that together produce profound hypoperfusion.[2,3] Regardless of the mechanism, all shock states share the common pathophysiology of inadequate oxygen delivery to meet cellular oxygen demands.

PATHOLOGY AND STAGES OF SHOCK

Initial Stage

During the initial stage of shock, cardiac output is decreased, leading to decreased tissue perfusion. Without adequate oxygen, the cells switch to anaerobic metabolism as their energy source. Lactic acid is a by-product of this inefficient form of metabolism, and the buildup of this acid can lead to further cellular insult.

Compensatory Stage

The compensatory mechanisms of the body attempt to improve tissue perfusion. Catecholamine release causes progressive vasoconstriction, which redistributes blood from the skin, muscles, and viscera to preserve blood flow to the heart, brain, and kidneys. Other effects of catecholamine release include increased heart rate and myocardial contractility, which improves cardiac output and increases blood pressure. Hormonal responses include the release of renin and stimulation of the anterior pituitary and adrenal medulla. These responses lead to a cascade of events ultimately leading to sodium and water retention, a rise in blood glucose levels, and release of epinephrine and norepinephrine.

Progressive Stage

In the progressive stage the compensatory mechanisms have peaked and start to fail. Prolonged anaerobic metabolism leads to a buildup of toxic waste products. These waste products act as potent vasodilators, further decreasing critical blood flow to the tissues. The integrity of the capillary membrane is weakened, and fluid shifts from the intravascular space to the interstitial space, which contributes to additional decreased venous blood return to the heart. On the cellular level the cell membrane loses its ability to maintain a normal electrical gradient.

Sodium and water enter the cell, causing swelling, progressive damage, and ultimately cellular death. Although the patient can be resuscitated hemodynamically at this stage, there are profound systemic toxic effects from the ischemia and reperfusion. Sequelae include acute respiratory distress syndrome that can lead quickly to gastrointestinal dysfunction, cardiac failure, renal failure, and immunosuppression.

Refractory Stage

The refractory stage is a lethal state of ongoing hemorrhage with associated coagulopathies from which the patient cannot survive.

NONHEMORRHAGIC SHOCK IN THE INJURED PATIENT

The American College of Surgeons Committee on Trauma divides shock in a trauma patient into two major categories: hemorrhagic and nonhemorrhagic.[1] Hemorrhagic is the most commonly seen type of shock in trauma. Nonhemorrhagic categories of shock seen in the injured patient include cardiogenic, neurogenic, inflammatory, and obstructive.

Cardiogenic Shock

Cardiogenic shock occurs when the heart is unable to pump blood effectively. This dysfunction can occur when the right ventricle fails to pump venous blood into the pulmonary system or when the left ventricle fails to pump oxygenated blood into the systemic circulation. Causes of cardiogenic shock include myocardial infarction, mechanical complications such as cardiac valve rupture, and end-stage cardiac disease.

Specific markers may include the following:

- Cardiac dysrhythmias
- Elevated cardiac isoenzymes
- Electrocardiogram changes indicative of myocardial infarction

Treatment considerations include the following:

- Early central venous pressure monitoring to help guide fluid resuscitation
- Inotropic agents to increase cardiac output and coronary artery perfusion
- Pain control

Neurogenic Shock

Neurogenic shock is a "pipe" problem caused by vasodilation. Neurogenic shock may be the result of a severe brainstem injury, an injury to the spinal cord, or spinal anesthesia. The cause of neurogenic shock is a loss of sympathetic tone, causing peripheral vasodilation and hypotension. This patient typically has flat, nondistended jugular neck veins.

Neurogenic shock may mask signs and symptoms of other types of shock. If neurogenic shock is present, there should be a heightened index of suspicion for undetected sources of hemorrhage. Any sources of ongoing blood loss should be identified, and hemorrhage control measures should be initiated. Specific markers may include the following:

- Decreased blood pressure
- Rapid, shallow respirations or no respirations

- Bradycardia
- Paraplegia or quadriplegia
- History of recent spinal anesthesia
- History of recent major head trauma
- Priapism (sustained erection) indicating spinal cord injury
- Cool, clammy skin *above* the level of the spinal cord lesion
- Possible diaphoresis *below* the level of the lesion

Treatment considerations include central venous pressure monitoring to guide fluid resuscitation.

Inflammatory Shock

Inflammatory (septic) shock is a "pipe" problem caused by vasodilation. Inflammatory shock is caused by an overwhelming infection and may be the result of a suppressed immune system, a massive burn injury, or any other condition that can introduce an infecting organism into a compromised victim. The organism enters the vascular system and promotes the release of endotoxins, which cause an interstitial fluid leak, increased vascular permeability, and vasodilation (also known as *volume shunting*), which leads to shock.

Specific markers may include the following:

- Normal blood pressure with widened pulse pressure or decreased blood pressure
- Tachycardia
- Hyperpyrexia
- Chills or tremors
- Warm, dry skin
- Positive blood cultures

Treatment considerations include the following:

- Appropriate antibiotics
- Inotropic agents

Obstructive Shock

Obstructive shock occurs when a mechanical obstruction impedes venous return to the heart. This decreased venous return prevents adequate cardiac filling and leads to decreased cardiac output. The two most common obstructions are tension pneumothorax and cardiac tamponade. Distended jugular veins may indicate increased intrathoracic pressure, which forces blood to "backflow" into the jugular veins and decreases filling of the right side of the heart. Central venous pressure (CVP) values are typically greater than 10 cm H_2O in obstructive shock.[4] However, if the patient has lost a significant amount of blood as well, the jugular veins may be flat and the CVP may be normal or even decreased.

Specific markers may include the following:

- Distended neck veins
- Shortness of breath
- Muffled heart sounds

Treatment considerations include placement of a needle in the pericardial sac (tamponade) or pleural space (tension pneumothorax) as an immediate temporizing measure to relieve pressure.

HEMORRHAGIC SHOCK

Clinical Signs of Hemorrhagic Shock

Taken individually, the clinical signs of hemorrhagic shock are relatively nonspecific. Looked at together with the patient history and mechanism of injury, the signs have significantly increased usefulness.

Pulse

As shock worsens, the pulse increases as a compensatory mechanism until catecholamines are depleted, and then bradycardia signals a terminal event. Tachycardia may not be seen in an elderly patient whose catecholamine release and subsequent cardiac response are limited. Tachycardia is defined as follows[1]:

Infants	Greater than 160 beats/min
Preschool-age children	Greater than 140 beats/min
Preschool- to puberty-age children	Greater than 120 beats/min
Adults	Greater than 100 beats/min

Respirations

As the shock state worsens, respirations become more rapid and shallower. This is a mechanism to improve oxygenation and compensate for the metabolic acidosis associated with shock.

Blood Pressure

Blood pressure is not a reliable indicator of shock in the early stages because compensatory mechanisms may cause the blood pressure to remain at a normal level for a time. Hypotension results from significant fluid loss with compensatory mechanism failure and is usually a late sign of shock.

Skin

Sympathetic nervous system activation results in peripheral vasoconstriction. The patient's skin becomes pale, cool, and clammy.

Jugular Veins

Flat jugular veins typically indicate hypovolemia.

Level of Consciousness

Patients in early shock may exhibit restlessness or anxiety. As the shock state worsens, brain tissue perfusion is compromised, resulting in a decreased level of consciousness.

Arterial Blood Gas Values

Early blood gas findings may show respiratory alkalosis caused by the patient's compensatory tachypnea. This can be followed by metabolic acidosis caused by anaerobic metabolism from inadequate tissue perfusion and the production of lactate.

Central Venous Pressure

CVP, which is a measurement of pressure of the right side of the heart, indirectly reflects blood volume, vascular tone, and pump effectiveness. A normal CVP measurement is 4 to 10 cm H_2O pressure. A value of less than 4 cm H_2O may indicate hypovolemia. A CVP reading may be falsely elevated because of use of the pneumatic antishock garment (PASG).

Pulmonary Artery Wedge Pressure

Pulmonary artery wedge pressure is an indirect measurement of left atrial and ventricular pressure. Normal values are 6 to 12 cm H_2O. Values less than 6 cm H_2O may indicate hypovolemia.

Urinary Output

The average adult hourly urine output is 0.5 to 1 mg/kg. Less than 35 mL per hour may indicate decreased renal perfusion.[1,4] In the pediatric population, 1 mL/kg per hour is an adequate urinary output.[1]

Classifications of Hemorrhagic Shock

The average amount of blood in an adult is 7% to 8% of the person's ideal body weight. A child's blood volume is calculated as approximately 8% to 9% of ideal body weight. Shock can be classified into four categories based on the amount of blood loss[1]:

Class I: Less Than 15% Blood Loss

Typical clinical findings include the following:

- Slight tachycardia
- Normal blood pressure
- Normal pulse pressure
- Normal respiratory rate and depth
- Normal skin findings (color, temperature, moisture)
- Normal urinary output

Class II: 15% to 30% Blood Loss

Typical clinical findings include the following:

- Tachycardia
- Increased respiratory rate or no change in depth
- Decreased pulse pressure or increase in diastolic pressure
- Slightly cool skin
- Slightly decreased urine output
- Mildly anxious

Class III: 30% to 40% Blood Loss

Typical clinical findings include the following:

- Tachycardia
- Anxiety, confusion

- Cool, clammy extremities
- Tachypnea
- Narrow pulse pressure
- Decreased blood pressure
- Significantly decreased urinary output
- Decreased CVP
- Decreased pulmonary artery wedge pressure

Class IV: Greater Than 40% Blood Loss

Typical clinical findings include the following:

- Decreased level of consciousness
- Marked tachycardia
- Cool, clammy skin
- Severely decreased blood pressure
- Significantly decreased urinary output to anuria
- Decreased CVP
- Decreased pulmonary artery wedge pressure (less than 4 mm Hg); may be decreased before Class IV
- Arterial blood gas values: metabolic acidosis and respiratory alkalosis

Treatment of Hemorrhagic Shock

Treatment of shock starts first with the recognition of the condition and then with directed therapy to maintain critical tissue oxygenation and organ perfusion. Intervening before the patient progresses to decompensated shock can mean the difference between life and death. The degree of shock depends on the amount of blood lost, the age and general physical condition of the patient, the amount and type of injuries sustained, and the patient's ability to activate compensatory mechanisms. Treatment must be individualized and reassessed continually. The general objectives of shock management are as follows:

1. Providing adequate oxygenation
2. Providing adequate ventilation
3. Recognizing and controlling hemorrhage
4. Providing appropriate fluids to combat cellular dysfunction

Management of airway and breathing issues are well described in Chapter 11. After ensuring that the airway and breathing are being maintained adequately, controlling hemorrhage takes center stage. Key interventions include applying direct pressure to bleeding wounds, reducing pelvic volume by use of sling/sheet or PASG in patients with pelvic fractures, applying traction splints for long-bone fractures, and early operative interventions.

Pneumatic Antishock Garment

The use of the PASG remains controversial, and clinicians should follow local protocol regarding the use of the device. The most common indication cited for the PASG is in the case of suspected pelvic fractures with hypotension (defined as a systolic blood pressure less than 90 mm Hg).[5]

The Prehospital Trauma Life Support Committee of the National Association of Emergency Medical Technicians offers six specific contraindications for PASG use:[5]

1. Penetrating thoracic trauma
2. Splinting of lower extremity fractures
3. Evisceration of abdominal organs
4. Impaled objects in the abdomen
5. Pregnancy
6. Traumatic cardiopulmonary arrest

Fluid Replacement

Fluid replacement is not benign. Injudicious fluid replacement can cause electrolyte imbalances, dilutional coagulopathies, and secondary clot disruption with increased bleeding. Deliberate decision making is critical to choose the appropriate type and amount of fluid to give to the patient.

Gaining vascular access can be challenging in the injured patient. Poiseuille's law states the rate of flow is proportional to the fourth power of the radius of the cannula and is inversely related to its length. Therefore, clinical personnel should use the largest-gauge and shortest-length cannula possible to ensure the most rapid infusion of large volumes of fluid. Access options include peripheral forearm and antecubital veins; central venous access via the femoral, jugular, or subclavian veins; saphenous vein cutdown; and intraosseous needle for the pediatric patient.

Types of Tubing

- Standard *macrodrip* tubing or high-volume trauma tubing is capable of administering blood; *microdrip* tubing should not be used.
- In-line manual pumping devices are helpful to speed the delivery of the fluid to the patient.
- Extension tubing is controversial because it slows the rate of delivery of fluid to the venous system.

Adjunct Devices

- Pressure cuffs speed the rate of delivery.
- Hypothermia is a significant risk with the delivery of crystalloids and colloids. All intravenous solutions should be warmed to 37° to 40° C (98.6° to 104° F).[1] High-volume fluid warmers allow the fluid to be warmed and delivered quickly.

Types of Fluids. The debate of the most appropriate type and amount of resuscitation fluid to use continues to spark controversy.[2] Isotonic Ringer's lactate solution approximates plasma electrolyte composition and osmolality and is the recommended crystalloid solution to use for the initial resuscitation. Normal saline solution may be used, but because it may cause hyperchloremic acidosis if large volumes are given, it is recommended as a "second choice."[1] Solutions containing glucose should be avoided because hyperglycemia aggravates central nervous system injury.[6] The use of colloids, such as human albumin, in the initial resuscitation is not recommended.[2]

As an initial guideline, the dosing of isotonic fluid is 20 mL/kg for a pediatric patient and 1 to 2 L for an adult.[1] The American College of Surgeons Committee on Trauma offers the recommendation of a "3 for 1" ratio, where 1 mL of blood loss requires 3 mL of crystalloid fluid replacement. The patient should be monitored frequently, and further fluid therapies should be based on the patient's response to the fluid.

Blood and Blood Components. The purpose of giving blood is to restore the oxygen-carrying capacity of the intravascular volume. The risks of giving blood must be considered carefully. Transfusion-transmitted diseases include viral infection, bacterial contamination, acute and delayed hemolytic reactions, and transfusion-related acute lung injury. Hepatitis B and hepatitis C are the most frequent infectious complications posttransfusion, occurring in 1 in 30,000 to 1 in 250,000 transfusions, respectively.[2]

The decision to transfuse should be individualized, based on the rate and magnitude of the blood loss, the patient's medical condition (such as patient age, the degree of cardiopulmonary reserve, and the presence of atherosclerotic disease), and potential for ongoing blood loss. In general, anemia is fairly well tolerated, especially in the previously healthy, young trauma patient. A rough guideline is to use hemoglobin of 7 to 8 g/dL as a transfusion trigger.[2] Patients who remain unstable or have preexisting cardiovascular or pulmonary disease may require a higher threshold.

Red Blood Cells (Packed Red Cells). Packed red blood cells (RBCs) are units of whole blood with most of the plasma removed. One unit of packed RBCs has a hematocrit of 65% to 80%. In general, one unit of packed RBCs will raise the recipient's hematocrit by 3% (or hemoglobin level by approximately 1 g/dL).

Crossmatched, type-specific blood offers the least risk to the patient but can take up to an hour to process. Type-specific, uncrossmatched blood generally is available within 10 minutes, and the risk of hemolytic transfusion reaction is low.

If blood is required *immediately,* O-negative packed RBCs can be given until type-specific or type and crossmatched blood is available. O-negative packed RBCs have no major antigens and can be given reasonably safely to patients of any blood type. Because of limited supplies of O-negative blood, many institutions have adopted a policy of giving O-positive blood to male patients and reserving O-negative blood for women of childbearing age.

Massive Transfusion. Massive transfusion is the complete replacement of a patient's blood volume as a result of exsanguination or a transfusion replacing the patient's blood volume within a 24-hour period.[2] Several problems are associated with massive transfusion, including electrolyte imbalances, such as hyperkalemia and hypocalcemia, and blood pH imbalances. These issues may be more theoretically than clinically significant. However, hypothermia and coagulopathies are of major concern. Coagulopathy can occur because of dilution, infusion of thrombogenic substances, and hypothermia. Deloughery[7] recommends tight and repeated monitoring of five laboratory tests that reflect the basic parameters essential for blood volume and hemostasis. The tests are hematocrit, platelet count, international normalized ratio, activated partial thromboplastin time, and fibrinogen level. Table 12-1 provides general recommendations for component replacement therapy.

Hypothermia can result from delivering cold blood to the patient and can and should be prevented by warming the blood. Hypothermia leads to an increased affinity of hemoglobin

Table 12–1   General Guidelines for Blood Component Replacement

Test	Level	Provide
Hematocrit	Less than 21-24%	3+ units packed red blood cells
Platelet count	Less than 50,000-70,000	6-8 packs platelets
International normalized ratio	Greater than 2 and increased activated partial thromboplastin time	2-4 units of fresh frozen plasma
Activated partial thromboplastin time	Greater than 1.5 times normal	2-4 units of fresh frozen plasma
Fibrinogen	Less than 100 mg/dL	10 units cryoprecipitate

for oxygen, and it impairs clotting function. Packed RBCs commonly are stored at 4° C, and the infusion of just one unwarmed unit can lower a patient's body temperature by 0.25° C.[7] Hypothermia affects clotting in the following ways:

- Enzyme reactions necessary for clot formation are muted.
- Platelet function declines.
- Fibrinolysis is stimulated, which leads to more bleeding.

Recent reports cite the benefit of using recombinant activated factor VIIa for the massively bleeding trauma patient.[7] Recombinant activated factor VIIa binds to the tissue factor exposed at the site of injury and stimulates coagulation. This drug is currently expensive, and there are no definite recommendations for its use because clinical trials are ongoing. However, this factor is available and may be an option in the severely bleeding patient who is not responding to traditional blood product replacement therapy.

Autotransfusion. Autotransfusion may be a useful adjunct in an emergency department when there is massive blood loss into the thoracic cavity. Autotransfusion is not used routinely to collect blood from other body cavities in the emergency setting because blood other than blood from the chest is considered contaminated. Also, if there is a known coagulation defect or if the patient has cancer, shed blood from any cavity should not be used. With autotransfusion, blood from the chest cavity is collected, filtered, anticoagulated, and reinfused into the vascular system. Patients receiving cell-saver blood should have their coagulation status frequently monitored.

Additional Transfusion Considerations. Some patients may refuse to accept blood products because of cultural and religious considerations. This can pose a challenge to the trauma team if the patient is in hemorrhagic shock. Institutional policies and protocols can help delineate treatment alternatives.

The cost of used blood products in apparently futile attempts to resuscitate nonsurvival trauma victims is enormous. The trauma team easily can exhaust the local supply of blood on one patient. As with all facets of trauma care, the team's decision to initiate a massive transfusion protocol must reflect sound clinical judgment, carefully assessing all the risks and benefits.

Endpoints in Resuscitation. Knowing when to stop giving fluids can be a difficult question. The goal of blood and crystalloid infusion is to improve circulation and organ perfusion. Recent studies are evaluating the measurement of blood flow to the gastrointestinal tract as a direct indicator of circulating blood volume.[8] These researchers used a prototype spectroscopy gastric probe concurrently to measure tissue oxygen saturation of the splanchnic bed. Monitoring regional tissue oxygenation in critically ill patients could augment traditional clinical endpoints, such as arterial blood pressure and urine output. Evaluation of regional oxygen delivery and utilization also could aid the clinician in assessing the adequacy of resuscitation techniques. Until these technologies become widely available, we are left with using indirect measures. Indirect indicators include the following:

- Improved mental status
- Increased pulse pressure
- Increased urine output
- Resolution of lactic acidosis and base deficit
- Improved mixed venous oxygen content and saturation

References

1. Committee on Trauma, American College of Surgeons: *Advanced trauma life support instructor manual,* ed 6, Chicago, 1997, The College.
2. Harbecht B, Alarcon L, Peitzman A: Management of shock. In Moore EE, Feliciano DV, Mattox KL, editors: *Trauma,* ed 5, New York, 2004, McGraw-Hill.
3. Scalea TM, Boswell SA: Initial management of traumatic shock. In McQuillan KA, VonRueden KT, Hartsock RL et al, editors: *Trauma nursing from resuscitation through rehabilitation,* ed 3, Philadelphia, 2002, WB Saunders.
4. Peterson SR, Weinberg JA: Transfusion, autotransfusion, and blood substitutes. In Moore EE, Feliciano DV, Mattox KL, editors: *Trauma,* ed 5, New York, 2004, McGraw-Hill.
5. Prehospital Trauma Life Support Committee, National Association of Emergency Medical Technicians: *PHTLS basic and advanced prehospital trauma life support manual,* St Louis, 2003, Mosby.
6. Lam AM, Winn HR, Cullen BF et al: Hyperglycemia and neurological outcome in patients with head injury, *J Neurosurg* 75:545, 1991.
7. Deloughery TG: Coagulation defects in trauma patients: etiology, recognition, and therapy, *Crit Care Clin* 20:12-24, 2004.
8. Cohn SM, Varela JE, Giannotti G et al: Splanchnic perfusion evaluation during hemorrhage and resuscitation with gastric near-infrared spectroscopy, *J Trauma* 50(4):629-635, 2001.

Suggested Readings

Johnson K: Shock states. In Kidd PS, Wagner KD, editors: *High acuity nursing,* Upper Saddle River, NJ, 2001, Prentice Hall.

Mikhail J: Massive transfusion in trauma: process and outcomes, *J Trauma Nurs* 11(2):55-60, 2004.

Stacy KM, Fitzsimmons L: Shock and multiple organ dysfunction syndrome. In Urden LD, Stacy KM, Lough ME, editors: *Priorities in critical care nursing,* St Louis, 2004, Mosby.

Vary T, McLean B, VonRueden KT: Shock and multiple organ dysfunction syndrome. In McQuillan KA, VonRueden KT, Hartsock RL et al: editors: *Trauma nursing from resuscitation through rehabilitation,* ed 3, Philadelphia, 2002, WB Saunders.

PAIN MANAGEMENT

GAIL M. WILKES AND JOAN MEUNIER-SHAM

Pain is a complex phenomenon that almost all persons experience in their lifetime. Pain is a protective mechanism that warns the person of actual or impending harm to the body. The person experiencing pain is the *expert* on the pain experience, and only that person can describe the intensity of the pain and whether it is relieved by interventions.[1] How a person responds to pain, or pain behaviors, is a result of physical, psychological, social, and cultural factors. However, undertreated pain has become an epidemic in the United States. Although a common human experience, pain has become a major health problem because of provider and patient barriers. These include provider attitudes, lack of knowledge, and lack of accurate pain assessment and patient fear of opioid dependency or side effects. After a more in-depth review of the barriers to effective pain control, this chapter reviews the physiology of pain, types of pain, principles of pain assessment, nursing interventions, and patient/family education about pain.

EFFECTIVE PAIN CONTROL IN THE EMERGENCY DEPARTMENT

Pain is the most common reason that patients seek emergency medical attention. In the emergency department (ED), patients with trauma-related pain may experience distress for a long time, causing intense physiologic and emotional responses that may challenge the nurse. Studies have shown that pain is underestimated by many providers and is undertreated, resulting in needless patient suffering. Whipple et al.[2] studied the use of intravenously administered morphine in trauma patients at multiple institutions, using an observational prospective study design from 1992 to1993. In this study, 141 trauma patients were admitted to the surgical intensive care unit and received morphine intravenously. The most frequently ordered dose of morphine by the surgeon was 2 to 4 mg IV every hour as necessary. No correlation existed between the ordered dose and injury severity. The authors found that of the 1257 doses ordered and administered, 44% were at or below the minimum amount prescribed by the surgeons, and 33% doses were received late, at, or after a 3-hour interval.

As a result of this national problem, pain management has become a priority for national and professional organizations. The Joint Commission on Accreditation of Healthcare Organizations (JCAHO) implemented standards on pain in 2001 so that now all hospitals, in order to meet JCAHO standards, must have an effective pain management program that meets the following criteria[3]:

1. It recognizes the *right* of patients to appropriate assessment and management.
2. It identifies pain during an initial *assessment* and, as appropriate, in ongoing reassessments.
3. It develops a *plan* to control the pain.
4. It *educates patients* and their families about pain management.

EDs are working to reduce patient wait times. Next to waiting too long, unrelieved pain is the next priority concern of patients. The American College of Emergency Physicians advocates the following policy key points[4]:

- ED patients should receive expeditious pain management, avoiding delays such as those related to diagnostic testing or consultation.
- Hospitals should develop unique strategies that optimize ED patient pain management using opioid and nonopioid medications.
- ED policies and procedures should support the safe use and prescription writing of pain medications in the ED.
- Effective physician and patient educational strategies should be developed regarding pain management, including the use of pain therapy adjuncts and how to minimize pain after disposition from the ED.
- Ongoing research in the area of ED pain management should be conducted.

Barriers to Effective Pain Management

The intellectual, or knowledge, component of developing an effective pain management plan is simple. The barriers are what interfere with the process. One barrier is provider attitudes. Many providers believe that they are the expert in determining the amount of pain a person is experiencing, when of course, the patient is the expert. In addition, providers may be biased in treating patients. In a study at a Midwestern university, physician prescriptions of opioid analgesics were highly variable when the physicians were faced with identical case scenarios, such as if a patient asked for "something strong" for the pain, where 10% of physicians were influenced positively and 10% influenced negatively, with the rest in between.[5] Studies of elderly patients with extremity fractures showed that the elderly were less likely to receive analgesics compared with younger patients with similar fractures. The ED nurse should use an unbiased assessment to assess patients accurately and should help the physician colleague to develop an effective plan for the patient in pain.

Ethnic bias, another barrier, may prevent nurses and physicians from accurately assessing and providing an effective plan of care. In a Southern university study, 74% of white patients with long-bone fractures received pain medicine, whereas only 57% of black patients received pain medication.[6] A similar study in 1993 showed that in a Los Angeles urban ED, Hispanic patients with isolated long-bone fractures were twice as likely as non-Hispanic white patients to receive no pain medicine.[7] Other groups of patients who receive less or no analgesics compared with similar patients are those with sickle cell disease, a history of intravenous drug use, the elderly, and patients with a cultural background or language different from the nurse or physician.

Physicians may underprescribe appropriate analgesics, and nurses may give less than the prescribed dose—both barriers to effective pain management. Nurses may assume that patients do not have pain, which in itself is a bias. Nurses commonly believe that patients, who are receiving methadone maintenance to prevent withdrawal from opiate dependency, do not need additional opiates for a painful procedure or injury. This is untrue because methadone only prevents withdrawal and does nothing to reduce pain. In addition, the patient who has been or is dependent on opioids will be tolerant to opioids and will require higher than usual doses of an opioid compared with an opioid-naive patient with a similar pain stimulus or cause. Providers may fear that administration of an opioid will cause the patient to become an addict. This occurs rarely, if at all.

The nurse should keep in mind the following key terms:

- *Addiction:* Psychological dependency, seeking the opioid for its psychological effect, not for pain relief

- *Tolerance:* Loss of drug effect over time, requiring a larger dose of an opioid to relieve the pain given a similar stimulus, compared with previously
- *Physical dependency:* Dependency such that withdrawal will occur if the opioid is stopped; this is a physical phenomenon

Other providers may fear that opioid administration will result in respiratory depression or contribute to further instability in an otherwise ill patient. Respiratory depression may occur if a large, inappropriate opioid dose is given to an opioid-naive patient, but this is uncommon with appropriate dosing. Unrelieved pain, however, can lead to further instability. Unrelieved pain causes significant, *harmful* physiologic sequelae[8]:

- Tachycardia, hypotension or hypertension, vasoconstriction
- Increased cardiac output, increased cardiac workload, increased myocardial oxygen demand
- Increased sympathetic response to pain with the potential to increase myocardial ischemia
- Impaired ventilation (lowered tidal volume, vital capacity, functional residual capacity, and alveolar ventilation), depending on the site of pain, with hypoxemia.

Inaccurate pain assessment is a barrier to effective pain management. Many studies have shown that physicians and nurses underestimate the intensity and severity of a patient's pain. A study of ED nurses' pain assessment scores of intensity compared with patients' self-reports revealed a large discrepancy with significant underestimation by triage and treating ED nurses.[9] Clearly, inaccurate assessment leads to inadequate pain intervention and increased patient distress. Thus, the first step in solving the pain management problem is an accurate pain assessment.

PHYSIOLOGY OF PAIN

Pain Transmission

Nociception is the perception of the pain stimulus sent from the peripheral nerves. Nociceptors, or pain receptors, are free nerve endings of the peripheral (afferent) nerves. They are located in the skin, subcutaneous tissues, muscles, viscera, fascia, and the covering of the bones (periosteum), joint surfaces, and artery walls. These afferent nerve fibers are A delta or C fibers. A delta are small, myelinated fibers that carry the pain impulse quickly to the spinal cord, whereas C fibers are smaller and nonmyelinated and carry the impulse slowly. A delta fibers are stimulated by mechanical injury and carry impulses that result in sharp, pricking sensations. C fibers are stimulated by mechanical, thermal, and chemical injury to the skin or deep tissues and result in dull, aching, and burning sensations. These nociceptors are stimulated by chemicals released at the site of injury and send the impulse along the afferent nerves to the dorsal horn of the spinal cord, where the impulse then is sent up to the higher brain centers (thalamus and postcentral gyrus) for interpretation. The dorsal root ganglion contains first-order neurons, which relay the pain signal from the receptor to the spinal cord, whereas second-order neurons in the gray matter of the spinal cord or brain stem relay the signal to the thalamus. Third-order neurons in the thalamus relay the signal to the cerebral cortex.

Pain Intensity

The intensity of the pain stimulus is modulated by substances descending from the midbrain and brainstem, such as endogenous opioids and serotonin, which block or modify the intensity. The pain impulse also can be modulated in the periphery. The gate-control theory of pain transmission supposes that a gate exists between the periphery and central nervous system (CNS) at the dorsal horn. The nociceptive impulse is transmitted from the periphery to the gate (e.g., dorsal horn of the spinal column or between the first-order neurons and the transmission cells in the lamina V) where, if the gate is open, the impulse enters unchanged; if the gate is partially open, the pain intensity is reduced; and if the gate is closed, no pain is felt. The gate can be closed partially or completely by descending modulators from the midbrain and brainstem, or peripherally by inhibitory neurotransmitters released from A delta and C fibers.

Types of Pain

Nociceptors are involved in acute and chronic pain. Pain caused by inflammation and activation of bony nociceptors, such as pain from arthritis or bony metastasis, is called *somatic pain.* The patient is able to localize the pain when asked and may describe it as aching, squeezing, throbbing, or stabbing. Stimulation of nociceptors in the viscera produce *visceral pain,* which is generalized and vague and may be described as cramping or gnawing. Visceral pain may be associated with referred pain, such as jaw or shoulder pain from myocardial infarction, shoulder pain from liver metastases, back pain from pancreatitis, or pain between the scapula related to bile duct blockage.[10] Chronic pain results from chronic inflammation. Chronic pain may result from secondary changes to the nerves caused by tissue injury and may involve sensitization of the nociceptors so that the activation at the site of injury continues to send pain impulses to the spinal cord. Neuropathic pain is related to changes in the peripheral or CNS from injury that is independent of the original injury or tissue damage. Neuropathic pain often is described as electric shocks (lancinating) superimposed on a burning sensation.

Many patients come to the ED for treatment of injury. Trauma causes tissue damage, such as stretching, tearing, or compression. This stimulates mechanical and polymodal nociceptors. The severity of the pain impulse is related to the number of nociceptors stimulated. The tissue injury releases chemical mediators—such as bradykinin, serotonin, norepinephrine, leukokinins, acetylcholine, and substance P—that activate the nociceptors. Prostaglandins increase the nociceptive stimulation by lowering the threshold of the nociceptors to the chemical mediators. These chemical mediators start the pain impulse transmission by depolarization of the nociceptor nerve endings. In addition, the chemical mediators can increase the number of nociceptors and stimulate chemoreceptors that intensify the pain sensation. An example is the pain of inflammation, including the uninjured area around the tissue injury.

Ischemic pain, caused by inadequate blood perfusion, results from the accumulation of lactic acid, bradykinin, and proteolytic enzymes that stimulate nociceptors and occurs more quickly if the tissue metabolic rate is high. Muscle spasms result from stimulation of motor (efferent) fibers and sympathetic reflexes and stimulate the chemoreceptors, heightening the perceived pain intensity. If muscle activity is increased because of injury, the metabolic rate increases, with the accumulation of lactic acid, further increasing tissue ischemia. Because pain intensity and the rate of tissue damage are closely related, a patient who has an acute injury may perceive intense pain.[11]

Other Factors That Influence the Pain Experience

Psychological factors influence pain perception. Anxiety or depression lowers the pain threshold, so that providing a calm, supportive environment for the patient with an acute, painful injury may decrease pain perception. Also, offering reassurance and showing efficient teamwork helps reduce anxiety. A person's past experience with pain can influence whether the gate is open or closed: if in past the patient has had repeated exposures to pain or if the pain was uncontrolled, the patient's threshold will be lowered, with increased sensitivity to the painful stimulus. Once the nociceptors have been sensitized or overstimulated, it takes only a small stimulus to produce an intense, painful impulse.[11] Cultural beliefs can help close the gate so that painful impulses are modulated. For example, a person who says prayers

| Box 13-1 | FACTORS INCREASING OR REDUCING PAIN THRESHOLD |

Factors increasing pain threshold

Relief of symptoms
Sleep, rest
Relaxation therapy
Explanation/support
Understanding/empathy
Diversional activity
Companionship
Active listening
Understanding the meaning and significance of pain
Mood elevation

Factors decreasing pain threshold

Anxiety or depression
Discomfort
Fatigue
Insomnia, lack of sleep
Anger, boredom
Fear
Sadness
Social abandonment
Introversion
Mental isolation

(Modified from Twycross R, Lack SA: *Symptom control in advanced cancer,* London, 1984, Pitman Books.)

because this is an important cultural coping strategy can report less intense pain. Conversely, the provider's culture can impair the plan if the nurse or physician's cultural beliefs prevent a complete pain assessment. Factors that increase or decrease pain tolerance are shown in Box 13-1.

ACUTE AND CHRONIC PAIN

Acute pain is the pain most commonly encountered in the ED, but patients with chronic pain also are seen. *Acute pain* is defined as lasting less than 6 months and is removed when the stimulus is removed, such as healing of a fracture. Because pain is a protective response, a warning to the person that life or limb is threatened, it is associated with the fight-or-flight response. An outpouring of catecholamines, such as epinephrine and norepinephrine, occurs. Thus in acute pain, signs and symptoms of autonomic nervous system arousal are seen, such as tachycardia, hypertension, grimacing, and diaphoresis. Acute pain often is associated with anxiety. In contrast, *chronic pain* is pain that lasts longer than 6 months, and the stimulus cannot be removed. The body could not support the continual outpouring of catecholamines, so the signs and symptoms of pain seen with acute pain are absent. Thus, it is especially important for the nurse to respect the patient as the expert about his or her pain and to believe the patient. Chronic pain often is associated with depression. This has implications for the use of adjuvant medications, such as an antidepressant together with an analgesic for chronic pain. Unfortunately, nursing studies have shown that nurses are more likely to "believe" that the patient is in pain when changes in vital signs or facial grimacing are present and therefore to undermedicate or not to medicate patients who do not show these signs or symptoms.

PAIN AND THE NURSING PROCESS

Patients have a right to rapid, efficient assessment and the development of an effective plan for pain control. A commonly used mnemonic developed by the consensus group of the Agency for Health Care Policy and Research on acute pain can be helpful: *ABCDE* for Pain Assessment and Management:

- *A*sk about pain regularly. *A*ssess pain systematically.
- *B*elieve the patient and family in their reports of pain and what relieves it.
- *C*hoose pain control options appropriate for the patient, family, and setting.
- *D*eliver interventions in timely, logical, and coordinated fashion.
- *E*mpower patients and their families. *E*nable them to control their course to the greatest extent possible.

Assessment of Pain

A complete assessment considers physical, psychosociocultural, and environmental factors. All patients should be asked if they have pain, not only the patients with injury or cancer. Many institutions have instituted pain assessment as the fifth "vital sign" so that pain is assessed along with temperature, pulse, oxygen saturation, and blood pressure. Patients with pain should have a complete pain assessment, and then the pain should be reassessed with documentation after intervention and at regular intervals. The initial pain assessment should characterize a patient's pain as to the following:

- Onset: when did the pain begin
- Location(s)
- Intensity
- What makes it better; what makes it worse
- Whether the pain is constant or comes and goes (intermittent)
- Factors that lower pain threshold, such as lack of sleep and anxiety
- If pain has been a problem before, history including medications used and their effect
- Effect of pain on patient's ability to function and perform activities of daily living
- Physical exam (as appropriate)

Medical history and the chief complaint help give context to the possible cause of pain, such as trauma. A number of pain assessment tools are available, as shown in Figure 13-1. The patient's verbal report of pain is the most valid and reliable indicator of pain. Encourage the patient to describe what the pain feels like.

Most nurses use a 0-to-10 numeric rating scale, where 0 is "no pain" and 10 is the "worst pain ever," or the Wong-Baker FACES scale. Others may use a visual analog scale with anchors of "no pain" and "worst pain ever." The patient is asked to place a finger at a place on a straight 10-cm (100-mm) line between descriptor anchors of "no pain" and "worst pain ever," reflecting pain intensity. The advantage of the visual analog scale is that the scale is not

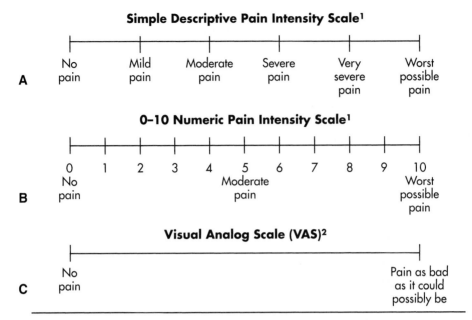

Simple Descriptive Pain Intensity Scale[1]

| No pain | Mild pain | Moderate pain | Severe pain | Very severe pain | Worst possible pain |

A

0-10 Numeric Pain Intensity Scale[1]

0 No pain   1   2   3   4   5 Moderate pain   6   7   8   9   10 Worst possible pain

B

Visual Analog Scale (VAS)[2]

No pain   Pain as bad as it could possibly be

C

[1]If used as a graphic rating scale, a 10-cm baseline is recommended.
[2]A 10-cm baseline is recommended for VAS scales.

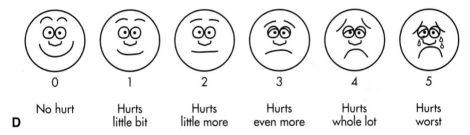

| 0 | 1 | 2 | 3 | 4 | 5 |
| No hurt | Hurts little bit | Hurts little more | Hurts even more | Hurts whole lot | Hurts worst |

D

Figure 13-1. Pain intensity assessment tools. **A,** Simple descriptive pain intensity scale. **B,** 0-10 numeric pain intensity scale. **C,** Visual analog scale. **D,** Wong-Baker FACES scale. *(A, B, and C from Management of cancer pain: clinical practice guideline no.9, Pub No AHCPR 94-0592, Rockville, Md, 2004, Agency for Health Care Policy and Research, Public Health Service, US Department of Health and Human Services. D from Hockenberry MJ, Wilson D, Winkelstein ML: Wong's essentials of pediatric nursing, ed 7, St Louis, 2005, Mosby. Used with permission. E, Copyright© 2002, The Regents of the University of Michigan)* *Continued*

limited to the 10 levels of intensity. A difference of 13 to 16 mm is considered significant. All have shown reliability and validity when tested in adults. In at least one study comparing the three scales in adult patient populations, patients preferred the FACES scale as easiest to use, compared with the visual analog scales (too abstract) or the simple numeric scale (difficulty selecting a number that reflected their pain intensity). The FACES scale is also accurate for patients who are experiencing stress, who are mildly cognitively impaired, or who do not speak

The FLACC Behavioral Pain Assessment Scale*

Categories	Scoring		
	0	**1**	**2**
Face	No particular expression or smile	Occasional grimace or frown; withdrawn, disinterested	Frequent to constant frown, clenched jaw, quivering chin
Legs	Normal position or relaxed	Uneasy, restless, tense	Kicking or legs drawn up
Activity	Lying quietly, normal position, moves easily	Squirming, shifting back and forth, tense	Arched, rigid, or jerking
Cry	No cry (awake or asleep)	Moans or whimpers, occasional complaint	Crying steadily, screams or sobs; frequent complaints
Consolability	Content, relaxed	Reassured by occasional touching, hugging, or being talked to; distractable	Difficult to console or comfort

*Each of the five categories is scored from 0-2, resulting in a total score between 0 and 10.

E

Figure 13–1, *cont'd*, **E**, FLACC scale.

English.[12] This scale is also appropriate for use with children beginning at age 5 to 6 years. Before this age, the ability to self-report may be difficult for most children.

A reliable and valid pain scale for young, preverbal children is the FLACC scale. The nurse uses this scale to rate the child's pain objectively after an observation period of several minutes. The child is rated from 0 to 2 on the expression of pain related to five physical parameters: *F*ace, *L*egs, *A*rms, *C*ry, *C*onsolability.[13] Whichever scale is used, it is imperative that the same scale be used by all providers interacting with the patient. As mentioned, special attention should be given to the assessment of vulnerable patient populations who are at risk for ineffective pain management plans: infants and children, the elderly, patients who do not speak English or who have a cultural background different from the nurse or physician, and patients with a history of substance abuse. In addition, patients with cancer or human immunodeficiency virus infection may have severe pain that requires higher than usual opioid doses, especially if they are tolerant to high doses of opioids (have been taking them for a long time for chronic pain).

Pain Management

Pain-relieving strategies can be divided broadly into pharmacologic—nonopioid or opioid—and nonpharmacologic, involving distraction, relaxation, reiki, and other nurse-driven interventions. The goals for pain management are to relieve pain and improve function. Historically, pain management strategies in ED settings have been inconsistent and often ineffective, related to practice and attitude barriers. Improvements involve the following[14]:

- Educational emphasis on pain management practices in nursing and medical schools
- Clinical quality improvement activities evaluating pain management in the ED
- Rigorous studies of patients with special needs to identify ways to improve the pain management of the elderly and very young in the ED
- Strategies to help clinicians change attitudes about addiction, which currently results in inappropriate diagnosis of drug-seeking behavior, fear of addiction, and fear of prescribing opioids (opiophobia)
- Strategies to help clinicians change attitudes/remove bias in terms of ethnic and racial stereotyping
- Educational programs to help clinicians realize the safety of opioids compared with nonsteroidal antiinflammatory drugs (NSAIDs), so that providers feel comfortable prescribing opioids appropriately

ED nurses and physicians identify four myths that explain in a large measure why pain is undertreated in the ED[15]:

1. Fear of adverse reactions of opioids. It has been established in multiple studies that adverse reactions are rare (2.2%), and when they occur, they are not serious.
2. Will mask exam findings: Six prospective studies have disproved this.
3. Will cause addiction to opioids: Boston study showed incidence is 1 in 3000 patients.
4. Patients will tell us if they are in pain: 70% of patients will not request treatment despite pain.

Pharmacologic Strategies

In the ED setting, pharmacologic management is the cornerstone of the pain management plan. Routine assessment of pain should identify patients in pain, especially with painful conditions such as trauma, so that they can receive quick and effective relief of their pain. Because of the need for timely analgesia, intravenous administration is preferred to intramuscular administration, which takes longer and is painful in itself. In addition, the intravenous route allows rapid titration of analgesics as needed and should always be used for patients in moderate to severe pain. NSAIDs have a prominent place in slight to mild pain but are not always benign. Meperidine should not be used because the accumulation of the metabolite normeperidine, which lowers the seizure threshold. Fentanyl, hydromorphone, and morphine are the opioids of choice. Finally, combination therapy most often is needed, especially in managing patients with severe pain, to modulate different pain pathways; for example[15]:

- Opioids: stimulate endogenous opioid receptors in the CNS
- NSAIDs: block prostaglandins, chemical mediators of inflammation
- Local anesthetics: block transmission of the pain impulse to the CNS
- Tricyclic antidepressants: stimulate descending serotonin modulation pathways
- Transcutaneous nerve stimulation, acupuncture, massage, relaxation: "close gate" at dorsal horn so intensity of pain impulse is modulated
- Anxiolytics: raise pain threshold; help in pain interpretation

Much controversy has surrounded the use of opioids to control pain in a patient with an acute condition of the abdomen. In a government initiative to make health care safer, Brownfield[16] reviewed the literature to determine the strength of the evidence of studies showing potential masking of the patient's diagnosis or potential for harm. She found that appropriate use of analgesics in patients with acute abdominal pain effectively decreases pain and does not interfere with the diagnosis or treatment.

Nonopioids. The World Health Organization recommends that initially or for slight to mild pain, nonopioids with or without adjuvants (such as an anxiolytic or antidepressant) be used, as shown in Figure 13-2. NSAIDs are the drug of choice for musculoskeletal injuries because they are antiinflammatory and antipyretic. NSAIDs decrease the synthesis of prostaglandins, which otherwise would sensitize the nociceptors and increase the pain stimulus. NSAIDs work primarily in the periphery, in contrast to acetaminophen, which primarily acts in the CNS. NSAIDs are equally efficacious, and their side effect profile directs selection. Each of the NSAIDs is limited by the specific drug toxicity profile. As a class, NSAIDs inhibit cyclooxygenase-1 and so can cause gastrointestinal distress, ulceration, and bleeding; renal dysfunction or failure; bleeding; and rarely, increase the incidence and severity of congestive heart failure. Cyclooxygenase-1 enzymes are important in maintaining normal function of the stomach, intestines, kidneys, and platelets.

Opioids. Morphine 10 mg is the cornerstone of opioid equianalgesic dose calculations, and the rule of 10 often is used for relative equivalent potencies. The following dosages are therefore equivalent to 10 mg of morphine[15]:

- 0.1 mg of fentanyl
- 1 mg of hydromorphone
- 100 mg of meperidine

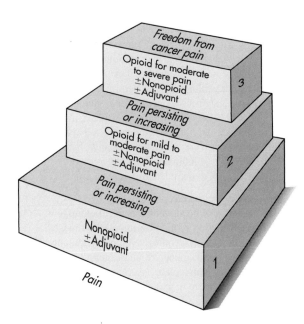

Figure 13-2. WHO's Pain Relief Ladder. (*World Health Organization: WHO's Pain Relief Ladder. Retrieved July 12, 2004, from www.who.int/cancer/palliative/painladder/en/*)

The current strategy in EDs across the country is to use fentanyl for early, rapid control of pain, titrated intravenously with a limited total dose. Hydromorphone then is used for maintenance, starting 5 to 30 minutes after fentanyl is administered, without any maximum dose but titrated to the patient's response, for example, pain relief.

In the past, meperidine (Demerol) was a popular drug, but now it is used infrequently. Meperidine is in the same opioid class as fentanyl; therefore, fentanyl can be used if the patient is allergic (e.g., develops hives or angioedema) to morphine and hydromorphone. Often patients say they are allergic to morphine; however, it is important to determine what the patient reports as an allergic response, for example, nausea and vomiting or hives. Nausea and vomiting are expected side effects of opioids and can be prevented by the coadministration of an antiemetic agent. Meperidine is not commonly used because it is inferior to the other opioids given its toxicity profile: metabolism prolonged in patients with renal or hepatic disease, metabolite that lowers seizure threshold, and the highest level of associated euphoria.

Morphine is considered the gold standard, and many clinicians feel comfortable prescribing this drug. However, its peak effect is 15 to 20 minutes after intravenous administration. Morphine is a potent respiratory depressant, is associated with more of a histamine release than other opioids, causes nausea frequently, and leads to the accumulation of active metabolites in patients with renal dysfunction.[15] However, in the management of chronic pain, such as cancer pain, morphine has demonstrated safety and usefulness. Opioids have no ceiling effect; therefore the dose can be titrated as necessary to relieve pain.

Hydromorphone (Dilaudid) has similar pharmacokinetics to morphine but has no active metabolites, and the drug does not accumulate with repeated doses. Hydromorphone is potent and highly soluble, requires smaller injection volumes, and is well tolerated.

Fentanyl offers the most rapid onset and elimination from the body. Fentanyl has an onset of 1 minute, peaks at 3 to 5 minutes, and has a half-life of 30 to 90 minutes. Fentanyl is called a "clean drug" because it has no histamine release and no active metabolites and causes no hemodynamic instability.[15] The usual dose is 1 to 3 mcg/kg. Rarely, the drug can cause glottic spasm and chest rigidity when given at high doses (greater than 10 mcg/kg). The drug can accumulate in fat tissue with repeated doses, which is why it is so effective in a transdermal patch used for chronic pain.

Other oral opioids that may be used in the ED are hydrocodone, codeine, propoxyphene, and mixed analgesic/antagonists. Codeine is converted by the P_{450} microenzyme system in the liver to morphine; however, 2% to 15% of patients have polymorphisms, so they receive no analgesic effect. Codeine and hydrocodone have similar half-lives (3 to 4 hours); codeine is less effective and causes more gastrointestinal upset. Thus, hydrocodone should be used rather than codeine.[15] Propoxyphene (Darvon) causes respiratory depression and dysphoria, especially in elderly patients, and so should be used cautiously if at all. Nalbuphine, butorphanol, and pentazocine are mixed analgesics/antagonists, can cause dysphoria, and should never be given to a patient receiving opioids because they can precipitate withdrawal.

Injections of local anesthetics at trigger points may help reduce pain in patients with headaches. Regional anesthesia, such as femoral nerve blocks, may be useful in the treatment of fractures of the femoral shaft, as well as neck or knee injuries. Intercostal nerve blocks can be useful for patients with fractured ribs, flail chest, or thoracic injuries that are so painful, they interfere with respiration.

Newer pharmacologic strategies being studied in the ED are patient-controlled analgesia, nitrous oxide,[17] moderate procedural sedation, and deep procedural sedation.[15] A study of propofol and fentanyl compared with ketamine and midazolam for emergency orthopedic procedural sedation showed that propofol and fentanyl significantly reduced the recovery time for patients undergoing pediatric orthopedic procedures. Both regimens were equally efficacious in relieving and/or preventing pain.[18]

Topical Anesthetic Options for Trauma-Related Procedures. Although trauma related injuries are a common cause of pain in ED settings, interventions for traumatic injuries in themselves can cause pain that can and should be prevented. Painless placement of intravenous lines, nasogastric tubes, indwelling urinary catheters, arterial punctures, and even tetanus administration can be facilitated by the application of topical anesthetic agents for adult and pediatric patients. Although the gold standard of topical anesthetics, lidocaine/prilocaine (EMLA) cream, may have little utility in the context of major trauma because of an application time of 60 to 90 minutes, there are several other topical anesthetics that are time-appropriate options.

Vapocoolants are a group of skin refrigerants that may be used to reduce the pain associated with venipuncture, intravenous catheter placement, arterial line placement or blood gas sampling, and tetanus toxoid administration. Vapocoolants are applied under pressure to an intact skin surface. The preparation is sprayed on for 3 to 9 seconds, or until the skin turns white.[19] The vapocoolants provide an immediate cooling that only lasts for 5 to 10 seconds. Therefore, immediately following application, the area should be cleansed with an alcohol swab followed by the needlestick. In a pediatric study, vapocoolant provided relief that was equivalent to EMLA when pain scales were done by the child, parent, and nurse and later by a blinded observer via videotape.[20] Currently, three preparations of vapocoolants are available for clinical use: Gebauer's Ethyl Chloride, Gebauer's Spray and Stretch (previously Gebauer's Fluori-Methane), and Gebauer's Fluro-Ethyl.[19] The different preparations vary by administration time, degree of coldness, flammability, risk to the ozone layer, and available forms. Ethyl chloride, the longest standing of the vapocoolants, is flammable and may not be allowed in some clinical areas. Spray and Stretch and Fluro-Ethyl are nonflammable and often are preferred for this reason.

Two procedures rated by patients as the most painful are nasogastric tube and urinary catheter placement.[21] The pain caused by these procedures can be attenuated with the timely use of 4% lidocaine jelly. The jelly should be applied to the urinary meatus or nasal nares for 5 minutes before tube insertion. Because of absorption risks, 4% lidocaine jelly should be used sparingly if used on infants.

For less serious traumatic injuries such as isolated fractures, adequate time may be available for the application of a topical anesthetic such as ELA-Max before placement of an intravenous catheter required for procedural sedation. ELA-Max, a 4% lidocaine cream in a liposomal base, is an important medication for topical anesthesia. The drug permeates the dermis to a depth of 4 mm and provides topical anesthesia within 30 minutes. In a pediatric study comparing ELA-Max with EMLA , no significant difference was found between a 30-minute ELA-Max application time and a 60-minute EMLA application time when the child, parent, and a blinded observer rated pain.[22] ELA-Max has not been studied in infants; therefore, current use should be restricted to children 12 months of age and older.

Adjuvant Medications. Adjuvant medications for pain relief used in the ED are anxiolytics, anticonvulsants, antidepressants, and skeletal muscle relaxants. Benzodiazepines are useful to reduce anxiety and pain related to muscle injury and spasms. Anticonvulsants such as gabapentin and tricyclic antidepressants such as amitriptyline can help relieve chronic, neuropathic pain. Muscle relaxants such as cyclobenzaprine (Flexeril) can help reduce muscle spasms in patients with chronic back pain exacerbated by muscle spasms.

Other medications used to treat the cause of pain are targeted drugs for headaches, gouty arthritis, and fractures. Ergotamines and 5-hydroxytryptamine$_1$ receptor antagonists are used to treat migraine and cluster headaches; colchicine is used to treat acute gout; and calcitonin is used to treat acute vertebral fractures related to osteoporosis. Corticosteroids are used to decrease bone, visceral, and neuropathic pain.[23]

Nonpharmacologic Strategies

Nurses should not underestimate the important nonpharmacologic pain management practices that they use daily. The use of rest, ice, immobilization, and elevation help prevent further injury but also significantly reduce the pain experienced by patients with fractures and sprains by limiting and/or reducing edema and bone movement. The approach that nurses take toward caring for a trauma patient plays a significant role in decreasing pain and anxiety. The calming, reassuring voice of a nurse explaining what is happening or will happen to a frightened trauma patient is often what patients recall about their care. Many nurses have expanded their repertoire of nursing skills to include the techniques of relaxation, breathing techniques, guided imagery, emotive imagery, and even reiki. Box 13-2 depicts scripts for relaxation exercises and guided imagery. These techniques can be used in adults and pediatric patients.

Evaluation of the Analgesic Plan

Once an analgesic plan has been developed and analgesics administered, it is imperative to evaluate the patient's response and satisfaction with the plan. If the plan is ineffective, it must

Box 13-2	RELAXATION EXERCISES

Example 1: Deep breath/tense, exhale/relax, yawn for quick relaxation

1. Clench your fists; breathe in deeply and hold it a moment.
2. Breathe out slowly and go limp as a rag doll.
3. Start yawning.

Additional points: Yawning becomes spontaneous. Yawning is also contagious, so others may begin yawning and relaxing too.

Example 2: Slow rhythmic breathing for relaxation

1. Breathe in slowly and deeply.
2. As you breathe out slowly, feel yourself beginning to relax; feel the tension leaving your body.
3. Now breathe in and out slowly and regularly, at whatever rate is comfortable for you. You may wish to try abdominal breathing. If you do not know how to do abdominal breathing, ask your nurse for help.
4. To help you focus on your breathing and breathe slowly and rhythmically: Breathe in as you say silently to yourself, "in, two, three." Breathe out as you say silently to yourself, "out, two, three," or each time you breathe out, say silently to yourself a word such as *peace* or *relax.*
5. You may imagine that you are doing this in a place you have found very calming and relaxing for you, such as lying in the sun at the beach.
6. Do steps 1 through 4 only once, or repeat steps 3 and 4 for up to 20 minutes.
7. End with a slow deep breath. As you breathe out, say to yourself, "I feel alert and relaxed."

Additional points: If you intend to do this for more than a few seconds, try to get in a comfortable position in a quiet environment; you may close your eyes or focus on an object. This technique has the advantage of being adaptable in that it may be used for only a few seconds or for up to 20 minutes.

Continued

Box 13–2	RELAXATION EXERCISES—cont'd

Example 3: Peaceful past

Something may have happened to you a while ago that brought you peace and comfort. You may be able to draw on that past experience to bring you peace or comfort now. Think about these questions:

1. Can you remember any situation, even when you were a child, when you felt calm, peaceful, secure, hopeful, and comfortable?
2. Have you ever daydreamed about something peaceful? What were you thinking of?
3. Do you get a dreamy feeling when you listen to music? Do you have any favorite music?
4. Do you have any favorite poetry that you find uplifting or reassuring?
5. Have you ever been religiously active? Do you have favorite readings, hymns, or prayers?

Even if you have not heard or thought of them for many years, childhood religious experiences still may be soothing.

Additional points: Very likely some of the things you think of in answer to these questions can be recorded for you, such as your favorite music or a prayer. Then you can listen to the tape whenever you wish. Or, if your memory is strong, you may simply close your eyes and recall the events or words.

(Adapted with permission from McCaffery M, Beebe A: *Pain: clinical manual for nursing practice,* St Louis, 1989, Mosby.)

be revised. The dose should be increased or the drug changed to a more effective agent, and then following administration, the patient should be assessed again for pain relief. Alternatively, the addition of an adjuvant medication may improve the efficacy of the analgesic as well. Although analgesia should be individualized, it is important in the setting of long-bone fractures or crush injuries to remember that a patient's report of pain that is more intense than expected or pain that is unrelieved by the usual range of analgesic dosing may indicate the development of compartment syndrome. Such patients require further assessment regarding the neurovascular status of the affected extremity.

Of special concern is the area of nursing documentation not only of the pain assessment and intervention but also most importantly of the reassessment of pain after the intervention so that the patient's response to the intervention is known. If the intervention is ineffective or does not achieve adequate pain relief, then the plan must be revised, reimplemented, and reassessed. The JCAHO has made this a major focus of hospital accreditation surveys.

Patient and Family Education

Patients must be taught how to use a pain assessment tool, such as the numeric pain intensity scale, because the patient will be an integral part of the plan. Once pain relief has been achieved, then providing maintenance analgesia to prevent the development of severe pain is a priority. Pain is easier to prevent than to treat, and it takes significantly more analgesic drug to relieve severe pain than it does to prevent pain. If the patient is discharged, then patient teaching focuses on the importance of filling the analgesic prescription to prevent or minimize pain at home. Self-care instructions include potential side effects of the medicines, care of the injured body part and possible complications, self-administration instructions, and who to call if the pain becomes severe or if any unforeseen problems occur.

If the patient is admitted, then it is important to communicate the analgesic care plan to ensure that the work the nurse has done to bring about pain relief is carried along during the next step of the patient's care. If significant pain relief has not been achieved, then the goal of improved pain control should be emphasized.

References

1. McCaffery M: *Nursing practice theories related to cognition, bodily pain, and man-environment interactions,* Los Angeles, 1968, University of California at Los Angeles Students' Store.
2. Whipple JK, Lewis KS, Quebbeman EJ et al: Analysis of pain management in critically ill patients, *Pharmacotherapy* 15:592-599, 1995.
3. Joint Commission on Accreditation of Healthcare Organizations: *Comprehensive accreditation manual for hospitals: the official handbook,* Oakbrook Terrace, Ill, 2006, Joint Commission Resources.
4. American College of Emergency Physicians: *Pain management in the emergency department,* 2004. Retrieved July 10, 2004, from www.acep.org/webportal/PracticeResources/PolicyStatements/pracmgt/PainManagementintheEmergencyDepartment.htm
5. Tamayo-Sarver JH, Dawson NV, Cydulka RK et al: Variability in emergency physician decision making about prescribing opioid analgesics, *Ann Emerg Med* 43(4):483-493, 2004.
6. Todd KH, Deaton C, D'Adamo AP et al: Ethnicity and analgesic practice, *Ann Emerg Med* 35(1):11-16, 2004.
7. Todd KH, Samaroo N, Hoffman JR: Ethnicity as a risk factor for inadequate emergency department analgesia, *JAMA* 269(12):1537-1544, 1993.
8. Puntillo K: Pain experiences of intensive care unit patients, *Heart Lung* 19(5):526-533, 1990.
9. Puntillo K, Neighbor M, O'Neill N et al: Accuracy of emergency nurses in assessment of patients' pain, *Pain Manag Nurs* 4(4):171-175, 2003.
10. American Medical Association: *Pain management: pathophysiology of pain and pain assessment,* 2003. Retrieved July 10, 2004, from www.ama-cmeonline.com/pain_mgmt/module01/
11. Emergency Nurses Association: *Trauma nursing core course,* ed 5, 2000, Des Plaines, Ill.
12. Berg DM: *Pain assessment tool preferences among adults* [Wong on the Web], 2002. Retrieved July 12, 2004, from www3.us.elsevierhealth.com/WOW/faces16Berg.html
13. Merkel S, Voepel-Lewis T, Malviya S: A behavioral scale for scoring postoperative pain in young children, *Pediatr Nurs* 23(3):293-297, 1997.
14. Rupp T, Delaney KA: Inadequate analgesia in emergency medicine, *Ann Emerg Med* 43(4):494-503, 2004.
15. Panaccek EA: *Review of ED therapeutics for patient pain management.* Retrieved July 10, 2004, from www.ferne.org/Lectures/saem0504/panacek_therapeutics_pain_mgmt_ saem0504.htm
16. Brownfield E: Pain management: use of analgesics in the acute abdomen. In University of California at San Francisco–Stanford University Evidence-based Practice Center: *Making health care safer: a critical analysis of patient safety practices,* Evidence Report/Technology Assessment, No. 43, AHRQ Pub 01-E058, Rockville, Md, 2001, Agency for Healthcare Research and Quality, US Department of Health and Human Services. Retrieved October 31, 2006, from http://www.ahrq.gov/clinic/ptsafety/
17. Gregory PR, Sullivan JA: Nitrous oxide compared with intravenous regional anesthesia in pediatric forearm fracture manipulation, *J Pediatr Orthop* 16(2):187-191, 1996.

18. Godambe SA, Elliott V, Matheny D et al: Comparison of profofol/fentanyl versus ketamine/ midazolam for brief orthopedic procedural sedation in a pediatric emergency department, *Pediatrics* 112(1):116-123, 2003.

19. *Gebauer's ethyl chloride: prescribing information,* Cleveland, 2005, Gebauer. Retrieved October 31, 2006, from www.gebauerco.com

20. *Gebauer's fluro-ethyl: prescribing information,* Cleveland, 2004, Gebauer. Retrieved October 31, 2006, from www.gebauerco.com

21. *Gebauer's Spray and Stretch,* Cleveland, 2004, Gebauer. Retrieved October 31, 2006, from www.gebauerco.com

22. Cohen Reis E, Holubkov R: Vapocoolant spray is equally effective as EMLA™ cream in reducing immunization pain in school-aged children, *Pediatrics* 100(6):ed 5, 1997.

23. Singer AJ, Richman PB, Kowalska A et al: Comparison of patient and practitioner assessments of pain from commonly performed emergency department procedures, *Ann Emerg Med* 33:652-658, 1999.

24. Eichenfield LF, Funk A, Fallon-Friedlander S et al: A clinical study to evaluate the efficacy of ELA-Max (4% liposomal lidocaine) as compared to eutectic mixture of local anesthetics cream for pain reduction of venipunctures in chidren, *Pediatrics* 109(6):1093-1099, 2002.

25. Zun L: Innovations in process management: optimizing patient management. Retrieved July 12, 2004, from www.ferne.org/Lectures/saem0504/un_process_mgmt_saem0504.htm

Suggested Readings

American Medical Association: *Pain management: the online series,* 2005-2006. Retrieved October 31, 2006, from www.ama-cmeonline.com/

Jacob E: Pain management in sickle cell disease, *Pain Manag Nurs* 2(4):121-131, 2001.

Kamin RA, Nowicki TA, Courtney DS et al: Pearls and pitfalls in the emergency department evaluation of abdominal pain, *Emerg Med Clin North Am* 21(1):61-72, 2003.

Passik SD, Kirsch KL: Opioid therapy in patients with a history of substance abuse, *CNS Drugs* 18(1):13-25, 2004.

Tanabe P, Buschmann M: A prospective study of ED pain management practices and the patient's perspective, *J Emerg Nurs* 25(3):171-177, 1999.

Wilsey B, Fishman S, Rose JS et al: Pain management in the ED, *Am J Emerg Med* 22(1):51-57, 2004.

CHAPTER 14

WOUNDS AND WOUND MANAGEMENT

PAMELA W. BOURG

Proper attention to traumatic wounds in the early phases of injury management is vital to achieving the goals of obtaining hemostasis, avoiding complications such as impaired healing and wound infection, and maximizing functional recovery and optimum cosmetic appearance. The same conscientious attention should be paid to all wounds, regardless of whether they are minor or major, because any wound infection affects the patient's overall recovery and functional outcome. Providers also should be aware that wound-related complaints are the fourth most common cause of malpractice complaints against emergency care providers.[1]

Distracting wounds, such as major lacerations or degloving injuries, are well-named because they can distract clinical personnel from managing the ABCs (airway, breathing, circulation) primarily. The ABC priorities of evaluation and resuscitative management of trauma patients should always be maintained, and the caregiver must be careful not to be distracted by dramatic wounds. The risk of infection also should be given careful consideration, and appropriate initial treatment should be begun. In addition to the therapeutic interventions outlined in this chapter, content coverage includes the strict adherence to standard precautions (gown, mask, eye protection, and gloves) for all caregivers with direct access to the patient. Breaks in the skin integrity, no matter the cause, provide access to foreign pathogens that potentially can cause serious infection.

THE SKIN, INJURY, AND WOUND HEALING

The two major layers of the skin are the epidermis and the dermis. The epidermis, the outermost layer, and the underlying dermis protect the body from external pressure and injuring forces. The dermal layer also provides the skin with its strength and elasticity and is the key layer for ultimate healing of skin wounds.

Beneath the dermis lies the subcutaneous tissue. The subcutaneous tissue plays an important role in traumatic injury because of its shock absorption, insulation, nutrient storage, and body "shaping" functions. The subcutaneous tissue is vulnerable to decreases in vascular supply when blood is shunted to vital organs and therefore can be at a higher risk for impaired healing and infection. Beneath the subcutaneous tissue lies the fascia and muscle tissues.

Wounds are classified as superficial (involving the epidermal layer) or full thickness (involving the epidermal, dermal, and perhaps the subcutaneous tissue, muscle, and bone layers).

Tissue Response and Healing in Injury

Vasoconstriction occurs immediately at the time of injury, followed by vasodilation 5 to 10 minutes later. Vasodilation results in redness with subepithelial swelling (inflammation) and hemostasis through the processes of the intrinsic and extrinsic coagulation cascade. Over the next 24 to 36 hours, the wound is cleared of cellular debris, and epithelial cells begin to migrate. Fibrin also begins to layer in the wound (fibroblast proliferation). The wound then is fortified with collagen over the next several months (epithelialization, contraction, remodeling).

Factors Affecting Wound Healing

The following factors affect would healing:

- Age (especially the elderly)
- Impaired tissue oxygenation and perfusion
- Wound infection, contamination, or systemic sepsis
- Anemia (hemorrhagic and chronic)
- Nutritional status (malnutrition/obesity; vitamins A or C, zinc, iron, or copper deficiencies)
- Electrolyte imbalance
- Stress (physical and psychological)
- Preexisting conditions (liver failure, vascular disease, diabetes mellitus, chronic obstructive pulmonary disease, uremia, cancer, chronic alcohol use, immunologic depression)
- Medications (especially steroids)
- Radiation, chemotherapy
- Sutures, drains, foreign bodies, packings or dressings
- Patient compliance with treatment regimen

WOUND ASSESSMENT AND MANAGEMENT

The only element of the primary survey related to wounds is to control major hemorrhage. This usually can be accomplished by using sterile pressure dressings. The sterile dressings also protect against further contamination or injury. After the primary survey and management of life-threatening injuries is completed, clinical personnel can assess all wounds quickly and decide how to manage them.

Assessment of Traumatic Wounds

Whether the patient's wounds are isolated or a result of multiple trauma, the care provider must attempt to obtain as much information as possible concerning the circumstances of the injury, because this information will guide wound management decisions.

History (from the prehospital report, the patient, family, or witnesses) should include the following[2]:

- How did the wound occur?
- What type of object caused it? Was this a high-velocity missile?
- In what environment did the wound occur (type and degree of contamination, such as feces, fresh water, road dirt, and human versus mammalian bites)?
- What interventions or treatments have been provided already?
- When did the wound occur?
- What is the patient's general physical condition? Medical history (smoking and alcohol use, medications, allergies)? Detailed history is important even in routine wound evaluation.
- What is the tetanus prophylaxis status? (See Prevention of Infection on page 10.)
- What type of work does the patient do?

- Which is the dominant hand?

Wound assessment and documentation of information should include the following:

- Where is the wound located?
- Describe the wound using appropriate wound terminology (length, depth, and appearance).
- Is there bleeding or exudate?
- Are there any foreign bodies?
- What do the peripheral tissues look like? Can the wound edges be approximated?
- Are there any obvious underlying or associated injuries (e.g., fractures or tendon or vessel injuries)?
- Document the neurovascular status distal to the wound and the cranial nerve status in facial injuries.

Wound Management Considerations

Therapeutic decisions about wound management are influenced by the answers to the following questions[2]:

- Does the wound require management in the operating room?
- Are there associated injuries that will require other interventions, such as underlying fractures, visceral injuries, or brain injuries?
- Are there preexisting conditions that will impair healing?
- How should the wound be closed to best minimize infection risk and optimize healing (primary, secondary, or tertiary intention healing)?
- Will the patient require antibiotic therapy?
- What type of dressing care, splints, activity restrictions, and home care will the management plan require?

Wound Closure Options

Options for wound closure include closure by suture, tape, tissue adhesives, or staples (primary intention healing, or primary closure); leaving the wound open to granulate and close on its own (secondary intention healing); leaving the wound open and then closing it primarily a few days after injury (delayed primary closure, or tertiary intention healing); or closing the wound using a skin graft or tissue flap (the timing of this procedure varies depending on the wound).

The decision whether to close a wound primarily is determined by the degree and type of contamination and the length of time from injury to treatment. If a wound is heavily contaminated (all traumatic wounds are considered contaminated), especially with the bacteria contained in feces or saliva, it may be wiser to allow the wound to heal by secondary intention. A carefully managed open wound is less likely to develop infection than a heavily contaminated, inadequately cleansed and débrided closed wound. Generally, wounds that are treated within 6 to 8 hours of injury are considered for primary closure. Wounds that have occurred more than 8 hours earlier should be considered for second-intention healing or delayed primary closure. Wounds of the face and scalp may be an exception to this rule because a better vascular supply to these areas reduces infection risk and because of the cosmetic considerations. Wounds that exhibit extensive soft tissue loss and cannot be closed primarily require skin grafting or flap closure.

ANESTHESIA FOR WOUND CLEANSING AND REPAIR

Several types of anesthesia are used for the cleansing, débridement, and repair of traumatic injuries. This chapter focuses on the anesthetics commonly used in the emergency department. Documentation of neurovascular status before tissue is anesthetized is important.

Local and Topical Anesthetics

The most common form of anesthetic is local anesthesia delivered by subcutaneous infiltration. Commonly used agents include the following:

- Lidocaine hydrochloride (Xylocaine): the most common agent used for local anesthesia; available with or without epinephrine; lidocaine has a rapid onset and a 30- to 120-minute duration

NOTE: Epinephrine should not be used around the ears, nose, fingers, toes, or penis. Its use should be avoided in patients with severe peripheral vascular disease. Epinephrine has been implicated in contributing to the risk of wound infection and delayed healing.

- Bupivicaine (Marcaine): slower onset than lidocaine but still rapid onset; 3 to 7 hours' duration; not recommended for children under the age of 12
- Procaine (Novocaine): onset 2 to 5 minutes; 1 to 1½ hours' duration
- Mepivacaine (Carbocaine): rapid onset; 2 to 2½ hours' duration
- LET (mixture of lidocaine 1% to 4%, epinephrine 1:1000 to 1:2000, and tetracaine): topical anesthetic; onset 20 to 30 minutes. Apply directly to laceration with saturated cotton ball, cover with transparent film dressing; expect white ring around wound caused by epinephrine-induced vasoconstriction.
- EMLA (eutectic mixture of local anesthetics; lidocaine and prilocaine): topical used to produce anesthesia of wounds; onset 20 to 30 minutes.

Note that for LET and EMLA, the onset of effect is often greater than 30 minutes, thus potentially limiting use in emergency departments with heavy volume and need for rapid turnover.

Regional Anesthetics

Regional blocks are a useful alternative to local anesthetics for extremity wounds and are preferable for wounds innervated by one superficial nerve. When local anesthetics are injected at the site, the wound may swell and landmarks can distort. Regional blocks avoid this disadvantage. They are also less painful, provide better anesthesia for the patient, and require a smaller volume of anesthetic agent. Regional blocks are administered by applying a tourniquet near the wound proximal to the body and injecting an anesthetic agent intravenously distal to the wound. Digital nerve blocks are an injection of an anesthetic agent along a nerve course.

Sedation and Inhalation Agents

Sedation may be used in the emergency department for the management of painful wound cleansing or repair of lacerations. A combination of intravenous fentanyl (Sublimaze) and midazolam (Versed) commonly is used, but staff should adhere to institutional protocols. Continuous vital sign and oxygenation monitoring are essential.

A mixture of 50% nitrous oxide and 50% oxygen (Nitronox, Entonox) is an inhalational agent that the patient self-administers. This agent is particularly useful when a procedure will be short but may be painful, such as scrubbing or débridement of abrasions or burn wounds. If intravenous opioids are used concurrently, the potential problems of oversedation are not as great because the patient self-administers the gas.

WOUND CLEANSING AND DÉBRIDEMENT

The importance of appropriate and thorough wound cleansing cannot be overemphasized. The quality of the cleansing is important. All traumatic wounds are contaminated. The risk of developing a wound infection is related directly to the adequacy of cleansing, irrigation, and débridement.

In general, the procedure is as follows:

1. Irrigation with 0.9% normal saline solution (the choice of solutions is debated, but normal saline is believed to be the least toxic to tissues, followed by surfactant cleansers) under pressure. Irrigation methods include the following:
   - A liter bag of saline intravenous solution with the intravenous tubing attached via a stopcock to a 22-gauge angiocath and a 30-mL syringe, allowing the solution to be delivered under pressure[1,2]
   - A plastic liter bottle of normal saline irrigation solution with 8 to 12 holes cut in the sterile plastic cap, ejecting the fluid with firm pressure[1,2]
   - Commercially available irrigation systems
   - Especially important is to keep facial wounds moist. If the wound edges dry out, this can cause difficulty with repair.
2. Surfactant cleansers (ShurClens, Pluronic F68) are nontoxic substances that may be packaged with the agent impregnated in a sponge. These cleansers are useful for irrigation or for cleaning abrasions.

NOTE: High-pressure irrigation greater than 7 psi is an important key to proper cleansing.[1] Irrigation with a bulb syringe does not remove bacteria and microscopic debris adequately, nor does simple gravity flow of fluid via intravenous tubing.

3. Débridement of any nonviable or necrotic tissue using a scalpel and normal saline irrigation. This may require a physician.
4. Achievement of complete wound hemostasis. The development of hematomas is a risk factor for infection. Hematomas may require a pressure dressing, closed-suction drainage, or operating room management.
5. Change wet, contaminated drapes and gloves for closure.
6. The number of wound examinations should be kept to a minimum.
7. Body, facial, and scalp hair usually is removed as necessary to clean and examine a wound (except never remove eyebrows). Hair removal is aimed at preventing hair from becoming a foreign body in a wound while minimizing the skin injury inherent in hair removal technique. When hair does not need to be removed, it should be left in place; when hair needs to be removed, it should be removed in the least traumatic way possible.[2] Generally, hair should not be shaved; rather it should be clipped or cut short in the area immediately surrounding the wound.
8. Concentrated providone-iodine, hydrogen peroxide, and detergent solutions can cause significant tissue toxicity and are not recommended for internal wound irrigation.

FOREIGN BODY ASSESSMENT

All wounds should be assessed carefully for the presence of foreign bodies. No surefire way exists to identify and remove foreign matter from wounds. Glass pieces can be visualized when greater than 1 mm thick. Standard radiography is usually not helpful. Computed tomography scans are excellent for identifying foreign substances but are expensive.[1] Follow-up with the patient is paramount. If foreign bodies are suspected, the physician should be informed.

SUTURES AND OTHER CLOSURE MATERIALS

The type of closure material selected is influenced by the location of the wound, the type of wound, the amount of tension that is applied to the wound, and the desired cosmetic result. In the acute phase of trauma management, the need to control significant external bleeding takes priority over these other factors. Skin staples commonly are used for this purpose in areas in which cosmesis is not a concern.

Suture Material

Sutures are available as absorbable or nonabsorbable and monofilament or multifilament. Absorbable sutures dissolve on their own (they retain tensile strength for about 60 days), and nonabsorbable sutures need to be removed within a prescribed period. Absorbable, monofilament sutures are used on the deeper layers of tissue to provide closure and decrease tension on the skin surface. Nonabsorbable, monofilament sutures such as prolene, nylon, and stainless steel are the sutures of choice for primary closure of the skin because they produce less skin reaction.

General guidelines for suture removal are as follows:

Eyelids	2 to 3 days
Face	3 to 4 days
Scalp, abdomen, chest, trunk	7 to 10 days
Hands, arms, legs, feet	10 to 14 days (1 to 2 weeks longer if over an active area)
Joints	14 days

Skin Staples

Skin staples allow rapid skin closure for linear wounds. If the wound requires accurate approximation of tissues, then staples are not the appropriate choice. Staples most commonly are used in the trauma setting to control rapid bleeding and in patients who are unstable and who will not be able to have their wounds further addressed for several hours. Staples can leave significant skin marks if not removed in 7 days or less.

Tape Closure

Closure of wounds with adhesive tapes (e.g., SteriStrips) is another option that does not require anesthesia, is less time consuming, and does not leave needle marks. However, wound edge approximation may be less precise, keeping the area clean is more difficult, and patient compliance (especially in children) may be an issue. Applying tincture of benzoin around the wound before applying the tapes enhances adhesion. The tapes are applied in rows perpendicularly across the wound; they may be reinforced with additional tapes in a cross-hatching pattern if needed.

Tissue Adhesives

Tissue adhesives (2-octylcyanoacrylate) have advantages because they can be applied quickly and easily without patient discomfort. These agents are applied after the bleeding has stopped. Tissue adhesives should be avoided on the palms of the hands and soles of the feet because these are areas of high moisture. Adhesives are not recommended for use on hands or joints because of their high tension and repetitive movements. Because the adhesive quality and tensile strength are less than that of traditional sutures, tissue adhesives can be used only for routine, uncomplicated lacerations. Tissue adhesives serve as their own dressings.

WOUND DRESSINGS

Many wound dressings are available for use in the emergency care setting today. Although the type of dressing may vary depending on the type of wound and treatment plan, the general principles and goals have remained constant. These include decreasing contamination and dehydration of the wound, providing support to the wound during granulation, and stabilizing the reapproximated wound edges.

In general, wound dressing materials can be broken down into major groups[1,2]:

- Gauze (fluffs, 4 × 4s): adherent, absorbent, occlusive; can be painful to remove
- Impregnated gauzes (e.g., Xeroform and Vaseline): nonadherent, absorbent, occlusive
- Hydrocolloids (e.g., Duoderm, Comfeel, Tegasorb, and Biofilm): maintain a moist environment; nonadherent, absorbent, occlusive
- Alginates (e.g., Sorbsan, Tegagel, and Kaltostat): absorbent, occlusive, may be used in infected or contaminated wounds.
- Films (e.g., Op Site, Tegaderm, and Bioclusive): nonabsorbent, occlusive

Traditionally, a sterile, occlusive, normal saline-moistened wet-to-dry gauze dressing has been applied to open wounds, and a dry, sterile dressing to sutured or stapled wounds. Although these methods still are used widely and are effective, the hydrocolloid and alginate dressings are gaining popularity for use with primary closure and second-intention wounds. Proponents cite the advantages of more rapid healing, less frequent dressing changes, and increased ease of management.

SPECIFIC TYPES OF WOUNDS AND WOUND MANAGEMENT

Wounds are categorized by their mechanism of injury and/or depth of injury. The major types of wounds include abrasions, avulsions, amputations, contusions, crush injuries, lacerations, and punctures.

Abrasion

An abrasion is the loss of the epithelial layer with exposure of the dermal and epidermal layers (partial-thickness skin loss) caused by friction of the skin against a hard surface or object. Abrasions sometimes are referred to as *road rash* when the mechanism involves a motorcycle or bicycle crash.

ASSESSMENT

- Assess the amount of fluid loss in large wounds.
- Assess functional capabilities.

- Assess pain control.
- Assess tetanus prophylaxis status.

THERAPEUTIC INTERVENTIONS

- Consider pain management with parenteral sedation or local infiltrative, topical, or general anesthesia for wound cleansing.
- Cleanse wounds thoroughly by scrubbing with normal saline or surfactant-soaked sponge or brush and irrigation. Be sure to remove all debris and foreign bodies to avoid traumatic tattooing.
- Apply antibiotic ointment.
- Leave wound uncovered, or cover with nonadherent, occlusive dressing (reduces pain but increases infection risk).

PATIENT EDUCATION

Teach the patient to do the following:

- Take systemic antibiotics as directed.
- Take pain medication as directed.
- Cleanse wounds (or shower) with mild (nonperfumed) soap and water at least twice daily and as necessary to keep clean. Scarring and tattooing may be increased if crust and debris are allowed to accumulate.
- Pat wound dry, and apply antibiotic ointment each time.
- Call physician or return for check for presence of pus, bleeding, redness, warmth around wound, or fever that occurs after the first several days.
- Return for wound check as directed.
- Keep wound lightly covered with clothing if out in direct sunlight. After wounds are completely healed, continue to cover or apply sunscreen for 6 months to 1 year to avoid hyperpigmentation.

Avulsion

An avulsion is a full-thickness skin loss in which wound edges cannot be approximated, usually as a result of a tearing or gouging mechanism. Degloving or flap injuries are avulsions. Sometimes the skin will appear still to be attached because it has moved around the limb like a glove.

ASSESSMENT

- Assess amount of tissue loss, depth, functional loss, and pain status.
- Assess tetanus prophylaxis status.

THERAPEUTIC INTERVENTIONS

- Control bleeding by direct pressure.
- Administer appropriate pain medication.

- Cleanse wound thoroughly as described before.
- Physician will débride nonviable tissues, repair viable underlying structures, and repair and/or refer for split-thickness skin graft or flap closure.
- Cover wound with appropriate sterile dressing, splints, and/or ointments depending on location of wound and closure versus second-intention healing.
- Provide tetanus prophylaxis and systemic antibiotics as appropriate.

PATIENT EDUCATION

Teach the patient to do the following:

- Take antibiotics as prescribed.
- Take pain medication as directed.
- Perform daily dressing changes (type and frequency determined by wound depth, location, degree of contamination, closure versus open management), and wound check if the patient is discharged home. Dressings must stay clean and dry. Determine the need for home nursing visits and physical therapy if an extremity is involved.
- Return or call before scheduled follow-up for increased pain, fever, wound redness, swelling, heat or drainage (pus), and development of numbness, coolness, or cyanosis if an extremity injury.

Amputation

An amputation is an avulsion or crushing type of injury in which a body part is partially or completely severed or torn from the body.

ASSESSMENT

- Assess for amount of blood loss, continued bleeding, neurovascular status, and pain control. ABCs are a top priority.

NOTE: Time (sometimes up to 6 to 12 hours postinjury) and degree of damage to vascular and nerve structures are critical factors in replantation.

- Assess tetanus prophylaxis status.

THERAPEUTIC INTERVENTIONS

- Control bleeding from the proximal part with direct pressure and elevation.
- Apply moist, sterile dressing over amputation stump.
- Amputated part should be wrapped in moist, sterile dressing; placed in plastic bag; and placed *over* ice in an insulated cooler (do not freeze or place in water or other solutions). Assessment of amputated part for viability by a reconstructive surgeon should occur immediately.
- Administer pain medication and tetanus prophylaxis as directed.
- Partial and complete amputations require operative irrigation and débridement, repair of injury to underlying structures, and revision of stump.

PATIENT EDUCATION

- Most patients with partial or complete amputations of body parts require an inpatient stay for operative repair and/or a replantation attempt, followed by rehabilitative therapy.

See Chapter 20 for further discussion of amputation.

Bite

A bite is breakage of the skin caused by animal or human teeth. All bite wounds are considered contaminated.

ASSESSMENT

- Assess the nature of bite: human or animal; type of animal.
- Assess time of bite and location of wound (hand wounds, deep puncture wounds, and old wounds are at increased risk for infection).
- Assess tetanus prophylaxis status.
- Assess rabies exposure risk for animal bites (see Prevention of Infection, page 148).

THERAPEUTIC INTERVENTIONS

- For human bites, copiously irrigate the wound, débride devitalized tissue, and apply a bulky dressing. The wound initially is left open. Antibiotics should be given within 3 hours of arrival.
- For animal bites, perform irrigation and débridement as for human bites. Small wounds are closed. Prophylactic antibiotics are recommended for high-risk patients.
- Antibiotic therapy and tetanus and rabies prophylaxis as indicated.

PATIENT EDUCATION

Teach the patient to do the following:

- Take antibiotics as prescribed.
- Perform wound care and dressing changes as directed.
- Return for wound checks as directed. Return or call before scheduled follow-up for increased pain, fever, wound redness, swelling, heat, or drainage (pus).

Burn

See Chapter 25 for discussion of burn wounds.

Contusion

A contusion is the formation of a hematoma beneath unbroken skin because of the rupture of small blood vessels and is caused by blunt trauma. The damage results in classic bluish purple skin discoloration.

ASSESSMENT

- Assess for depth of hematoma and potential damage to underlying vascular, nerve, and bony structures. Test circulation, sensation, and motor function.
- Is the patient currently receiving anticoagulation therapy?
- Assess need for analgesia.

THERAPEUTIC INTERVENTIONS

- Apply ice pack to affected area.
- Elevate contused area or extremity.
- Observe progression of swelling and discoloration. Monitor circulation, sensation, and motor function.

PATIENT EDUCATION

Teach the patient to do the following:

- Take analgesia as prescribed. Avoid aspirin or aspirin-containing products.
- Keep affected area elevated, with ice pack to affected area (20 minutes on and 20 minutes off) as necessary for the first 24 hours.
- Return or call if affected area or limb becomes significantly more painful; normal function is affected from significant swelling; limbs become numb, cool, cyanotic, or insensate; fever develops; or hematoma becomes significantly larger and fluctuant. Tell the patient that hematomas take 2 to 3 weeks to resolve, but very large hematomas may need to be drained after 1 to 2 weeks for patient comfort and function or to decrease the risk of infection.

Crush Injury

A crush injury is an injury to multiple tissues, muscle, or bone in which there is a blunt, high-energy exchange, such as in a fall, pedestrian versus motor vehicle incident, or an industrial injury. The force applied essentially squashes the tissues. Crush injuries carry a higher risk of infection because of the amount of devitalized tissue present. They also present the risk of compartment syndrome and rhabdomyolysis.

ASSESSMENT

- Assess for blood loss, tissues involved, wound depth, neurovascular status of the affected area.
- Assess need for analgesia.
- Assess tetanus prophylaxis status.
- Because the patient likely will require surgical intervention for further evaluation, irrigation and débridement, fasciotomy, amputation or fracture repair, prepare for surgery (e.g., place intravenous line, assess time of last meal, and withhold fluids by mouth).

THERAPEUTIC INTERVENTIONS

- Control bleeding by direct pressure.
- Apply dry, sterile dressing (pressure dressing if bleeding).
- Elevate extremity.
- Administer pain medication as needed.

- Administer antibiotics as directed.
- Monitor for signs and symptoms of compartment syndrome. These include pain, firmness of the muscle compartment, and paresthesia.
- Apply dressing type as determined by the injury and treatment plan.

PATIENT EDUCATION

Teach the patient to do the following:

- Take antibiotics as prescribed.
- Take pain medication as directed.
- Keep the affected extremity elevated above the level of the heart to decrease swelling and pain.
- Keep the wound and dressing clean and dry at all times.
- Change dressings daily as directed.
- Return sooner than scheduled follow-up if redness, swelling, increased pain, numbness, coolness, blue discoloration of fingers or toes, fever, or wound drainage (pus) develop.

See Chapter 20 for further discussion of crush injuries, compartment syndrome, and rhabdomyolysis.

Laceration

A laceration is a cut or tear of the skin that may involve the epidermis and dermis (superficial) or deeper structures (deep); it may be caused by blunt or sharp objects.

ASSESSMENT

- Assess age of wound, depth, degree/type of contamination, associated injuries, neurovascular status distal to wound.
- Assess need for analgesia.
- Assess tetanus prophylaxis status.

THERAPEUTIC INTERVENTIONS

- Control bleeding with direct pressure.
- Apply local anesthetic as prescribed.
- Cleanse and irrigate thoroughly. Be certain to remove all debris and foreign bodies. Wound may require physician exploration/débridement.
- Provide wound closure by suture, skin staples, tape, or tissue adhesive if indicated.
- Apply dressing/immobilization appropriate to wound type, location, and closure versus nonclosure treatment plan (see section on wound dressings). Assess need for home nursing services for wound care.
- Administer tetanus prophylaxis and systemic or topical antibiotics as prescribed.

PATIENT EDUCATION

Teach the patient to do the following:

- Apply topical antibiotic ointment twice daily as directed
- Take analgesia as prescribed
- Keep sutures clean and dry

- Change dressings as directed
- It is not necessary to cover sutured wounds after 24 hours
- Leave adhesive tapes attached until they fall off
- Leave tissue adhesive in place until it peels off by itself
- Return for wound check sooner than scheduled appointment if wound becomes reddened, hot, or swollen, or if drainage (pus) or fever develops
- Return for suture removal in the prescribed number of days (Suture removal is determined by wound location [see section on suture material]).
- Keep wound lightly covered with clothing if out in direct sunlight and, after wounds are completely healed, to continue to cover or apply sunscreen to wound for 6 months to 1 year to avoid hyperpigmentation
- Scars take 6 to 12 months to develop into their final cosmetic appearance

Puncture

A puncture is a wound created by a small-diameter sharp object that externally may not produce a large defect but may penetrate superficial and/or deeper tissues.

ASSESSMENT

- Assess for presence of foreign bodies/materials, impaled objects, depth of tissue penetration, underlying structural damage, type/degree of contamination, and need for analgesia.
- Assess tetanus prophylaxis status.

THERAPEUTIC INTERVENTIONS

- Control bleeding by direct pressure.
- Secure any impaled objects.
- Administer local and/or systemic analgesia as necessary.
- Soak the wound in isotonic solution for several minutes.
- Remove any easily dislodged debris, necrotic tissue, or foreign bodies. This may require physician intervention and placement of drains.
- Cleanse and irrigate the wound (see section on wound cleansing).
- Apply appropriate dressing (may include loose packing).
- Administer systemic or topical antibiotics and tetanus prophylaxis as prescribed.

PATIENT EDUCATION

Teach the patient to do the following:

- Take antibiotics as directed.
- Take analgesia as directed.
- Keep wound clean and dry.
- Change dressings as directed.
- Assess need for home nursing services for wound care and checks.
- Observe for retained foreign bodies or material.
- Return before scheduled follow-up if wound becomes reddened, swollen, hot to touch, begins to drain pus, or if fever develops.

PREVENTION OF INFECTION

Antibiotic Therapy in Trauma

Prophylactically administered antibiotics usually are not indicated for minor, uncomplicated wounds with low contamination or for those wounds in which there has been adequate and appropriate cleansing, débridement, and closure. In certain situations it generally is believed that antibiotics are indicated, considering that the morbidity of a wound or systemic infection can be significant or even life or limb threatening. These situations include the following[2]:

- Open joint, tendon, nerve, or fracture injuries (including teeth)
- Heavily contaminated wounds (e.g., soil or mammalian bites)
- Wounds with major soft tissue injury or losses (e.g., degloving injuries)
- Premorbid conditions, such as valvular disease or replacement, immunosuppression, or diabetes mellitus
- Delays in wound management such as cleansing, débridement, and repair

Antibiotics must be present in adequate tissue levels before wound closure and during operative management to be effective; therefore the timing of administration in trauma is important. The specific antibiotic for a particular wound is determined by the age of the wound and the type, location, and degree of contamination.

Tetanus Prophylaxis in Trauma

Clostridium tetani, the causative organism of the disease tetanus, exists in animal and human excreta and is found in soil and dust. This organism enters the human body through an open wound. Tetanus is prevented easily through appropriate vaccination, immunization, and wound care. Table 14-1 outlines current recommendations for tetanus prophylaxis.[3]

The need for immunization after injury depends on the condition of the wound and the patient's vaccination history. In addition to the most recent dose of tetanus toxoid, it is important to ascertain whether patients have ever received the full primary vaccination series of three doses. Patients with unknown or uncertain vaccination histories should be considered to have had no previous tetanus toxoid doses. Those who have served in U.S. military forces at any time since 1941 usually have received the complete primary series. Patients 60 years of age or older are most at risk of being unvaccinated or inadequately vaccinated.[3]

Rabies Prophylaxis in Trauma

Rabies, a rare but fatal disease, is preventable through proper wound care and postexposure prophylaxis. Rabies is transmitted when the virus, carried in the saliva of an infected animal, is introduced into open cuts or wounds in the victim's skin or mucous membranes. More than half of recent cases in the United States have been traced to bats. Other cases have been attributed to carnivorous wild animals, especially skunks, raccoons, and foxes; woodchucks; exotic pets; and dogs and cats.[4,5]

The risk of rabies infection and the need for prophylaxis vary with the nature and extent of exposure. Wounds are categorized as bite wounds or nonbite wounds. Nonbite exposures (scratches, abrasions, open wounds, or mucous membrane contacts) rarely cause rabies. Bat exposures are a special category: seemingly insignificant physical contact with bats may result in viral transmission. Therefore rabies postexposure prophylaxis should be considered in all situations in which there is reasonable probability of contact with a bat, unless the bat is tested and the result is negative. In addition to known bites, scratches, and mucous membrane

Table 14-1 Summary Guide to Tetanus Prophylaxis* in Routine Wound Management, United States

Previous tetanus toxoid doses	Clean, minor wounds		All other wounds[†]	
	Td[§]	TIG[¶]	Td[§]	TIG
Uncertain or <3	Yes	No	Yes	Yes
>3**	No[††]	No	No[§§]	No

From Centers for Disease Control and Prevention: Update on adult immunization: recommendations of the Immunization Practices Advisory Committee (ACIP), *MMWR* 40(RR-12):70, 1991, and from Centers for Disease Control and Prevention: Preventing tetanus, diphtheria, and pertussis among adolescents: use of tetanus toxoid, reduced diphtheria toxoid and acellular pertussis vaccines: recommendations of the Advisory Committee on Immunization Practices (ACIP), MMWR 55(RR-03);1-43, 2006.

*See also the CDC National Immunization Program website, www.cdc.gov/nip/publications/vis/ for current and detailed information on vaccines or toxoids, including contraindications, precautions, dosages, side effects, adverse reactions, and special considerations.

[†]Such as, but not limited to: wounds contaminated with dirt, feces, and saliva; puncture wounds; avulsions; and wounds resulting from missiles, crushing, burns, and frostbite.

[§]Td = Tetanus and diphtheria toxoids, adsorbed (for adult use). For children <7 years old, DTP (DT, if pertussis vaccine is contraindicated) is preferred to tetanus toxoid (TT) alone. For persons aged 7-10 years or over age 18, Td is preferred to tetanus toxoid alone. For adolescents aged 11-18 years, tetanus toxoid, reduced diphtheria toxoid, and acellular pertussis vaccine (Tdap) is preferred to Td for adolescents who have never received Tdap. Td is preferred to TT for adolescents who received Tdap previously or when Tdap is not available (if TT and TIG are both used, Tetanus Toxoid Adsorbed rather than Tetanus Toxoid for Booster Use Only [fluid vaccine] should be used).

[¶]TIG = Tetanus immune globulin.

**If only three doses of fluid toxoid have been received, a fourth dose of toxoid, preferably an adsorbed toxoid, should be given.

[††]Yes, >10 years since last dose.

[§§]Yes, >5 years since last dose. (More frequent boosters are not needed and can accentuate side effects.)

contacts, examples of potential contact include a sleeping person awakening to find a bat in a room or a person finding a bat in a room with an unattended child or a mentally disabled or intoxicated person.[4,5]

Patient management begins with appropriate wound care. A decision then should be made concerning the need for postexposure prophylaxis (Table 14-2). If needed, rabies vaccine and rabies immune globulin are given according to a standard regimen (Table 14-3). State or local health departments should be consulted for additional advice regarding prophylaxis.[4,5]

Table 14-2   **Rabies Postexposure Prophylaxis Guide, United States, 1999**

Animal Type	Evaluation and Disposition of Animal	Postexposure Prophylaxis Recommendations
Dogs and cats	Healthy and available for 10 days' observation	Should not begin prophylaxis unless animal develops symptoms of rabies*
	Rabid or suspected rabid	Immediate vaccination
	Unknown (escaped)	Consult public health officials
Skunks, raccoons, bats, foxes, and most other carnivores; woodchucks	Regarded as rabid unless geographic area is known to be free of rabies or until animal is proved negative by laboratory tests†	Immediate vaccination
Livestock, rodents, and lagomorphs (rabbits and hares)	Consider individually	Consult public health officials. Bites of squirrels, hamsters, guinea pigs, gerbils, chipmunks, rats, mice, other rodents, rabbits, and hares almost never require antirabies treatment

Centers for Disease Control: Human rabies prevention—United States, 1999: recommendations of the Advisory Committee on Immunization Practices (ACIP), *MMWR* 48(RR-1):1-23, 1999.
*During the 10-day holding period, begin treatment at first sign of rabies in a dog or cat that has bitten someone. The symptomatic animal should be killed immediately and tested.
†The animal should be killed and tested as soon as possible. Holding for observation is not recommended. Discontinue vaccine if immunofluorescence test results of the animal are negative.

Table 14-3   Rabies Postexposure Prophylaxis Schedule, United States, 2000

Vaccination Status	Treatment	Regimen*
Not previously vaccinated	Local wound cleansing	All postexposure treatment should begin with immediate thorough cleansing of all wounds with soap and water.
	HRIG	20 units/kg body mass. If anatomically feasible, up to one half the dose should be infiltrated around the wound(s) and the rest should be administered intramuscularly in the gluteal area. HRIG should not be administered in the same syringe or into the same anatomic site as the vaccine. Because HRIG may partially suppress active production of antibody, no more than the recommended dose should be given.
	Vaccine	HDCV or RVA, 1 mL IM (deltoid area†), one each on days 0, 3, 7, 14, and 28.
Previously vaccinated‡	Local wound cleansing	All postexposure treatment should begin with immediate thorough cleansing of all wounds with soap and water.
	HRIG	HRIG should not be administered.
	Vaccine	HDCV or RVA, 1 mL IM (deltoid area†), one each on days 0 and 3.

Centers for Disease Control: Human rabies prevention—United States, 1991: recommendations of the Advisory Committee on Immunization Practices (ACIP), *MMWR* 40(RR-1):1-21, 1999.
HRIG, Human rabies immunoglobulin; *HDCV,* human diploid cell vaccine; *RVA,* rabies vaccine absorbed.
*These regimens are applicable for all age groups, including children.
†The deltoid area is the only acceptable site of vaccination for adults and older children. For younger children, the outer aspect of the thigh may be used. Vaccine should never be administered in the gluteal area.
‡Any person with a history of preexposure vaccination with HDCV or RVA, prior postexposure prophylaxis with HDCV or RVA, or previous vaccination with any other type of rabies vaccine and a documented history of antibody response to the prior vaccination.

References

1. Simon B, Hern H: Wound management principles. In Marx J, editor: *Rosen's emergency medicine,* vol 1, ed 5, St Louis, 2002, Mosby.
2. Stewart RM, Meyers J, Dent D: Wounds, bites, and stings. In Feliciano DV, Moore EE, Mattox KL, editors: *Trauma,* ed 4, Stamford, Conn, 2004, McGraw-Hill.
3. Immunization Action Coalition: *Summary of recommendations for adult immunization,* August 2005. Retrieved January 30, 2006 from www.immunize.org/catg.d/p2011b.pdf
4. Centers for Disease Control: Rabies prevention—United States, 1999: recommendations of Immunization Practices Advisory Committee (ACIP), *MMWR* 48(RR-1):1-23, 1999.
5. Rabies: Prevention and Control. Retrieved November 1, 2006, from www.cdc.gov/ncidod/dvrd/rabies/prevention&control/ preventi./htm

Suggested Readings

Flynn MB: Burn and wound care, *Crit Care Nurs Clin North Am* 16(1):1-177, 2004.

Flynn MB: Host defense systems. In Emergency Nurses Association: *Course in advanced trauma nursing—II: a conceptual approach to injury and illness (CATN II),* ed 2, Dubuque, Iowa, 2003, Kendell Hunt.

Herman ML, Newberry L: Wound management. In Emergency Nurses Association: *Sheehy's emergency nursing: principles and practice,* ed 5, St Louis, 2004, Mosby.

McQuillian K, Von Rueden K, Hartsock R et al, editors: *Trauma nursing: from resuscitation through rehabilitation,* ed 3, Philadelphia, 2002, Saunders.

Robson M, Steed D, Franz G: Wound healing: biologic features and approaches to maximize healing trajectories, *Curr Probl Surg* 38(2):61-140, 2001.

Steed D, editor: Wound healing [entire issue], *Surg Clin North Am* 83(3):463-726, 2003.

Trott AT: *Wounds and lacerations: emergency care and closure,* ed 3, Philadelphia, 2005, Mosby.

CLINICAL PRACTICE

CHAPTER 15

HEAD TRAUMA

NICKI GILBOY

Head trauma is a major cause of morbidity and mortality in the United States and accounts for up to 30% of all trauma-related deaths.[1] Each year, approximately 1.6 million Americans sustain head injuries. More than a million of those injured are treated and released from emergency departments. Approximately 60,000 die, and more than 250,000 are hospitalized and survive. More than 70,000 suffer some degree of irreversible loss of neurologic function. The highest injury rate occurs in males between the ages of 15 and 30 and persons over age 75. In approximately 40% of all severe head injuries, alcohol has been shown to be a contributing factor.[2]

The three most common mechanisms of injury are motor vehicle crashes, violence, and falls.[3] In the 75 years and older age group, the leading cause of death from head trauma is falls.[4] Penetrating head trauma, usually caused by an assault, is a significant problem in the United States. Penetrating head trauma is responsible for 35% of all deaths caused by head trauma.[5]

ANATOMY OF THE HEAD

The brain is well protected by the hair, scalp, skull, meninges, and cerebrospinal fluid (Figure 15-1).

The scalp itself is composed of five layers of tissue: skin, subcutaneous tissue, aponeurosa, ligaments, and periosteum.

The skull is a bony structure the main purpose of which is to protect the brain. The skull is divided into four main areas: the frontal area, the parietal area, the occipital area, and the temporal areas. The skull also is divided into two major sections: the calvaria or cranial vault (which houses the brain) and the base (which provides an opening for the spinal cord to enter the cervical area). The bones of the skull are united at immovable joints called sutures.

Three meningeal layers provide protection (or padding) for the brain and the spinal cord. From the surface of the brain outward, the layers are the pia mater, the arachnoid mater, and the dura mater. The pia mater is thin and mucouslike and adheres to the cortex of the brain. The arachnoidal layer is thin, vascular, and spiderlike (hence the term *arachnoid*). The subarachnoid space lies between the arachnoid mater and pia mater (Figure 15-2). The dura mater (Latin words translating as "tough mother") adheres to the inner surface of the skull. In the area where the dura mater forms the tentorial notch, the tissue is knifelike and can cause severe damage to the brain when there is anterior-posterior movement of the brain.

The meningeal arteries are between the internal surface of the skull and the dura mater in an area known as the epidural (above the dura mater) space.

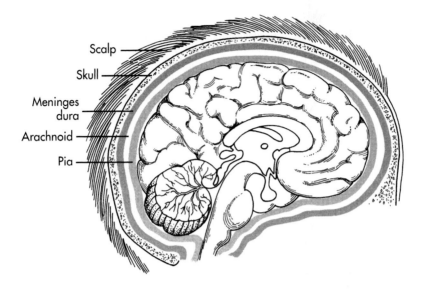

Figure 15–1. The anatomy of the head.

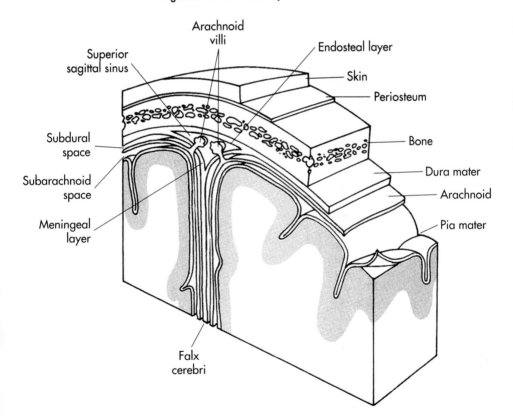

Figure 15–2. Coronal section of the skull and brain. *(From Barker E:* Neuroscience nursing: a spectrum of care, *ed 2, St Louis, 2002, Mosby.)*

Cerebrospinal Fluid

Cerebrospinal fluid (CSF) is produced continuously at a rate of approximately 20 mL per hour in the ventricles of the brain. CSF passes from the lateral ventricles to the third and then the fourth ventricle into the subarachnoid space. The arachnoidal villi provide the outlet for CSF to flow into the venous system. The function of CSF is to provide a cushion for the brain and the spinal cord, thereby minimizing damage from mechanical trauma.

Brain

The body of the brain is a fluid-filled collection of delicate tissues (Figure 15-3) and water, which composes 80% to 85% of the cranial mass. The bulk of the brain is the cerebrum, which is divided into the right and left hemispheres. Each hemisphere is subdivided into four lobes: frontal, parietal, occipital, and temporal, named the same as their overlying skull sections.

The function of the frontal lobe is to conceptualize, think abstractly, and form judgments. When this lobe of the brain is injured, judgment and reasoning may become impaired, and the patient may begin to shout out obscene and foul language. This is known as being *frontal lobish.*

The parietal lobe is the area in which the highest integration and coordination of perception and interpretation of sensory phenomena occur. Injury to this area of the brain may cause the patient to have difficulty with receptive communication.

The occipital lobe is the area of the brain that is responsible for vision. Injury to this area of the brain may cause blurred vision, diplopia (double vision), or even blindness.

The temporal lobes (one is located on each side of the brain) resemble the thumbs of a boxing glove. These lobes frequently are injured because they are enclosed in relatively bony chambers. Injury to the temporal lobe or lobes may cause temporary or permanent memory loss.

The brainstem contains the reticular activating system and is responsible for consciousness. The medulla, which is the lower part of the brainstem, contains the cardiorespiratory centers.

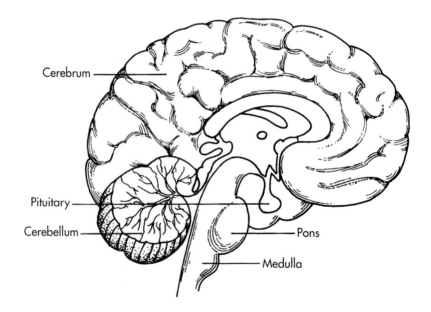

Figure 15-3. The brain is a collection of delicate tissues.

The cerebellum is located next to the brainstem, under the cerebrum. The cerebellum is responsible for movement and coordination. The area where the cerebrum and midbrain meet is the tentorial notch. The tentorial notch is formed by a separation of the dura mater and has extremely sharp edges; sudden contact with the brain may cause severe damage to the brain. This is also an area where brain herniation may occur.

Cranial Nerves

Connected to the brain are 12 pairs of cranial nerves.

Olfactory (I)

The olfactory nerve is responsible for the sense of smell. To test this nerve, the patient is instructed to close both eyes, occlude one nostril, and identify the odor from a common substance that has been placed under the open nostril. This procedure is repeated with the opposite nostril. Testing usually is deferred unless an anterior fossa mass is suspected.

Optic (II)

The optic nerve controls visual acuity and the visual fields. Gross visual acuity is measured by instructing the patient to cover one eye and identify the number of fingers held up by the examiner. The procedure is repeated with the other eye.

Oculomotor (III), Trochlear (IV), and Abducens (VI)

The third, fourth, and sixth cranial nerves have much to do with the function and movement of the eye. They are tested by checking pupil size, shape, and reactivity to light. Extraocular movement also can be assessed by having the patient follow a moving finger with his or her eyes without moving the head: up, down, to the right, and to the left. The third cranial nerve (oculomotor) passes through the tentorial notch. Brainstem herniation causes pressure to be placed on this nerve and will cause pupil dilation on the ipsilateral (same) side as the herniation. Clinical personnel should be aware that a difference of 1 mm in pupil size may be a significant finding.

Trigeminal (V)

The trigeminal nerve controls facial sensation and jaw movement. This nerve is tested by checking for facial sensation, strength of mastication muscles, and movement of the jaw.

Facial (VII)

The facial nerve controls facial expression and taste in the anterior two thirds of the tongue (testing usually is deferred). The motor component is tested by having the patient raise the eyebrows, close the eyelids tightly to resistance, show the teeth, smile, frown, and puff up the cheeks. If there is peripheral ipsilateral injury, the upper and lower face will be involved. If there is a central injury, the brow of the contralateral (opposite side) will be spared.

The corneal reflex, an important brainstem reflex, can provide the examiner with important information on the functioning of cranial nerves V and VII. When the cornea is stimulated by lightly brushing a piece of cotton across it, the normal response is to briskly and immediately blink. No response indicates abnormality.

Acoustic/Auditory (VIII)

The eighth nerve is divided into two branches. The acoustic branch controls balance; it is tested by cold water calorics (usually deferred during the initial trauma assessment and contraindicated if the patient has a ruptured tympanic membrane or signs of a basilar skull fracture that may include otorrhea). The auditory branch controls hearing; it is tested by ascertaining the patient's response to a loud noise, such as a clap.

Glossopharyngeal (IX) and Vagus (X)

The glossopharyngeal and vagus nerves usually are evaluated together because of their close anatomic and functional relationships. The glossopharyngeal nerve controls taste in the posterior two thirds of the tongue and sensation in the nostrils and pharynx. The vagus nerve controls the soft palate, the pharynx and larynx muscles, the heart, the lungs, and the stomach. Both nerves are tested by checking for the presence of a gag and a swallow reflex and by assessing the patient's ability to distinguish between salty and sweet tastes.

Accessory (XI)

The accessory nerve controls movement of the sternocleidomastoid and trapezius muscles. This nerve is tested by asking the patient to turn his or her head against resistance or to shrug the shoulders.

NOTE: Before testing the accessory nerve, spinal cord injury or the potential for it must be ruled out.

Hypoglossal (XII)

The hypoglossal nerve controls movement of the tongue. This nerve is tested by asking the patient to stick out the tongue. If the tongue is in the midline position, the nerve is considered to be intact.

BRAIN PHYSIOLOGY AND TRAUMATIC INJURY

This section reviews a few important concepts related to brain physiology and traumatic injury.

Monroe-Kellie Doctrine

The skull is a rigid container that holds the brain, blood, CSF, and other components (tumor, hematoma). The sum of the components is fixed. As the volume of one component increases, a compensatory change is made in the volume of other components so that the pressure remains constant and within normal limits. Small changes in volume are tolerated, but at some point when compensatory mechanisms are exhausted, small increases in intracranial volume result in sharp increases in intracranial pressure (ICP).

Cerebral Blood Flow

The survival of the brain depends on its receiving an adequate amount of blood. Routinely the brain receives about 15% of the cardiac output. The brain has no capacity to store oxygen or glucose so that if an episode of hypotension or hypoxia occurs, the brain is deprived of essential substances.

Inflammation and Head Injury

Following an injury, the inflammatory response is initiated, with the release of cytokines, free radicals, excitatory amino acids, and other mediators. This inflammatory response causes an alteration in cerebral blood flow, cerebral edema, and an alteration in the permeability of the blood-brain barrier.

Cerebral Perfusion Pressure

In normal circumstances, cerebral blood flow is maintained at a constant rate. With injury and the resulting inflammation, these homeostatic mechanisms are impaired, and global and regional cerebral ischemia may result. If the homeostatic mechanisms are impaired, cerebral blood flow becomes dependent on systemic blood pressure. To ensure adequate cerebral blood flow, the cerebral perfusion pressure must be maintained at greater than or equal to 60 mm Hg.[6] Cerebral perfusion pressure is equal to the mean arterial pressure (MAP) minus ICP. MAP can be calculated but generally is derived from arterial monitoring. MAP equals diastolic pressure plus the difference of the systolic pressure and diastolic pressure, divided by 3. Box 15-1 gives an example. If cerebral perfusion pressure is not maintained, increased cerebral edema and increased ICP will occur.

Nursing care of the patient with a head injury is directed toward the manipulation of this equation. Nursing interventions can be directed toward the MAP or ICP, but the goal is to maintain cerebral perfusion pressure at greater than 60 mm Hg.

NEUROLOGIC ASSESSMENT

In the evaluation of a patient with a head injury, the extent of the neurologic assessment and reassessment depends on the patient's level of consciousness and stability of vital functions. Assessment and interventions for airway, breathing, and circulation are the priority. Patients who are awake, alert, and cooperative can have a detailed assessment performed; patients with a decreased level of consciousness should have a limited examination that includes the Glasgow Coma Scale (GCS) score, pupils, reflexes, and vital signs. Reassessment should be performed at regular intervals. The purpose of the neurologic assessment is to establish a baseline assessment of the patient and with repeat exams to be able to identify any changes in neurologic status. From the assessment data, changes in the plan of care can be made and the effect of interventions assessed. Nursing diagnoses frequently relevant to patients with head trauma are listed in the High-Frequency Nursing Diagnoses box.

Box 15-1	EXAMPLE OF CALCULATION OF CEREBRAL PERFUSION PRESSURE (CPP) FROM MEAN ARTERIAL PRESSURE (MAP) AND INTRACRANIAL PRESSURE (ICP)

CPP = MAP – ICP
MAP = 120
ICP = 24
120 – 24 = 96
CPP = 96

HIGH-FREQUENCY NURSING DIAGNOSES FOR PATIENTS WITH HEAD TRAUMA

- Ineffective airway clearance
- Risk for aspiration
- Ineffective breathing pattern
- Impaired gas exchange
- Ineffective tissue perfusion: cerebral
- Decreased adaptive capacity: intracranial
- Acute confusion
- Acute pain
- Impaired physical mobility
- Risk for infection
- Knowledge deficit: head injury aftercare

From NANDA International: *NANDA nursing diagnoses: definitions & classification, 2005-2006,* Philadelphia, 2006, The Association.

One must obtain a detailed history from the patient, bystanders, and prehospital personnel regarding the cause and mechanism of injury. Information about loss of consciousness, level of consciousness, and other events is the key.

Level of Consciousness

Consciousness can be defined as "a state of general awareness of self and the environment and the ability to produce a response."[4] Consciousness has two components: arousal or wakefulness (being aware of the environment) and content of consciousness, or cognition (demonstrating an understanding of a stimulus by responding to it). To determine level of consciousness, the examiner applies a stimulus and assesses the response. Consciousness is the most sensitive indicator of a change in neurologic status. Level of consciousness can be seen as a continuum, ranging from fully conscious to coma. No universally accepted definitions exist for the various levels of consciousness. The most useful terms are the following:

- Fully conscious: Awake, alert, and oriented to time, place, and person; responds appropriately to stimuli
- Confusion: Disoriented to time and/or place and/or person; difficulty with attention span and memory
- Coma: No response to an external stimulus; total absence of the awareness of self and the environment

Lethargy, obtunded, stuporous, and *semicomatose* are terms often used but difficult to discriminate between. A better practice is to avoid their use or supplement them with a more detailed description of the patient's status.

Responsiveness can be tested quickly by assessing the patient's response to a stimulus as one of the following:

- Purposeful
- Nonpurposeful
- Abnormal flexion (decorticate posturing; Figure 15-4): elbows are flexed, hands are pulled up toward the core. The lesion is higher in the brainstem, above the midbrain.

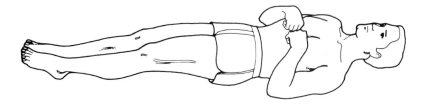

Figure 15–4. Abnormal flexion (decorticate position).

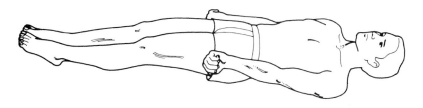

Figure 15–5. Abnormal extension (decerebrate position).

Box 15-2	**THE AVPU MNEMONIC FOR LEVEL OF CONSCIOUSNESS**	
A	Alert	The patient is awake, alert, and oriented to time, place, and person.
V	Verbal	The patient responds to verbal stimuli but is not fully oriented to time, place, and person.
P	Painful	The application of a painful stimulus is needed for the patient to respond.
U	Unresponsive	The patient does not respond to even a painful stimulus.

- Abnormal extension (decerebrate posturing; Figure 15-5): elbows are in extension, wrists point downward, with hands clenched, rotated outward. The lesion is at the level of the brainstem, below the midbrain.

The nurse must apply only one stimulus at a time and must wait to see whether there is a response. If verbal stimuli do not elicit a response, tactile, noxious, or painful stimuli should be applied. Documentation should describe the stimulus and the response.

The AVPU mnemonic (Box 15-2) can be used to conduct a brief assessment of the patient's level of consciousness. This mnemonic is useful to assess the patient's response to verbal and/or painful stimuli.[7]

Glasgow Coma Scale

The GCS has become a standard for the assessment of a patient's level of consciousness and a way of objectively measuring the severity of a head injury (Table 15-1). Patients are assessed

Table 15-1   Glasgow Coma Scale

Finding	Score
Eye opening	
Spontaneous	4
To voice	3
To pain	2
None	1
Best verbal response	
Oriented	5
Confused	4
Inappropriate words	3
Incomprehensible sounds	2
None	1
Best motor response	
Obeys commands	6
Purposeful movement (pain)	5
Withdraw (pain)	4
Flexion (pain)	3
Extension (pain)	2
None	1
POSSIBLE TOTAL SCORE	3-15

From Teasdale G, Jennett B: Assessment of coma and impaired consciousness, *Lancet* II: 81-84, 1974.

in three areas: eye opening, motor response, and verbal response. Clinical personnel should always use the patient's best score in each component. When testing motor response, the unaffected side of the body should be used if hemiplegia is present, and the head or face should be used if a spinal cord injury is present. A baseline score should be obtained before administering any medications. A neurologically intact patient would score the maximum possible score of 15. A patient with a score between 13 and 15 is classified as having no injury to having a mild head injury. A score between 9 and 12 indicates a moderate head injury. With a score of 8 or less, a severe injury is indicated. The lowest achievable score is 3 (i.e., one point in each area). The validity of the score depends on the absence of systemic abnormalities such as hypotension, hypoxia, hypothermia, hypoglycemia, and drugs that affect neurologic function.

Assessment of Motor Strength and Sensory Response

Assessment of a patient's motor strength is important for the nurse to understand how well the voluntary and involuntary motor pathways are functioning. The nurse needs to ask the patient to perform some activity using certain muscle groups and then evaluate the response. The evaluation is performed on the upper and lower extremities and includes a side-to-side comparison. For example, the nurse asks the patient to flex the arms at the elbows, and with

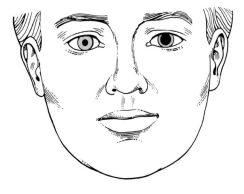

Figure 15-6. Unilateral fixed, dilated pupil suggests early third nerve involvement.

the nurse holding the elbows, the nurse first asks the patient to pull the hands toward the face. This can be repeated for various muscle groups of the upper and lower extremities. Also note any abnormal position of the limbs at rest. Motor strength cannot be tested in the unconscious patient, but spontaneous movement or movement in response to a noxious stimulus must be described in detail in the patient's medical record. Assess each limb individually by major muscle groups, grading from 0 to 5:

0—No motor function
1—Slight motion/flicker
2—Moves if gravity is neutralized
3—Moves against gravity
4—Strength diminished; able to pull or lift against moderate resistance
5—Normal function; able to pull or lift against resistance

For a sensory examination, if the patient is alert and cooperative and able to follow directions, the nurse can assess the response to a tactile stimulus applied to areas of the body. The patient should be able to tell the examiner where and what type of stimulus (sharp versus dull) is being applied.

Pupillary Response

Pupillary assessment can be performed in the conscious and unconscious patient. Look first at the size of the pupils before examination with a light; this is important. Normal resting pupil size is 2 to 6 mm, and normal pupils are round. When a bright light is shone into one eye from the side, both pupils should constrict. A brisk reaction is a rapid response. A sluggish response is one in which constriction occurs but more slowly than expected. Nonreactive pupils do not constrict or dilate and are described as fixed. Check the eyes for any extraocular movement. Note that up to 20% of the population may have minor differences in pupil size (anisocoria), but in these instances, both pupils will react to light.

Normally, pupils constrict to light; if pupils are fixed and pinpoint, consider possible opiate use or pontine herniation. A pupil that is dilated and fixed unilaterally may indicate early involvement of the third cranial nerve (Figure 15-6). Be sure to rule out direct eye trauma, cataracts, or use of medications that can cause pupillary dilation. Bilateral fixed dilated pupils indicate complete third cranial nerve involvement (Figure 15-7). Ptosis also indicates third cranial nerve involvement.

Figure 15–7. Bilateral fixed, dilated pupils indicate complete third nerve involvement.

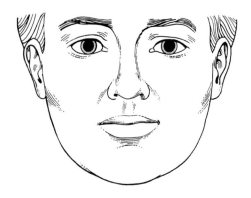

Vital Signs

As with any injured patient, monitor vital signs continuously. Vital signs should be evaluated relative to the patient's baseline values and the patient's medical history. All five vital signs should be monitored—temperature, pulse, respirations, blood pressure, and oxygen saturation—because changes in each value can indicate a deterioration or improvement in the patient's neurologic status.

Temperature is controlled by the hypothalamus. A rise in body temperature increases the metabolic rate throughout the body, including the brain.

Blood pressure and heart rate should be monitored for deviations from the patient's baseline. Knowledge of the patient's MAP is key to managing cerebral perfusion pressure. A decrease in blood pressure and an increase in heart rate may result from hypovolemic shock caused by other injuries. Hypertension and bradycardia may be due to increasing ICP. Cushing's triad, which includes bradycardia, hypertension, and irregular respirations, is a late sign of rising ICP and brain herniation.

Pay close attention to respiratory rate, rhythm, and depth. Increased ICP usually results in irregular, slow respirations. Patients with a severe head injury will be intubated and attached to a mechanical ventilator before or on arrival in the emergency department.

Reflexes

Reflex testing includes testing of pupils, corneal reflex, and gag reflex. These reflexes are described in previous sections. The other reflexes tested during neuroassessment are deep tendon reflexes and Babinski's reflex.

Deep Tendon Reflexes

Hypoactivity or absence of deep tendon reflexes indicates that there may be cerebellar involvement, peripheral nerve disease, or anterior horn cell disease. Hyperactivity indicates pyramidal tract lesions or psychogenic disorders.

Deep tendon reflexes are scored from 0 to 4:

0 = Absent
1 = Decreased
2 = Normal
3 = Increased
4 = Hyperactive

Babinski's Sign or Reflex

Babinski's sign or reflex is elicited by performing a cutaneous stimulation of the plantar surface of the foot. Normally, the toes flex. An abnormal response, called a *positive Babinski,* occurs when the great toe points cephalad (toward the head, to where the problem is) and the other toes fan out.

DIAGNOSTIC TESTS

Many diagnostic tests can be used when assessing the patient with a head injury. The more commonly used ones are presented in the following paragraphs. Clinical personnel should remember that some are more beneficial than others.

Computed Tomography

Computed tomography (CT), which can accurately detect 98% of intracranial injuries, now is used routinely for most patients with head injuries once initial resuscitation is complete and the patient is stable enough to be transported to the CT room. CT should be considered early when the patient has an altered level of consciousness, hemiparesis, or any type of aphasia.

Skull X-Ray Films

Skull x-ray films are no longer used as a routine diagnostic test. They have been superceded by CT scanning.

Angiography

Angiography is used when a vascular injury is suspected. Radiopaque contrast is injected, and serial images are obtained to visualize the blood vessels and cerebral circulation.

Nuclear Magnetic Resonance Imaging

Nuclear magnetic resonance imaging (MRI) is not useful in acute trauma situations because the procedure is time-consuming, the patient must be absolutely still, and access to the patient is limited during the procedure. MRI, however, may be useful in nonacute stages of trauma. MRI is particularly good at identifying soft tissue injuries, such as diffuse axonal injuries (shear injuries). Magnetic resonance angiography, a newer test, is being used to assess blood vessels and vessel injuries.

BRAIN INJURY

Head injury encompasses brain injury and injuries to the other structures of the head, including the scalp and skull. Brain injury, often referred to as traumatic brain injury, has been defined as "a physiological disruption of brain function resulting from trauma both external (an object striking the head or the head striking an object) and/or internal (the rapid acceleration/deceleration of the brain within the skullcap)."[9]

Brain Injury Severity

Traumatic brain injury has been classified by the Brain Injury Association of America as mild, moderate, and severe. The definitions used by the association follow.[9]

A mild brain injury is defined as an injury in which one of the following occurs:

- Any period of loss of consciousness
- Any amnesia for events immediately before or after the injury
- Any alteration in mental state at the time of the injury
- Transient or permanent focal neurologic deficit

Signs and symptoms of a mild brain injury can be classified as physical, cognitive, or behavioral. Physical symptoms can include headache, dizziness, nausea, sleep problems, and/or fatigue. Decrease in attention span, concentration, mental speed, and short-term memory are common cognitive signs. Behavioral signs include irritability, emotional lability, depression, and anxiety. The GCS also has been used to classify brain injury severity. A patient with a mild brain injury has a GCS of 13 to15.

A moderate brain injury is one that results in a loss of consciousness that lasts from a few minutes to a few hours, followed by days and/or weeks of confusion. An individual with a moderate brain injury can sustain physical, cognitive, or behavioral changes that can last for months or can become permanent. A person with a moderate brain injury has a GCS of 9 to 12.

With a severe brain injury, the patient is unconscious or in a coma for an extended time (days to months). A patient with a severe brain injury has a GCS of 3 to 8.

Brain Herniation

Herniation occurs when the brain protrudes through the tentorial notch and/or the foramen magnum, causing severe, permanent, neurologic deficits and alteration in cardiorespiratory function. Brain herniation is a result of increased ICP from an expanding hematoma or cerebral edema pushing the brain tissue toward the path of least resistance. The two types of herniation are transtentorial and central.

Transtentorial (Uncal) Herniation

A transtentorial herniation occurs when pressure on the lateral middle fossa or the temporal lobe causes the inner edge (basal edge) of the uncus and hippocampal gyrus to be pushed toward the midline and into the lateral edge of the tentorial notch. This movement causes pressure to build at the tentorial notch and pushes the midbrain into the opposite side of the tentorial notch. As a result, the third cranial nerve (oculomotor nerve) and the posterior cerebral artery may become caught between the part of the uncus that has herniated and the edge of the tentorial notch.

Early signs of transtentorial herniation are the following:

- Depth of coma: decreased level of consciousness
- Eyes: ipsilateral dilated pupil
- Respirations: Cheyne-Stokes respirations
- Motor and movement: contralateral hemiparesis and positive Babinski's reflex

Late signs of transtentorial herniation are the following:

- Depth of coma: severely decreased level of consciousness
- Eyes: midpoint and fixed pupils bilaterally

- Respirations: central neurogenic breathing (hyperventilation)
- Motor and movement: abnormal extension (decerebrate)

Central Herniation (Rostral-Caudal Deterioration)

When ICP is extremely high and uniformly distributed throughout the brain, the brain is forced downward and the cerebellar tonsils herniate through the foramen magnum. As this occurs, the medulla is compressed.

Early signs of central herniation are the following:

- Depth of coma: restlessness to lethargy
- Eyes: pupils equal and reactive but constricted
- Respirations: Cheyne-Stokes breathing with yawns and sighs that deteriorate to central neurogenic breathing
- Motor and movement: contralateral hemiparesis

Late signs and symptoms of central herniation are the following:

- Depth of coma: severely altered level of consciousness
- Eyes: nonreactive, midposition pupils
- Respirations: central neurogenic breathing deteriorating to ataxic breathing
- Motor and movement: posturing that deteriorates from abnormal flexion (decorticate) to abnormal extension (decerebrate)

Primary and Secondary Brain Injury

The concept of primary and secondary brain injury has become well accepted. The primary injury results from the initial insult, which leads to biomechanical changes in the brain. A primary injury causes focal or diffuse injuries that may lead to death of brain cells. The secondary brain injury occurs after the primary injury and may lead to further tissue damage. Secondary injuries are a result of physiologic events such as hypoxia, hypotension, cerebral edema, and increased ICP. Optimal initial management of the head-injured patient decreases the chance of secondary brain injury and therefore decrease morbidity and mortality.

Focal and Diffuse Brain Injuries

Brain injuries may be focal or diffuse. With focal injuries the damage is limited to a well-defined area and is the direct result of trauma to the tissues. Focal injuries account for about half of all brain injuries. Diffuse injuries produce damage throughout the brain resulting from widespread shearing and rotational forces. A general summary of therapeutic interventions is contained on p. 181. Specific interventions are discussed with each injury.

TYPES OF HEAD INJURY

Scalp Laceration

The most frequent type of head injury seen in practice is a scalp laceration. Scalp laceration is a common injury in children because their heads are large in relation to their bodies, they are relatively clumsy, and they have high activity levels. A scalp laceration can be caused by any blunt or penetrating force to the head. The scalp is extremely vascular, and a significant amount of blood can be lost from a scalp laceration.

ASSESSMENT

- Observe for profuse bleeding.
- Carefully examine the scalp with a gloved hand. Sometimes scalp lacerations are missed if hair is thick and bleeding is minimal.
- Check for concurrent neurologic injury.
- Check for other associated injuries.

THERAPEUTIC INTERVENTIONS

- Control bleeding with direct pressure.
- Apply ice.
- Clip hair around laceration for better visualization, but do not shave.
- Irrigate the wound with sterile normal saline.
- Inspect and palpate the wound.
- Devitalized tissue should be débrided. If bone fragments are present, a neurosurgical consultation is needed.
- The scalp should be sutured in layers. Close the galea first with 2-0 or 3-0 absorbable suture; then close the skin with nylon or Prolene suture. Skin staples are another option, especially for briskly bleeding wounds in unstable patients. For small lacerations, tissue adhesive can be used.
- Wound may be left open to air or covered with a small sterile dressing, depending on practitioner preference.
- Ensure tetanus prophylaxis.
- Provide the patient with verbal and written discharge instructions for wound care and closed head injury.

See Chapter 14 for more information on the care of lacerations.

Skull Fracture

Skull fracture is a common injury. The diagnosis of skull fracture may be made by physical findings or x-ray films. If a skull fracture is present, neurosurgical consult should occur.

The patient's scalp should be examined for bumps, defects, lacerations of the scalp, and bruises. In addition, neurologic status should be monitored. If the injury overlies the sinuses, profuse bleeding may occur. Also, the possibility of associated cervical spine injury and facial fractures should always be suspected, and appropriate precautions should be taken.

Although large forces are necessary to produce a skull fracture, the extent of underlying brain injury varies. Because a skull fracture indicates significant trauma, a thorough assessment is necessary. Patients with a basilar skull fracture also should be observed for the presence of a CSF leak.

Linear/Nondisplaced Skull Fracture

A linear/nondisplaced fracture is a fracture line in the skull that passes through its entire thickness. These fractures are not usually significant unless there are associated focal signs indicating underlying structural damage. These fractures usually are caused by a significant blow to the skull.

ASSESSMENT

- Difficult to palpate these fractures
- Seen on skull x-ray films (if obtained)

THERAPEUTIC INTERVENTIONS

- Usually no specific therapeutic intervention is required.
- Discharge instructions should include observation for signs and symptoms of a more severe head injury.
- If the fracture is across a vascular groove or a suture line, consider observation for 24 hours and neurosurgical consultation.

Depressed Skull Fracture

A depressed skull fracture is an actual depression of a fragment or fragments of the skull. The fracture may be open or closed. Great care should be taken for close observation of the presence or formation of an intracranial injury. These injuries often are associated with a contusion underlying the fracture.

ASSESSMENT

- Patient may be unconscious, unresponsive, and not breathing adequately.
- Palpate the skull depression gently.
- Verify the depressed fracture on x-ray film or CT scan.

THERAPEUTIC INTERVENTIONS

A closed depression requires the following:

- Neurosurgical consultation
- Hospital admission for close observation
- For depression greater than 5 mm, surgical intervention to elevate depressed segment

An open injury requires the following:

- Sterile wet-to-dry dressing over wound
- Neurosurgical consultation
- Surgical intervention to débride and elevate depressed segment
- Antibiotics
- Tetanus prophylaxis

Basilar Skull Fracture

A basilar skull fracture is a fracture of any of the bones that make up the base of the skull (frontal, ethmoid, sphenoid, temporal, or occipital). It may be a linear or a depressed fracture. This fracture could cause a CSF leak, which usually will close spontaneously but places the patient at risk for infection.

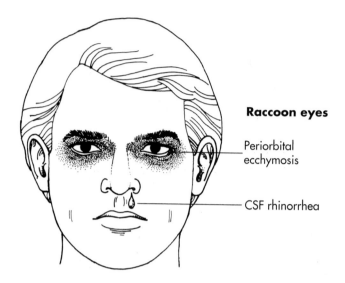

Figure 15–8. Basilar skull fracture: periorbital ecchymosis.

ASSESSMENT

- Presence of intracranial air or opaque sphenoid sinuses
- Possibly seen on a Waters' view (open-mouth) x-ray film
- Possibly seen on CT scan
- Patient may complain of severe headache
- Periorbital ecchymosis (Figure 15-8), also known as *raccoon eyes* or *owl eyes;* this type of intraorbital bleeding usually is seen with cribriform plate fracture or intraorbital root fracture
- Battle's sign (Figure 15-9), an ecchymosis behind the ear in the mastoid region that usually occurs 12 to 24 hours after injury
- Hemotympanum (blood behind the tympanic membrane), usually caused by fracture of temporal bone
- Patient complaint of salty taste at back of throat (CSF leak)
- Possible CSF otorrhea or CSF rhinorrhea

To test for this condition, if the drainage is bloody, drop some of the fluid onto a filter paper. The fluid may produce a finding known as a *ring sign,* a *halo,* or a *target sign,* where blood forms a central circle and CSF dissipates outward, forming a ring around the blood. Clear drainage may be tested for the presence of glucose, using a glucose reagent test strip. The CSF glucose level is approximately 25 mg/dL.

THERAPEUTIC INTERVENTIONS

- Admit patient for close observation.
- Avoid having the patient strain, which might exacerbate drainage (e.g., coughing or blowing nose).

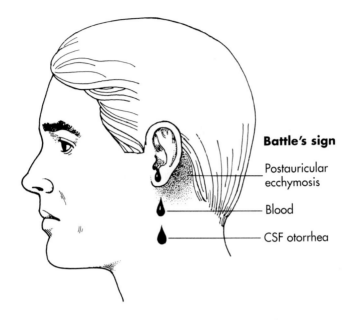

Battle's sign

Postauricular
ecchymosis

Blood

CSF otorrhea

Figure 15–9. Basilar skull fracture: Battle's sign.

- Monitor drainage.
- Ensure tetanus prophylaxis.
- Consider antibiotic therapy.

Focal Brain Injuries

Contusion

A contusion is a bruise of the cortex of the brain, causing tissue alteration and neurologic deficit without hematoma formation (Figure 15-10). A significant alteration in consciousness occurs without localizing signs. Contusion usually is caused by a severe acceleration/deceleration force or severe blunt trauma to the head.

ASSESSMENT

- Decreased level of consciousness
- Loss of consciousness longer than 5 minutes
- Nausea and vomiting
- Hemiparesis
- Confusion or restlessness
- Speech difficulties
- Seizures

Figure 15–10. Computed tomograph: contusion. *(Courtesy Laurence Cromsell, MD, Department of Radiology, Dartmouth-Hitchcock Medical Center, Lebanon, NH.)*

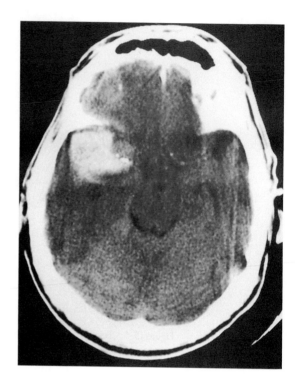

DIAGNOSIS

- History for event
- Clinical observation
- CT scan

THERAPEUTIC INTERVENTIONS

- Admit patient for close observation.
- Administer antiemetics as prescribed.
- Administer intravenous fluids judiciously to avoid fluid overload.

Intracranial Hemorrhage/Hematoma

An intracranial hemorrhage is bleeding between the skull and the meningeal layers or within the brain tissue itself. In all cases of head trauma, clinical personnel should observe the patient carefully for associated injuries.

Acute Epidural Hematoma

An epidural hematoma (below the skull and above the dura mater in the epidural space) is usually arterial (Figure 15-11). Epidural bleeding is a rare type of intracranial hemorrhage that occurs in approximately 2% of all persons with head injuries.[10] Epidural bleeding usually

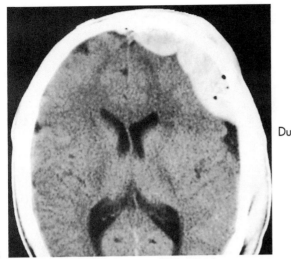
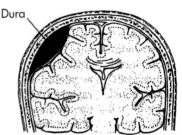

Dura

A

B

Figure 15–11. Acute epidural hematoma. **A,** CT scan (Computed tomograph). **B,** Schematic drawing. *(A courtesy Laurence Cromsell, MD, Department of Radiology, Dartmouth-Hitchcock Medical Center, Lebanon, NH. B From Urden LD, Stacy KM, Lough ME:* Thelan's critical care nursing: diagnosis and management, ed 5, *St Louis, 2006, Mosby.)*

results from rupture of the middle meningeal artery or from a tear of the dural sinus. Death may be rapid because the nature of the bleeding (arterial) precipitates an uncal herniation. An epidural hematoma may be associated with a skull fracture in the temporal or parietal region near the middle meningeal artery. Many patients, however, have no evidence of a skull fracture. The mortality is 25% to 50%; there is an equally high rate of morbidity.

ASSESSMENT

- Possibly loss of consciousness, followed by lucid interval, followed by another period of unconsciousness
- In conscious patient, complaint of severe headache
- Contralateral hemiparesis
- Possibly fixed, dilated pupil on ipsilateral side as hemorrhage
- Seizures
- Bradycardia
- Systolic hypertension

Acute Subdural Hematoma

A subdural hematoma results from bleeding between the dural and the arachnoidal layers of the meninges, usually caused by a torn bridging vein or cortical artery (Figure 15-12). Subdural hematoma is usually venous and may be life-threatening. This hematoma is the most frequently seen type of intracranial bleeding. Subdural hematoma may occur instantly (acute) or may develop over a period of days to weeks (subacute or chronic), and it usually results from a

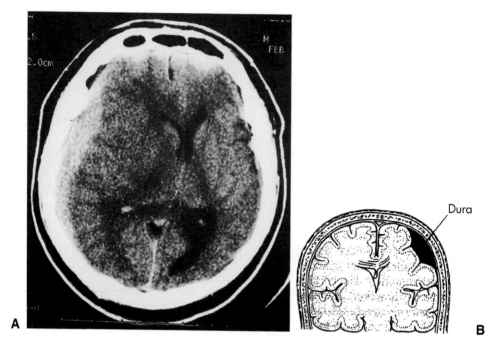

Figure 15–12. Acute subdural hematoma. **A,** Computed tomograph. **B,** Schematic drawing. (*A courtesy Laurence Cromsell, MD, Department of Radiology, Dartmouth-Hitchcock Medical Center, Lebanon, NH. B From Urden LD, Stacy KM, Lough ME:* Thelan's critical care nursing: diagnosis and management, ed 5, *St Louis, 2006, Mosby.)*

severe trauma to the head. Bleeding usually is gradual because the nature of the bleeding is venous. The brain is often extensively injured. If an acute subdural hemorrhage is detected in a child under 1 year of age, clinical personnel should suspect that the cause was severe shaking associated with child abuse (shaken baby syndrome). Elderly patients, chronic alcoholics, and those taking anticoagulant therapy are at high risk, even with a minor injury.

The prognosis for a patient with acute subdural hematoma is poor, with a 60% to 80% mortality rate. Mortality usually results from the severe underlying brain injury and extensive cerebral edema. If this condition is not treated rapidly, it will result in herniation and death.

ASSESSMENT

- Decreased level of consciousness
- Hypertension, bradycardia
- Fixed, dilated pupil or pupils
- Decreased motor function
- Hemiparesis
- Hyperreflexia
- Positive Babinski's reflex
- Possibly febrile in response to the inflammation caused by the injury

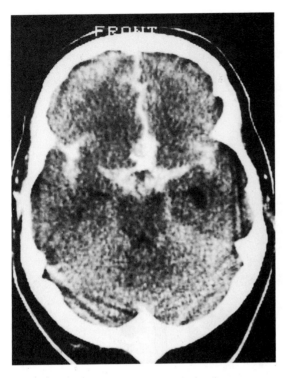

Figure 15–13. Computed tomograph: subarachnoid hemorrhage. *(Courtesy Laurence Cromsell, MD, Department of Radiology, Dartmouth-Hitchcock Medical Center, Lebanon, NH.)*

DIAGNOSIS

- CT scan

THERAPEUTIC INTERVENTIONS

- Surgical evacuation
- See summary on p. 181.

Subarachnoid Hemorrhage

A hemorrhage between the arachnoidal and pial meningeal layers is known as a subarachnoid hemorrhage (Figure 15-13). Subarachnoid hemorrhage may be the result of severe head trauma, severe hypertension, or a ruptured aneurysm. In head trauma, subarachnoid hemorrhage is often an incidental finding associated with other injuries. CSF will be bloody, and the patient will demonstrate signs of meningeal irritation.

ASSESSMENT

- Grand mal seizures
- Unconsciousness or restlessness
- Headache

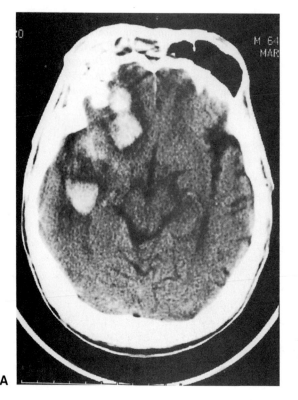

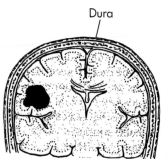

Figure 15-14. Intracerebral hemorrhage. **A,** Computed tomograph. **B,** Schematic drawing. *(A courtesy Laurence Cromsell, MD, Department of Radiology, Dartmouth-Hitchcock Medical Center, Lebanon, NH. B From Urden LD, Stacy KM, Lough ME:* Thelan's critical care nursing: diagnosis and management, ed 5, *St Louis, 2006, Mosby.)*

DIAGNOSIS

- CT scan

THERAPEUTIC INTERVENTIONS

- See summary on pp. 180-181.

Intracerebral (Brain) Hemorrhage

An intracerebral hemorrhage is a hemorrhage within the brain tissue itself (Figure 15-14). Intracerebral hemorrhage may occur at any location in the brain. The hemorrhage may result from a penetrating injury and may be a result of a laceration, especially in the basilar area where the skull has bony prominences, or may be a diffuse injury. With a closed head injury the hemorrhage is usually in the frontal or temporal lobe. Besides hemorrhage, there is usually an area of edema. Signs, symptoms, and prognosis depend on the size and location of the hemorrhage.

ASSESSMENT

- Hemiparesis
- Visual disturbances
- Unconsciousness
- Other neurologic findings

DIAGNOSIS

- CT scan

THERAPEUTIC INTERVENTIONS

- Minimize cerebral edema.
- See summary on pp. 180-181.

Diffuse Brain Injuries

Concussion

A concussion is an immediate and temporary disruption of the reticular activating system without structural defect and with possible microscopic bruising of the brain tissue (Figure 15-15). The mechanism of injury is an acceleration/deceleration force or a direct blow, usually resulting from blunt trauma. Temporary loss of consciousness results from the disruption of the reticular activating system. The patient with a concussion usually gives a history of unconsciousness or memory loss for the event, followed by consciousness. The period of unconsciousness is usually short.

ASSESSMENT

- History of head trauma
- Temporary amnesia for the event
- Complaint of headache
- Dizziness
- Nausea and vomiting
- Other neurologic deficits
- Identification of associated injuries

DIAGNOSIS

- History of event
- Clinical observation
- CT scan to rule out more serious injury

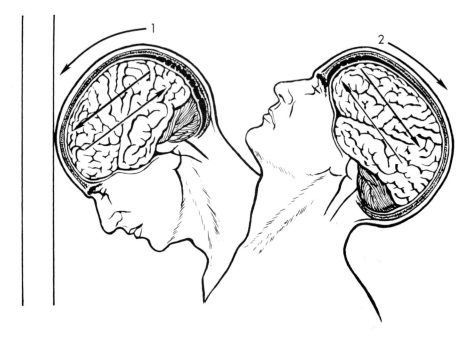

Figure 15–15. Coup *(1)*–contre coup *(2)* injury. *(Adapted from Urden LD, Stacy KM, Lough ME: Thelan's critical care nursing: diagnosis and management, ed 5, St Louis, 2006, Mosby.)*

THERAPEUTIC INTERVENTIONS

- Admit the patient for observation if the loss of consciousness is more than 5 minutes or if the patient is less than 12 years old. Otherwise, the patient may be sent home with careful aftercare instructions if there is someone reliable who can stay with the patient.
- Administer antiemetics, as required and prescribed.
- Administer nonnarcotic/nonaspirin analgesics, as prescribed.

Diffuse Axonal Injury (Shear Injury)

Diffuse axonal injury, also known as shear injury, is a tearing or shearing of axonal nerve fibers that results in diffuse brain damage. A more precise term is traumatic axonal injury because injury is scattered throughout the brain but not truly diffuse.[11] Coma usually occurs immediately and lasts for a prolonged period. The coma results from extensive damage to the white matter of the brain. Diffuse axonal injury has a high mortality rate, and the majority of survivors have major residual disabilities.[3]

ASSESSMENT

- History of head trauma with immediate decrease in level of consciousness
- Decerebrate/decorticate posturing
- Hypertension

- Hyperthermia
- Excessive sweating

DIAGNOSIS

- History
- Clinical observation
- MRI

THERAPEUTIC INTERVENTIONS

- Ensure airway, breathing, and circulation.
- Prevent secondary injury.
- See summary on pp. 180-181.

Penetrating Head Injuries

The incidence of penetrating head injuries is increasing. Gunshot wounds to the head have become a leading cause of death in many U.S. cities. Suicide by gunshot wound is another major problem. An impaled object, knife, or missile projected into the skull and cranial vault may or may not cause severe injury, depending on the type and velocity of the object causing the injury. The most common types of missile wounds are caused by bullets. These wounds are particularly devastating because the structural brain damage is extensive. The amount of damage depends on the site of the wound and the caliber, velocity, and angle of yaw of the missile. Lacerations, contusions, and destruction of tissue may occur from the missile itself or as a result of the energy dissipated by the missile. Bifrontal missile trajectories are almost inevitably fatal.

ASSESSMENT

- ABCs (airway, breathing, and circulation)
- Neurologic survey
- Examination for entrance and exit wounds
- Observation for associated injuries

DIAGNOSIS

- Physical examination
- CT scan

THERAPEUTIC INTERVENTIONS

- Maintain cervical spine alignment.
- Prevent movement.
- Do not remove the impaled object!

- Secure the impaled object.
- Control bleeding.
- Anticipate a neurosurgical consultation.
- Ensure tetanus prophylaxis.
- Administer antibiotics, as prescribed.

SUMMARY OF THERAPEUTIC INTERVENTIONS FOR ALL PATIENTS WITH SEVERE HEAD INJURIES

The initial priorities for any trauma patient are always airway with simultaneous cervical spine immobilization, breathing, and circulation. These ABC priorities are crucial for the head-injured patient. The goal is to maintain cerebral perfusion pressure at greater than 60 mm Hg and to prevent secondary injury from hypoxia or hypotension. Patients who experience episodes of hypotension or hypoxia or both have a significant increase in morbidity and mortality. Key interventions are summarized in this section and are based on recommendations of nationally accepted clinical guidelines.[6,8]

- Secure the airway, and ensure cervical spine immobilization.
- Endotracheal intubation using rapid-sequence technique is indicated in any patient with a GCS less than 8 or any patient who cannot protect his or her own airway.

This is the safest method of managing the airway for these patients. The drugs used for intubation should not affect ICP or cerebral perfusion pressure adversely. Induction agents that meet these criteria include thiopental, etomidate, and fentanyl. For paralysis, succinylcholine frequently is used, preceded by a dose of a nondepolarizing agent to prevent muscle fasciculations. Lidocaine 1.5 to 2 mg/kg IV push may be given 2 to 3 minutes before the succinylcholine to prevent an ICP surge during intubation.[4] Patients with a GCS of 9 or better should receive oxygen via a non-rebreather mask and should be monitored for early signs of hypoxemia and hypoventilation.

- Check mechanical ventilator settings.

The initial fraction of inspired oxygen should be 100%. The lowest possible level of positive end-expiratory pressure should be used because high levels can compromise cerebral venous return and therefore may increase ICP. The tidal volume should be set at 5 to 7 mL/kg. Maintain the partial pressure of carbon dioxide in arterial blood between 35 to 40 mm Hg. Hypoxia and hypercapnia must be avoided because of their negative effect on outcome.

- Obtain intravenous access, and initiate fluid replacement to correct or prevent hypotension, maintaining MAP at greater than 90 mm Hg.

The goal is to maintain adequate cerebral perfusion pressure. Intravenous fluids should include normal saline, lactated Ringer's solution, or packed red cells, and not 5% dextrose in water. Transfusions should be considered for a hematocrit less than 30%.

- Monitor neurologic status frequently, including GCS, pupillary response, level of consciousness, and vital signs. An arterial line may be placed to provide continuous monitoring of MAP.
- The use of prophylactic hyperventilation (pCO_2 less than 35 mm Hg) is no longer recommended.

Hyperventilation decreases ICP by causing cerebral vasoconstriction and subsequent decrease in cerebral blood flow. Cerebral blood flow during the first day after injury is less than half that of normal individuals; thus routine hyperventilation can compromise cerebral perfusion further and risk causing cerebral ischemia. Hyperventilation may be necessary for brief periods when there are signs of increased ICP. Mannitol, an osmotic diuretic, is recommended to reduce ICP. Mannitol has a plasma-expanding effect that decreases hematocrit, decreases blood viscosity, and increases cerebral blood flow and cerebral oxygen delivery. The maximum effect occurs 30 to 60 minutes after administration. Mannitol is more effective if administered in repeated boluses of 0.25 to 1 g/kg. Serum osmolarity should be kept below 320 mOsm/L, and serum electrolytes should be monitored closely. Loop diuretics, such as furosemide (Lasix), have been used as an adjunct to mannitol and are thought to decrease CSF production.[4] Steroids are no longer recommended for head injuries.

- Insert a urinary catheter, and record urine output hourly.
- Monitor laboratory results, especially those that can affect level of consciousness and seizure threshold (toxicology screen, electrolytes, and blood glucose).
- Maintain the patient's head in a midline position to ensure unobstructed jugular venous return. Elevate the head of the stretcher 15 to 30 degrees if possible to facilitate CSF drainage and decrease the incidence of ventilator-associated pneumonia.
- Prevent agitation and combativeness, which may lead to increased ICP.

Provide a quiet, low-stimulation environment. Administer intravenous sedation and/or pain medication. Monitor vital sign responses to medication. Consider the use of propofol, a sedative hypnotic agent with a rapid onset and short duration of action. This drug allows for periodic evaluations of the patient. Short-acting neuromuscular blocking agents also may be needed to prevent uncontrolled movement and straining.

- Control seizure activity.

For active seizures, lorazepam (Ativan) 2 to 4 mg may be given intravenously and titrated to effect. Phenytoin (Dilantin) 15 to 20 mg/kg may be administered for acute prophylaxis. Fosphenytoin (Cerebyx) may be used instead. Prophylactic anticonvulsant therapy is not recommended for the prevention of late posttraumatic seizures.[5]

- For patients with signs of increasing ICP, ICP monitoring will be needed and may be initiated in some emergency departments. The goal is to keep ICP less than 20 mm Hg. Use of an intraventricular catheter is the recommended monitoring modality. For the patient with increased ICP and a ventricular catheter, drainage of CSF will be instituted.
- Antibiotics are given to reduce the risk of infection in patients with open injuries.
- Blood glucose levels should be monitored closely and maintained between 80 to 120 mg/dL An elevated blood glucose level worsens cerebral edema.[4]
- Implement jugular bulb oximetry to measure the oxygen saturation in the jugular vein. This procedure involves the retrograde placement of a fiberoptic catheter and provides an indirect assessment of oxygen use by the brain (normal is greater than 55%). This procedure usually is reserved for the intensive care unit.
- Cautiously administer vasopressors to raise MAP and optimize cerebral perfusion pressure.
- Maintain normothermia. For every 1° C rise in body temperature, there is a 10% increase in metabolic rate.
- Two percent to 3% hypertonic saline at 30 to 50 mL/hr may be ordered to decrease ICP.[4] The solution pulls water out of the cells, decreases ICP, and increases cerebral perfusion pressure.
- Operative intervention may be necessary for definitive care and/or surgical decompression.
- Consider transfer to a facility that can provide more definitive care.

References

1. Myburgh JA: *Severe head injury.* Retrieved September 6, 2004, from www.harcourt-international.com/e-books/pdf/744.pdf
2. Marik P, Varon J, Trask T: Management of head trauma, *Chest* 122(2):699, 2002.
3. Langlois J, Kegler SR, Butler JA et al: Traumatic brain injury-related hospital discharges, *MMWR Surveill Summ* 52(4):1-20, 2003.
4. Bader M, Littlejohns L, editors: *AANN core curriculum for neuroscience nursing,* ed 4, St Louis, 2004, Saunders.
5. Vinas F, Pilitsis J: *Penetrating head trauma.* Retrieved April 3, 2005, from www.emedicine.com/med/topic2888.htm
6. *Guidelines for the management of severe traumatic brain injury: cerebral perfusion pressure,* New York, 2003, Brain Trauma Foundation. Retrieved November 2, 2006, from www2.braintrauma.org/guidelines/downloads/btf_guidelines_cpp_u1.pdf?BrainTrauma_Session=
7. Brain Injury Association of America: *Brain injury: the teenage years—understanding and preventing teenage brain injury.* Retrieved September 6, 2004, from www.biausa.org/publications/Teenage.Years%20_Edited_.pdf
8. Bullock MR, Chesnut RM, Clifton GL et al: *Management and prognosis of severe traumatic brain injury,* New York, 2000, Brain Trauma Foundation. Retrieved November 2, 2006, from www2.braintrauma.org/guidelines/downloads/btf_guidelines_management.pdf
9. Brain Injury Association of America: *Types of brain injury.* Retrieved April 5, 2004, from www.biausa.org/Pages/types_of_brain_injury.html
10. Liebeskind D: *Epidural hematoma.* Retrieved April 5, 2005, from www.emedicine.com/neuro/topic574.htm
11. Gaetz M: The neurophysiology of brain injury, *Clin Neurophysiol* 115:4-18, 2004.

Suggested Readings

Aarabi B, Alden TD, Chesnut RM et al: Management and prognosis of penetrating brain injury, *J Trauma* 51(2S):S1-S86, 2001.

Committee on Trauma, American College of Surgeons: Head trauma. In *Advanced trauma life support for doctors student manual,* ed 7, Chicago, 2004, The College.

Cushman JG, Nikhilesh A, Fabian TC et al: Practice management guidelines for the management of mild traumatic brain injury: the EAST Practice Management Guidelines Work Group, *J Trauma* 51:1016-1026, 2001.

Gabriel EJ, Ghajar J, Jagoda A et al: *Guidelines for prehospital management of traumatic brain injury,* New York, 2000, Brain Trauma Foundation. Retrieved November 2, 2006, from www2.braintrauma.org/guidelines/downloads/btf_guidelines_prehospital.pdf

Guidelines for the acute medical management of severe traumatic brain injury in infants, children, and adolescents, *Pediatr Crit Care Med* 4(3 suppl):S1-S71, 2003.

Hickey JV: Craniocerebral trauma. In Hickey JV, editor: *The clinical practice of neurological and neurosurgical nursing,* Philadelphia, 2003, Lippincott, Williams & Wilkins.

Howard PK: Head trauma. In Newberry L, editor: *Sheehy's emergency nursing principles and practice,* ed 5, St Louis, 2003, Mosby.

Josephson L: Management of increased intracranial pressure: a primer for the non-neuro critical care nurse, *Dimens Crit Care Nurs* 23:194-207, 2004.

CHAPTER 16

SPINE AND SPINAL CORD TRAUMA

DONNA W. LOUPUS AND CATHY M. GRAGG

Spine and spinal cord injuries can have profound implications. A spinal cord injury (SCI) with the resultant neurologic deficit is a catastrophic injury leading to enormous physical, psychological, social, and economic challenges for the patient, the affected family, and society. Although compared with other injuries, the incidence of spinal cord trauma is relatively low; it is estimated that between 7,600 and 10,000 persons are injured in the United States each year. Spinal cord injuries occur most often in males (82.1%) with the majority of injuries (57%) happening between the ages of 16 and 30. Most SCIs are associated with motor vehicle crashes. Falls, sports injuries, and assaults account for the remaining cases.[1]

Morbidity and mortality rates continue to improve for SCI patients but remain high. Mortality rates are significantly higher during the first year after injury. Factors that affect life expectancy include the level of the spinal cord lesion, the extent of the paralysis, the age of the patient at the time of injury, and the ability to survive the first few months after injury. The leading cause of death after SCI injury is respiratory complications, particularly pneumonia. Tetraplegic (quadriplegic) patients face a lifetime of complications, primarily those related to infection, respiratory compromise, and complications from decreased mobility.

Despite its low incidence, SCI remains a high-cost disability. For example, a person who sustains a complete quadriplegic injury at 25 years of age incurs an average of $710,275 in health care and living expenses in the first year after injury and an approximate lifetime direct cost of $2.8 million attributable to the injury. A person who sustains a complete paraplegic injury at 25 years of age incurs an average of $259,531 in first-year expenses and an average lifetime direct cost of $936,088.[2]

ANATOMIC CONSIDERATIONS

The function of the spinal column is to protect the spinal cord and provide vertical stability for walking. The spinal column is made up of 7 cervical, 12 thoracic, 5 lumbar, 5 fused sacral, and 4 fused coccygeal vertebrae (Figure 16-1). Although most of the vertebrae have similar structures, the first two are unique. The atlas, or C1, is a ringlike structure that articulates with the occiput and assists in providing for normal flexion and extension of the neck. The axis, or C2, articulates at the odontoid process with C1 and provides for some of the normal rotation of the head (Figure 16-2). The spine is supported by ligaments, which contribute significantly to spinal stability.

The spinal cord is a cylindric structure that passes through the bony spinal column. The spinal cord begins at the level of the foramen magnum and ends at the first or second lumbar vertebra. The cord is covered by the meningeal layers of dura mater, arachnoid mater, and pia mater and is protected by the meninges, vertebrae, and paravertebral muscles. Cerebrospinal fluid provides a cushioning effect for the spinal cord and provides a nutrient-rich environment

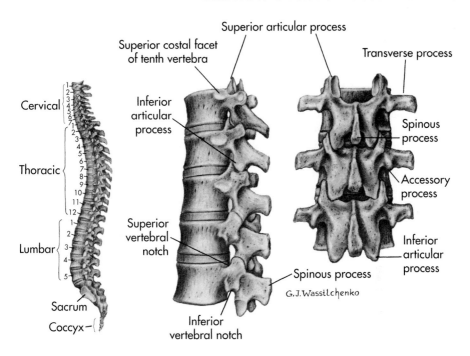

Figure 16-1. Vertebral column and anatomic structure of vertebrae. *(From Rudy EB:* Advanced neurological and neurosurgical nursing, *St Louis, 1984, Mosby.)*

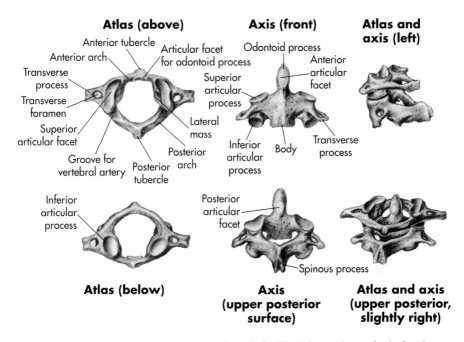

Figure 16-2. Atlas and axis vertebrae. *(From Ruby EB:* Advanced neurological and neurosurgical nursing, *St Louis, 1984, Mosby.)*

for nerve function. Spinal nerves, of which there are 31 pairs, exit the spinal cord bilaterally and consist of a ventral root (anterior) and dorsal root (posterior). The spinal nerves provide pathways for involuntary reactions in response to stimulation. The dorsal root is responsible for the transmission of sensory impulses. The ventral root transmits motor impulses. Therefore, each nerve is responsible for motor and sensory function. For example, the first cervical nerve supplies the sensory region of the occiput and is also partially responsible for motor function of the sternocleidomastoid muscle. The fourth cervical nerve involves sensation in the neck and shoulder region and is also partially responsible for diaphragmatic contraction. The thoracic nerves innervate portions of the upper arm, epigastrium, abdomen, and buttocks. Lumbar nerves are responsible for sensation and function of the lower extremities and also innervate the groin region. Sacral nerves supply the perianal muscles that control bowel and bladder function. The term *sacral sparing* refers to preservation of S3, S4, and S5 function. This is important because preservation of distal function indicates an incomplete injury and is associated with a more favorable prognosis.

Mechanism of Injury

Injury to the spinal cord and bony vertebrae can occur by a variety of mechanisms (Figure 16-3). Blunt trauma mechanisms are most common, though penetrating injuries are increasing in frequency. The predominant mechanisms of blunt trauma are as follows:

- Hyperextension: forcing the head posteriorly beyond normal limits, causing tension to the anterior longitudinal ligaments and compression of the posterior elements
- Compression (axial loading): the transmission of force in line with a straightened vertebral column

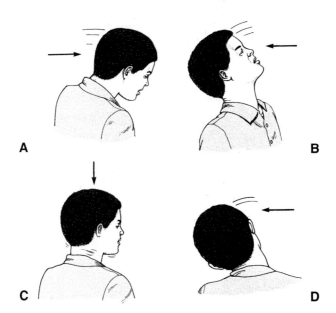

Figure 16-3. Injuries of the vertebrae and spinal cord may be caused by a variety of mechanisms of injury, forcing the head and neck into unusual positions. **A,** Hyperflexion. **B,** Hyperextension. **C,** Axial loading. **D,** Lateral bending.

- Flexion: forcing the head anteriorly beyond normal limits, causing compression of the bodies and disks anteriorly and disruption of the posterior ligaments and/or a posterior fracture
- Distraction: separation of the surfaces of the joint, resulting in a malalignment of the vertebrae
- Lateral bending: bending of the head and neck to one or both sides beyond normal limits

High-risk causes of injury include high-speed motor vehicle crashes or other high-energy blunt trauma, drowning or diving incidents, high falls (low falls in the elderly), or penetrating injuries to the spine.

SPINE INJURIES

Injuries can occur to the bony vertebrae from fracture, dislocation, and subluxation. Fractures generally are classified as simple, teardrop, compression, or comminuted. Definitions of common types of fractures follow:

- Simple fracture: usually occurs without neurologic compromise and affects spinous or transverse processes, pedicles, or facets
- Teardrop fracture: an avulsion of anteroinferior corner of cervical vertebral body by anterior ligament; often the result of diving into shallow water. This fracture is noted to be the most severe and unstable injury of the cervical spine.
- Compression fracture: occurs when a vertebral body is compressed, usually as a result of a hyperflexion injury
- Burst fracture/comminuted fracture: a shattering of the vertebral body. Because bone may be driven into the spinal cord, these fractures are more likely to result in neurologic compromise. Often, comminuted fractures result from axial loading in which the patient sustains a blow to the top of the head.
- Dislocation: dislocation of a vertebra occurs when one vertebra overrides another and is characterized by unilateral or bilateral facet dislocation. Atlantooccipital dislocations are produced by an avulsion of the atlas from the occiput and usually result in immediate death. Fractures can occur in association with dislocations, and in these serious injuries SCI is usually present.
- Subluxation: occurs when there is partial or incomplete dislocation of one vertebra over another. Partially dislocated vertebra often require placement of the patient into skeletal traction to realign the vertebrae.
- Jefferson fracture: a burst fracture of C1. This fracture may not result in any neurologic deficit but will require surgical intervention and stabilization.
- Hangman's fracture: a fracture through the arch of C1; named after the fractures characteristically found after a judicial hanging
- Odontoid fracture: involves the odontoid process of C2, also known as the *dens*.

ASSESSMENT

- Assess the airway, breathing, and circulation.
- Assess the injury event for high-risk characteristics. Assess the health history for preexisting spine disease or spinal surgery, which might place the spine at greater risk for injury.
- Palpate the entire spinal column, and check for pain, tenderness, deformity, and edema.
- Assess all four extremities for motor strength and weakness.
- Test for sensation of touch, pain, and proprioception. Note any areas of altered sensation.

HIGH-FREQUENCY NURSING DIAGNOSES FOR PATIENTS WITH SPINE OR SPINAL CORD TRAUMA

- Ineffective airway clearance
- Risk for aspiration
- Ineffective breathing pattern
- Ineffective tissue perfusion: spinal cord, generalized
- Ineffective thermoregulation
- Impaired urinary elimination
- Acute pain
- Disturbed sensory-perception: kinesthetic, tactile
- Risk for impaired skin integrity
- Impaired physical mobility
- Self-care deficit
- Risk for injury
- Risk for ineffective coping
- Risk for compromised family coping

From NANDA International: NANDA Nursing Diagnoses: Definitions & Classification, 2005-2006, Philadelphia, The Association.

- Consider the presence of associated injuries that increase the index of suspicion for spine injury, such as significant head/face injuries or altered mental status.
- For a list of common nursing diagnoses used for patients with spine and spinal cord trauma, see the Nursing Diagnoses box.

Clearance of the cervical spine to enable removal of immobilization paraphernalia has two components: clinical clearance and radiographic clearance. *Clinical clearance* is the process of assessing whether immobilization equipment can be removed based solely on clinical evaluation. Generally, only patients who are completely alert, oriented, and cooperative; have no spine pain or tenderness; do not have distracting injuries; and have a completely normal neurologic examination will not require radiographic clearance. Distracting injuries are difficult to define because every patient will have a unique threshold for what is considered "distracting." Typical distracting injuries include long-bone fractures, large lacerations or other major soft tissue injuries, large burns, and severe pain from any source. Two research-validated algorithms are available to guide clinical clearance decision making: the National Emergency X-Radiography Utilization Study (NEXUS) criteria[3] (Box 16-1) and the Canadian C-Spine Rule (CCR; Figure 16-4).[4] Radiographic clearance is based on the results of x-ray films, computed tomography scan, and/or magnetic resonance imaging.

DIAGNOSIS

- Clinical findings
- Radiographic clearance: Initial assessment begins with the lateral cervical spine film that must include all seven cervical vertebrae and the C7-T1 junction (Figure 16-5). However, a lateral cervical spine film alone is not sufficient to rule out injury. In addition, anteroposterior

Box 16-1	NEXUS CRITERIA FOR CERVICAL SPINE CLINICAL CLEARANCE

Does the patient have the following?
1. Absence of tenderness at the posterior midline of the cervical spine
2. Absence of a focal neurologic deficit
3. Normal level of alertness*
4. No evidence of intoxication*
5. Absence of clinically apparent pain that might distract the patient from the pain of a cervical spine injury*

•   •   •

If the patient satisfies all five criteria, the probability of cervical spine injury is low and x-ray films are not required.

(Data from Hoffman JR, Mower WR, Wolfson AB et al for the National Emergency X-Radiography Utilization Study Group: Validity of a set of clinical criteria to rule out injury to the cervical spine in patients with blunt trauma, *N Engl J Med* 343:95, 2000.)
*These criteria are not specifically defined; the examiner must use clinical judgment to evaluate the patient's ability to cooperate fully with the NEXUS assessment.

and odontoid views should be obtained. Anteroposterior views may best visualize injuries to the pedicles and facets; an odontoid, or open-mouth, view may best reveal fractures of the dens. If questions still exist regarding the stability of the cervical spine, computed tomography scans or flexion-extension films may be performed. Computed tomography scans provide superior fracture imaging. Flexion-extension views assist in identifying ligament damage but are contraindicated in patients with subluxation that has been identified in routine films, in patients with neurologic deficit, and in those not alert enough to cooperate during the test. Flexion-extension films should be used with caution during the acute stage of injury when spasm may mask ligament injury. Magnetic resonance imaging may assist in identifying soft tissue abnormalities resulting from hemorrhage, contusion, or compression of the cord. Patients with significant falls or jumps or those with a suggestive mechanism of injury should have thoracic and/or lumbar spine radiographs. If one spine fracture is identified, increased suspicion should be raised for the possibility of additional fractures, and the patient should undergo a radiograph of the entire spine.

THERAPEUTIC INTERVENTIONS

- Maintain spinal immobilization, or initiate immobilization if indicated, until a spinal column injury is ruled out. Complete immobilization includes a rigid cervical collar, bilateral head support devices (foam blocks or towel rolls), backboard, and straps to secure the patient in place. (See Chapter 28 for description of the immobilization procedure.)
- Note the time of placement on backboard and pad pressure points to prevent skin breakdown. Remove the backboard as soon as possible.
- Assist with placement of skeletal traction or definitive stabilization if needed.

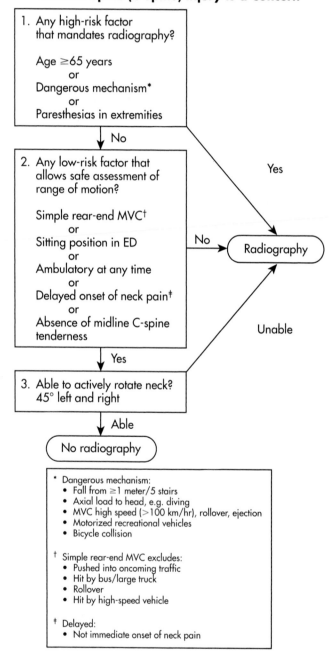

For Alert (Glasgow Coma Scale Score = 15) and Stable Trauma Patients Where Cervical Spine (C-Spine) Injury is a Concern

1. Any high-risk factor that mandates radiography?

   Age ≥65 years
   or
   Dangerous mechanism*
   or
   Paresthesias in extremities

   → No

2. Any low-risk factor that allows safe assessment of range of motion?

   Simple rear-end MVC†
   or
   Sitting position in ED
   or
   Ambulatory at any time
   or
   Delayed onset of neck pain‡
   or
   Absence of midline C-spine tenderness

   Yes

   No → Radiography

   → Yes

3. Able to actively rotate neck? 45° left and right

   Able

   No radiography

   Unable → Radiography

* Dangerous mechanism:
  • Fall from ≥1 meter/5 stairs
  • Axial load to head, e.g. diving
  • MVC high speed (>100 km/hr), rollover, ejection
  • Motorized recreational vehicles
  • Bicycle collision

† Simple rear-end MVC excludes:
  • Pushed into oncoming traffic
  • Hit by bus/large truck
  • Rollover
  • Hit by high-speed vehicle

‡ Delayed:
  • Not immediate onset of neck pain

Figure 16–4. The Canadian C-Spine Rule. *(From Stiell IG, Wells GA, Vandemheen KL et al: The Canadian C-Spine Rule for radiography in alert and stable trauma patients, JAMA 286:1846, 2001.)*

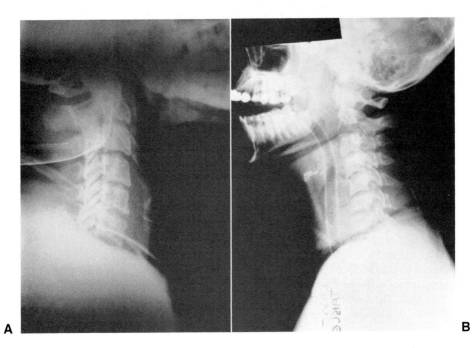

A   **B**

Figure 16–5 A, Inadequate cervical spine film: visualizing only six cervical vertebrae is inadequate. One must be able to visualize all seven cervical vertebrae. **B,** All seven cervical vertebrae can be seen here.

SPINAL CORD INJURIES

Injury to the spinal cord can occur following concussion, contusion, transection, or decreased perfusion resulting from blood vessel damage or hemodynamic instability. A direct effect of an SCI is spinal shock, which results in flaccid reflexes below the level of injury. Neurologic injury to the cord is described as complete or incomplete.

Complete Injury

A complete injury is defined as a total disruption of the motor and sensory function below the level of injury. This loss results from the interruption of the ascending and descending nerve tracts below the level of the lesion. Approximately 40% of all SCIs are complete. Complete SCI results in irreversible spinal cord damage; cervical injuries result in quadriplegia; and thoracic, lumbar, or sacral region injuries result in paraplegia.[1]

Incomplete Injury

An incomplete injury connotes some sparing of the sensory and/or motor fibers below the lesion. Incomplete lesions reflect a partial interruption of spinal cord function, manifested by a mixed loss of sensory or motor function. Multiple incomplete syndromes demonstrate varied neurologic deficits. The two most common incomplete cord lesions are the central cord syndrome and Brown-Séquard syndrome.

Figure 16–6. A, Central cord syndrome. **B,** Anterior cord syndrome. **C,** Brown-Séquard syndrome.

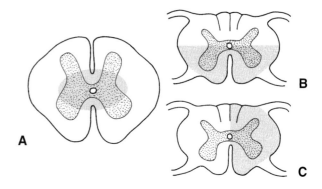

Central Cord Syndrome

Central cord syndrome results from injury to the central segments of the spinal cord in the cervical region (Figure 16-6, *A*). This syndrome commonly is seen in spinal injury in elderly patients who have cervical spinal canal stenosis and usually results from hyperextension. These patients have a motor deficit that is greater in the arms than in the legs and is most pronounced in the hands. The deficit may be subtle and easy to dismiss unless the examiner maintains a high index of suspicion. Sensory deficits vary, although greater sensory loss often is noted in the upper extremities. Bowel and bladder dysfunction also vary. Complete or partial recovery is possible, although residual neurologic dysfunction is common.

Anterior Cord Syndrome

The anterior spinal cord syndrome most commonly occurs with cervical cord injuries following flexion (Figure 16-6, *B*). Patients have loss of motor, pain, and temperature sensation below the level of the injury, but proprioception, sensory, and two-point discrimination remain intact.

Brown-Séquard Syndrome

Brown-Séquard syndrome most commonly is seen after a penetrating injury to the spinal cord (Figure 16-6, *C*). This syndrome is associated with a transverse hemisection of the spinal cord in which unilateral SCI occurs. The patient has loss of pain, tactile, and temperature sensation opposite the side of injury (contralateral) and loss of motor function, proprioception, sensory, and two-point discrimination on the same side as the injury (ipsilateral).

KEY CONCEPTS

Management of the patient with a real or suspected SCI includes reduction of the existing neurologic deficit and prevention of any further loss of function. Spinal injury should be suspected in patients who have sustained significant trauma, have an impaired level of consciousness after injury, complain of spinal pain or tenderness, or have motor or sensory impairment. The cervical spine is the most mobile portion of the spinal column and the most common site of SCI. If the cervical spine is unstable, it is at greater risk of causing SCI. Therefore, complete spinal immobilization of the injured patient is a paramount consideration. The patient's entire spine should be immobilized during the prehospital phase and throughout the assessment and resuscitation phases. Turning of these patients should be accomplished by logrolling while maintaining stabilization of the neck. Patients with SCI are at enormously high risk of skin breakdown because of the lack of sensory warning mechanisms, the inability to move, and circulatory changes. Therefore, immobilization time should be documented, and efforts to reduce this time should be implemented. Stabilization devices may be placed in the emergency department by the neurosurgical team. Several skeletal traction devices may be used to place the spine in alignment and relieve compression. These devices generally consist of tongs or rings attached to weights or of halo vest application. The tongs or rings are used in unaligned cervical injuries, whereas the halo vest is used in aligned cervical injuries. The amount of weight applied is determined by the location and type of injury. More permanent stabilization is achieved with surgical fixation/fusion. Rapid initiation or stabilization can relieve bony compression of the spinal cord and assist in maintaining spinal cord perfusion.

Respiratory compromise is a serious threat to the patient with a SCI. Cervical spine injuries have a high incidence of hypoxemia from hypoventilation. Hypoxemia can lead to further damage to the injured neurons and neuronal death. Patients who sustain an injury above the C4 level will have paralysis of the diaphragm and loss of phrenic nerve function. Patients with lesions in the upper cervical region often require early intubation and assisted ventilation. Patients with an injury within the C4-T9 levels may have respiratory compromise as a result of associated injuries, diaphragmatic or intercostal muscle paralysis, and/or aspiration. Increased cord edema, extension of injury, or fatigue may lead to respiratory compromise even in initially stable patients. The establishment of an airway in a patient with actual or potential SCI requires special consideration. Care must be taken not to manipulate the neck during establishment of the airway. Initially, a jaw thrust maneuver may be performed to open the airway. During intubation, an unstable cervical spine should be immobilized with manual immobilization. Complications from oral intubation are rare as long as manual, in-line stabilization is used. If available, fiberoptic bronchoscopy may be used.

Impairment of the sympathetic nervous system leads to loss of sympathetic innervation to the heart and loss of vasomotor tone and may cause neurogenic shock in patients with injuries above the T6 level. Vasodilation leads to pooling of blood intravascularly and consequently to hypotension. The loss of cardiac sympathetic tone leads to bradycardia. The combination of hypotension and bradycardia contributes to decreased spinal cord perfusion. This decrease in perfusion causes ischemia that can lead to further necrosis of the injured spinal cord segments. Therefore, management of neurogenic shock includes treating initial hypotension with fluid replacement and early use of vasopressors to reverse the loss of vasomotor tone. The absence of vasoconstriction and loss of the ability to shiver, conserve heat, and sweat results in an inability to control internal body temperature. The patient with SCI may exhibit poikilothermia, which is a condition in which the patient assumes the temperature of the environment.

Autonomic dysreflexia is an emergency in patients with SCI. Autonomic dysreflexia is a life-threatening condition that can occur in persons with SCI at T7 or above, resulting from an uninhibited sympathetic response of the nervous system to a noxious stimulus. The discharge of uninhibited sympathetic nervous system impulses as a result of noxious stimulation of sensory receptors below the level of SCI precipitates a hypersensitive episode (also known as autonomic hyperreflexia). Signs and symptoms may include sudden onset of hypertension with a systolic blood pressure greater than 15 mm Hg above baseline, severe headache, flushing, diaphoresis, piloerection, and congestion. Treatment may include placing the patient in the 90-degree sitting position, ensuring bladder emptying (check indwelling urinary catheter for kinking, or catheterize), evacuating the rectal vault, and checking skin for symptoms of breakdown. If there is no immediate resolution to the patient's condition, administer anti-hypertensive medication as directed. The syndrome usually is not a concern immediately after injury, but after that there is an ongoing risk of occurrence.

The patient who has sustained an SCI requires extensive psychological support. After SCI, many patients experience the same psychological stages as those noted in a dying patient.

Thus, patients and families may exhibit denial during the early phases of care. Those who ask about prognosis may be told that the patient has a serious injury and that it is too early to predict the long-term outcome because injury-related swelling obscures the true extent of injury and takes days to weeks (or longer) to resolve.

ASSESSMENT AND INTERVENTION

ASSESSMENT

- Assess the airway for patency and for the presence of edema, blood, vomitus, or foreign material.
- Determine respiratory rate, depth of breathing, tidal volume, use of accessory muscles, and oxygenation status.
- Check blood pressure and pulse rate.
- Check skin color, temperature, and moisture.
- Ascertain the mechanism of injury and the immediate history.
- Evaluate the entire spine for pain and tenderness.
- Evaluate motor strength and weakness using the standard five-point grading system (Box 16-2).
- Assess sensory changes, including sensation to touch, pain, temperature, presence of paresthesia, and proprioception. Begin at the area of no feeling and progress to the area of sensation (Figure 16-7).
- Evaluate rectal tone.
- Evaluate the patient for the presence of other injuries.
- Reassess the patient frequently for changes in vital signs or sensory-motor status.

NOTE: The strength of muscle groups of the upper and lower extremities should be graded systematically using a consistent scale to serve as a baseline for future neurologic assessment. When specifying the level of SCI, the accepted standard is to give the most caudal (inferior) location with normal motor and sensory function.

DIAGNOSIS

- Clinical evaluation
- Radiographic studies, especially magnetic resonance imaging
- Arterial blood gas

Box 16-2	MUSCLE STRENGTH GRADING SYSTEM

5 Normal
4 Active movement through range of motion against resistance
3 Active movement through range of motion against gravity
2 Active movement through range of motion with gravity eliminated
1 Palpable or visible contraction
0 Total paralysis

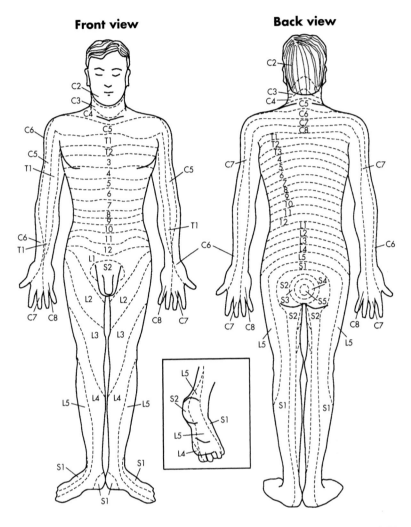

Figure 16-7. Dermatomes. *(From Cardona VD, Hurn PD, Bastnagel Mason PJ et al: Trauma nursing from resuscitation through rehabilitation, Philadelphia, 1994, Saunders.)*

THERAPEUTIC INTERVENTIONS

- Provide and/or maintain neck and spine immobilization.
- Maintain a patent airway; if needed, open the airway using a jaw thrust maneuver and suction.
- Provide supplemental oxygen, and consider early intubation to reduce the effects of hypoxemia.
- Provide aggressive respiratory therapy, including assisted coughing and suctioning to manage increased secretions.
- Maintain systolic blood pressure at greater than 90 mm Hg and mean arterial pressure at 85 to 90 mm Hg.

- Insert a urinary catheter, and monitor urinary output. (After SCI the bladder is areflexic-flaccid, and the patient will not be able to void.)
- Insert a nasogastric or orogastric tube to prevent abdominal distention and emesis and to reduce respiratory compromise and the possibility of aspiration of gastric contents. (After SCI an acute paralytic ileus may develop.)
- Administer methylprednisolone as soon as possible after injury, if consistent with local/institutional protocols. If the drug is initiated within 3 hours of injury, the initial dose is a 30 mg/kg bolus over 15 minutes followed 45 minutes later by 5.4 mg/kg per hour for 23 hours.[5,6] Between 3 and 8 hours after injury, the infusion should be continued for 48 hours.[6] After 8 hours, methylprednisolone is contraindicated.

NOTE: The risk-benefit analysis of high-dose methylprednisolone therapy is a matter of current debate. Those in favor of the regimen point out improvements in motor and sensory function, though small, identified by the large multicenter prospective randomized controlled trials (NASCIS, National Acute Spinal Cord Injury Study). Those opposed point out weaknesses in the original research, the questionable clinical significance of the minor improvements demonstrated, and the known adverse effects of steroids (increased incidence of pneumonia, wound infections, and sepsis). The "Guidelines for the Management of Acute Cervical Spine and Spinal Cord Injuries"[7] recommends methylprednisolone as "an option ... that should be undertaken only with the knowledge that the evidence suggesting harmful side effects is more consistent than any suggestion of clinical benefit." Some trauma centers have discontinued the use of high-dose methylprednisolone. Trauma clinicians should keep up to date by monitoring the literature on this topic.

- Document the time of placement on backboard, and pad pressure points to prevent skin breakdown. Minimize backboard time as much as possible.
- Maintain normothermia: cold patients should be warmed, hot patients cooled.
- Facilitate early neurosurgical consultation and more definitive stabilization.
- Provide psychological support.
- Anticipate transfer to a level I or II trauma center or SCI center.

FUTURE DIRECTIONS

Care of the patient with SCI has improved dramatically over the past 2 decades. Future therapy will include improved pharmacologic interventions aimed at increased preservation of neurologic function and enhanced neural regeneration. However, prevention will always be the most important strategy for addressing the problem of spine injuries and SCI.

References

1. Barker E: Consequences of traumatic spinal cord injury. In Nelson A, Zejdlik CP, Love L, editors: *Nursing practice related to spinal cord injury and disorders: a core curriculum,* Jackson Heights, NY, 2001, Eastern Paralyzed Veterans Association.
2. National Spinal Cord Injury Statistical Center: *Spinal cord injury: facts and figures at a glance, June 2005.* Retrieved January 10, 2006, from the Spinal Cord Injury Information Network, www.spinalcord.uab.edu/show.asp?durki=21446
3. Hoffman JR, Mower WR, Wolfson AB et al for the National Emergency X-Radiography Utilization Study Group: Validity of a set of clinical criteria to rule out injury to the cervical spine in patients with blunt trauma, *N Engl J Med* 343:95, 2000.
4. Stiell IG, Wells GA, Vandemheen KL et al: The Canadian C-Spine Rule for radiography in alert and stable trauma patients, *JAMA* 286:1846, 2001.

5. Bracken MB, Shepard MJ, Collins WF et al: A randomized, controlled trial of methylprednisolone or naloxone in the treatment of acute spinal-cord injury: results of the Second National Acute Spinal Cord Injury Study, *N Engl J Med* 322:1405-1411, 1990.

6. Bracken MB, Shepard MJ, Holford TR et al: Administration of methylprednisolone for 24 or 48 hours or tirilazad mesylate for 48 hours in the treatment of acute spinal cord injury, *JAMA* 277:1597-1604, 1997.

7. Guidelines for the management of acute cervical spine and spinal cord injuries, *Neurosurgery* 50(3 suppl):S1-S198, 63, 2002. Also available from www.spineuniverse.com/displayarticle.php/article2081.html

Suggested Readings

Hugenholtz H, Cass DE, Dvorak MF et al: High-dose methyprednisone for acute closed spinal cord injury: only a treatment option, *Can J Neurol Sci* 29:227-235, 2002.

Karlet MC: Acute management of the patient with spinal cord injury, *Int J Trauma Nurs* 7:43-48, 2001.

Kwon BK, Tetzlaff W, Grauer JN et al: Pathophysiology and pharmacologic treatment of acute spinal cord injury, *Spine J* 4:451-464, 2004.

Schreiber D: *Spinal cord injuries.* Retrieved January 10, 2006, from www.emedicine.com/emerg/topic553.htm

Facial and Eye, Ear, Nose, and Throat Trauma

Maureen M. Cullen

Facial Injuries

Facial injuries may cause severe airway obstruction and may be a major cause of deformity. Soft tissue and bone structure damage to the face may result from motor vehicle crashes (Figure 17-1), sports injuries, domestic violence, and other injuries that cause blunt and

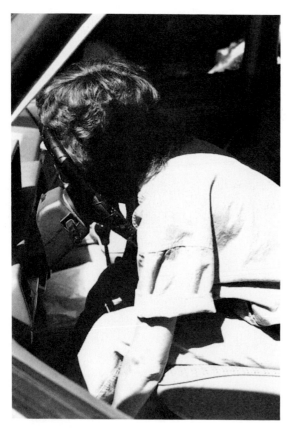

Figure 17–1. Soft tissue and bone structure damage of the face may result from motor vehicle crash.

penetrating trauma to the face. Patients who suffer maxillofacial injuries as a result of blunt trauma should be maintained with cervical spine immobilization until clearance is assured and should be monitored closely for airway patency.

ASSESSMENT

Clinical personnel should always conduct a thorough examination of the soft tissue and bony structures of the entire head and face, including the inside of the mouth, nose, and ears. Anticipate the following:

- Airway compromise with potential aspiration
- Cervical spine injury
- Hemorrhage
- Decreased level of consciousness because of intracranial bleeding and increased intracranial pressure
- Cerebrospinal fluid leak from the nose (rhinorrhea) or ear (otorrhea) or complaint of salty taste in throat
- Eye trauma
- Malocclusion of teeth
- Facial asymmetry
- Pain on palpation

Nursing diagnoses common to patients with facial or eye, ear, nose, and throat trauma are listed in the nursing diagnosis box.

DIAGNOSIS

- Clinical observation
- X-ray film or computed tomography (CT) scan

HIGH-FREQUENCY NURSING DIAGNOSES FOR PATIENTS WITH FACIAL OR EYE, EAR, NOSE, AND THROAT TRAUMA

- Ineffective airway clearance
- Risk for aspiration
- Impaired skin integrity
- Impaired tissue integrity
- Disturbed sensory-perception: visual
- Ineffective tissue perfusion: cerebral
- Acute pain
- Knowledge deficit: aftercare for injury
- Risk for infection
- Disturbed body image

From NANDA International: *NANDA nursing diagnoses: definitions & classification, 2005-2006*, Philadelphia, 2006, The Association.

THERAPEUTIC INTERVENTIONS

- Ensure the ABCs (airway, breathing, and circulation) while maintaining cervical spine immobilization.
- Monitor airway patency constantly, and maintain an open airway by suctioning as needed.
- Administer supplemental oxygen.
- Initiate intravenous therapy if indicated.
- Control bleeding with pressure dressings as needed.
- Provide tetanus prophylaxis and analgesia as prescribed.

Facial Lacerations

Blood loss can be significant from a facial laceration because of the dense vascularity of the soft tissue structures (Figure 17-2). The patient also may fear facial disfigurement as a result of this injury. Facial lacerations usually are caused by penetrating objects (such as glass, metal, and knives) or from severe, blunt trauma to the face.

ASSESSMENT

- Direct observation of the laceration
- Estimation of blood loss
- Exploration for foreign bodies
- Motor and sensory exam

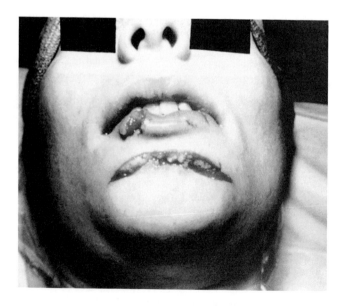

Figure 17-2. Facial laceration. *(Courtesy Daniel Cheney.)*

DIAGNOSIS

- Direct observation of the laceration
- X-ray exam for any retained foreign bodies

THERAPEUTIC INTERVENTIONS

- Apply local anesthesia (usually with epinephrine to control bleeding) as prescribed; regional anesthesia may be administered as appropriate.

NOTE: Do *not* use epinephrine for ear or nose lacerations. These areas are not highly vascularized and the vasoconstriction may cause *necrosis* because of the restriction of blood supply.

- Cleanse the wound with normal saline solution. If antibacterial solutions are used to cleanse the wound, be sure to rinse the wound thoroughly afterward.
- Carefully débride the wound to remove foreign substances, followed by suturing.
- Apply topical antibiotics as prescribed.
- Administer tetanus prophylaxis and analgesia as needed.
- Ensure that the patient understands discharge instructions.
- Consider discharge instructions regarding head trauma.

Special Considerations for Facial Trauma Patients

Patients with facial trauma require the following considerations:

- The vermilion border of the lips should be approximated carefully when sutured.
- Never shave eyebrows because they provide a landmark for repair and may not grow back.
- Approximate eyebrows as closely as possible before suturing.
- If a laceration is in the cheek area, the parotid duct and facial nerve should be checked carefully for disruption; if they are disrupted, they should be reanastomosed before the skin is sutured.
- Explain to the patient why sutures need to be reevaluated and removed on the prescribed day, because the patient may think it is better to leave them in longer, which may result in increased scarring.

For more information on lacerations, see Chapter 14.

Facial Fractures

In major multiple trauma, facial fractures are given a low priority except when a potential airway compromise is present. Cervical spine precautions and surveillance of the airway are paramount in the early assessment of facial trauma. The mechanism of injury is usually blunt trauma to the face caused by sports-related trauma, altercations, or motor vehicle crashes. Penetrating injury causes include gunshot wounds and stabbings.

Zygomatic Fractures (Tripod)

The zygomatic arch may be fractured in three places: at the arch, at the posterior half of the infraorbital rim, and at the zygomatic suture (Figure 17-3). This injury is caused by blunt trauma to the front and side of the face.

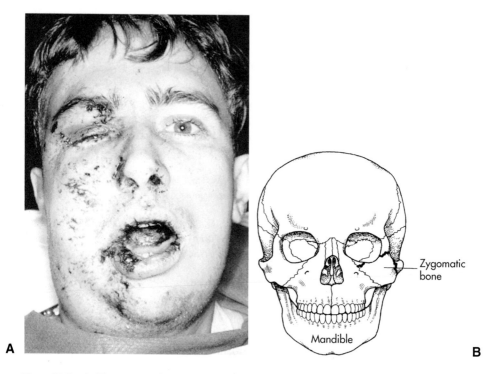

Figure 17-3. A, The zygoma frequently fractures in three places; this is known as a tripod fracture. **B,** Patient with a zygomatic fracture. *(Courtesy Daniel Cheney.)*

ASSESSMENT

- Primary survey, including spinal immobilization and neurologic function assessment
- Palpation of infraorbital rim fracture
- Step defect
- Periorbital ecchymosis
- Facial edema
- Exam for abnormality of ocular movements and visual acuity (may note an upward gaze)
- Enophthalmos (sunken globe)
- TIDES: *t*rismus, *i*nfraorbital hyperesthesia, *d*iplopia, *e*pistaxis (usually unilateral), and *s*ymmetry (absence of)
- Possible rhinorrhea
- Subconjunctival hemorrhage

DIAGNOSIS

- Palpable step defect of the inferior lateral orbital rim
- Clinical observation
- X-ray film (Water's view is best) or CT scan

THERAPEUTIC INTERVENTIONS

- Monitor the airway for patency.
- Elevate the head of the bed when spinal clearance is assured.
- Anticipate vomiting.
- Apply a cold pack.
- Consider preparing the patient for surgery.
- Administer tetanus prophylaxis and analgesia as needed.

Le Fort Fractures

Patients with Le Fort fractures often have a history of severe blunt trauma to the face, usually caused by a motor vehicle crash. Le Fort fractures may be bilateral or unilateral, and three types exist. Combination fracture patterns are not uncommon.

Le Fort I. A Le Fort I fracture is a fracture of the transverse alveolar process (Figure 17-4). Le Fort I is a horizontal fracture through the maxillary body that causes a detachment of the entire maxilla at the level of the nasal floor.

ASSESSMENT

- Epistaxis
- Malocclusion of teeth; possible fractured teeth
- History of blunt trauma to the midface, just below the nose
- Maxilla mobile with palpation (free floating maxilla)
- Laceration of the gingiva and/or lip

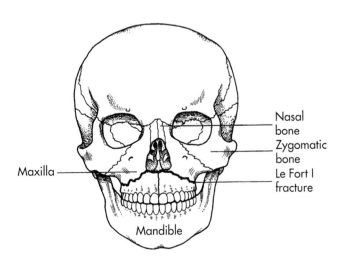

Figure 17–4. Le Fort I fracture.

DIAGNOSIS

- Clinical observation
- X-ray film or CT scan of facial bones

THERAPEUTIC INTERVENTIONS

- Check the ABCs (especially airway management).
- Apply a cold pack.
- Prepare the patient for surgery if internal fixation is needed.
- Place the patient in sitting position when spinal clearance is assured.
- Administer tetanus prophylaxis and analgesia as needed.

Le Fort II. A Le Fort II fracture is a pyramid-shaped, midfacial fracture segment extending up through the superior nasal area (in the shape of an oxygen delivery face mask; Figure 17-5).

ASSESSMENT

- Midface appears caved in
- If manipulated, nose moves with dental arch
- Nasal fracture with epistaxis
- Periorbital ecchymosis
- Telecanthus (widening between eyes)
- Subconjunctival hemorrhage
- Rhinorrhea
- History of blunt trauma to the midface

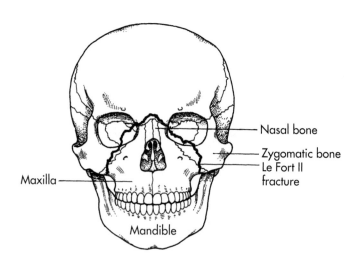

Figure 17–5. Le Fort II fracture.

DIAGNOSIS

- Clinical observation
- X-ray film (Water's view) or CT scan of facial bones

THERAPEUTIC INTERVENTIONS

- Check the ABCs (especially airway management) with cervical spine precautions.
- Apply a cold pack.
- Prepare the patient for surgery if open reduction and internal fixation is needed.
- Administer antibiotics intravenously, as prescribed, for infection prophylaxis.
- Administer tetanus prophylaxis and analgesia as needed.
- Place the patient in sitting position when spine clearance is assured.

Le Fort III. A Le Fort III fracture is a total craniofacial separation (Figure 17-6). Le Fort III is a potential airway emergency.

ASSESSMENT

- Flattened and elongated appearance of face
- Usually significant bleeding
- Massive facial edema and ecchymosis
- Patient often has loss of consciousness
- On manipulation, facial bones move without frontal bone movement
- Possible rhinorrhea
- History of blunt trauma to the face

DIAGNOSIS

- Clinical observation
- X-ray film (Water's view) and/or CT scan
- Extraocular muscle entrapment

THERAPEUTIC INTERVENTIONS

- Check the ABCs (especially airway management); consider securing airway patency with intubation as needed.
- Apply a cold pack.
- Prepare the patient for surgery if open reduction and internal fixation is needed.
- Administer antibiotics intravenously, as prescribed, for prophylaxis.
- Administer tetanus prophylaxis and analgesia as needed.

NOTE: Midface maxillofacial fractures also may be associated with cribriform plate fractures. Therefore, when a gastric tube is required, it should be placed orally.

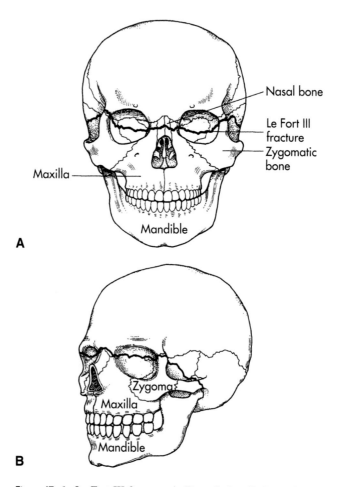

Figure 17–6. Le Fort III fracture. **A,** Frontal view. **B,** Lateral view.

Mandibular Fracture

Mandibular fractures are caused by severe blunt trauma commonly seen in sports-related injuries, motor vehicle crashes, altercations, and incidents of domestic violence (Figure 17-7). These fractures may affect any part of the mandible: the condyle, ramus, angle, body, symphysis, or the alveolar ridge. A mandibular fracture may be an open fracture if it involves the alveolar body. As a result of the shape of the mandible, more than 50% of the fractures are bilateral, so if one fracture is identified, one should always search for a second. Because the tongue is secured by muscles attached to the mandible, loss of control of the tongue and subsequent airway obstruction may occur. Trauma clinicians need to be scrupulous in the evaluation of the airway for compromise in patients with this injury. Keep in mind that the jaw is a strong joint and that if the mandible has been struck with enough force to fracture it, soft tissue injury and edema are probably significant.

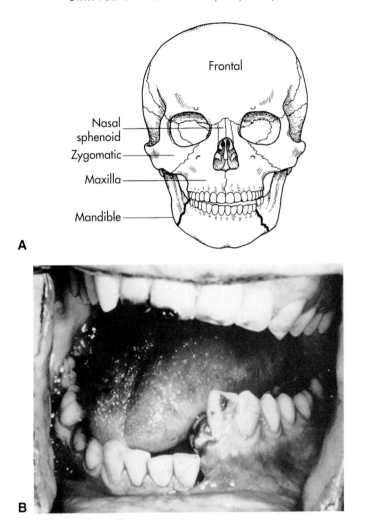

Figure 17-7. A, Mandible fracture. **B,** Fracture may be identified by gross deformity or more subtle malocclusion of teeth. *(Courtesy Daniel Cheney.)*

ASSESSMENT

- Airway compromise
- Observation of malocclusion of teeth
- Complaint of pain with jaw motion or tenderness on palpation
- Trismus
- Palpable fracture
- Soft tissue swelling with ecchymosis
- Malalignment of teeth and/or loose or missing teeth (risk of aspirated teeth)

DIAGNOSIS

- Clinical observation
- X-ray film, panoramic x-ray film, or CT scan
- Chest x-ray film as needed to observe for any aspirated teeth or dental fixtures

THERAPEUTIC INTERVENTIONS

- Check the ABCs (especially early airway management) with spinal immobilization.
- Provide frequent oral suctioning as needed.
- Apply a cold pack.
- Immobilize the patient with a Barton dressing (bulk wrap surrounding the head).
- Prepare the patient for surgery if open reduction and internal fixation is needed.
- Administer antibiotics intravenously, as prescribed, if an open fracture is present.
- Administer tetanus prophylaxis and analgesia as needed.

Dental Trauma

Chipped or Broken Teeth

Chipped or broken teeth most often are caused by direct trauma to the teeth. The teeth most commonly injured are the four front upper teeth.

ASSESSMENT

- Observations of chips or fractures
- Bleeding from the pulp
- Bleeding from the gums
- Associated head or facial trauma
- Observation for foreign bodies (teeth fragments) in airway or aspirated

THERAPEUTIC INTERVENTIONS

- Ensure airway clearance and check the ABCs.
- Cover exposed dental pulp to reduce pain.
- Obtain dental consultation, as ordered, if bleeding is from the pulp.

Avulsed Teeth

Teeth usually are avulsed or partially dislocated by blunt trauma to the mouth and directly to the teeth.

ASSESSMENT

- Absence of teeth or loose teeth with fresh wounds underlying

DIAGNOSIS

- Clinical observation
- Panoramic x-ray film

THERAPEUTIC INTERVENTIONS

- Ensure airway clearance and check the ABCs.
- Soak the tooth in milk, saline solution, or a commercially prepared tooth preservation solution, until dental consultation is available.
- A dental consult may be indicated for consideration of possible tooth reimplantation.

NOTE: If a tooth is missing as a result of trauma, a chest or abdominal radiograph is indicated to rule out aspiration or swallowing of the tooth (Figure 17-8).

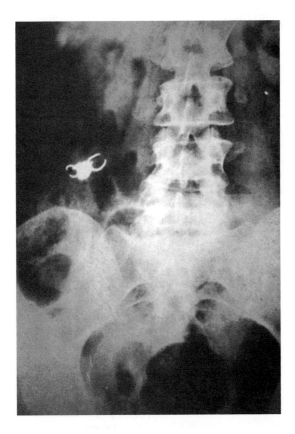

Figure 17–8. Look for dentures. Patient may swallow or aspirate dental appliances or fractured teeth. *(Courtesy Daniel Cheney.)*

EYE, EAR, NOSE, AND THROAT TRAUMA

Although not generally considered to be major trauma, injuries to the eyes, ears, and nose are common types of associated traumatic injuries. This chapter provides a brief review of some of the types of trauma that frequently are associated with major trauma.

Eye Trauma

If eye trauma is present, the patient should be assessed for other, more life-threatening injuries before focusing on the eye injury. The nurse may patch both eyes to minimize pain resulting from the trauma and to reduce the possibility of further injury by minimizing movement.

A majority of injuries to the eye are caused by industrial accidents that are blunt or penetrating. Other injuries may be caused by contact with an inflating air bag (Box 17-1). The nurse should obtain a thorough patient history; including mechanism of injury, the presence of foreign bodies or chemicals, the care given before arrival at the emergency department, presence of contact lenses, and any other medical history, especially that involving the eye, such as glaucoma or diabetes mellitus.

NOTE: Any patient involved in a motor vehicle collision with an air bag inflation should have visual acuity assessed, and eye irrigation may be required due to the exposure to the chemicals of the inflated air bag.

ASSESSMENT

- Assess visual acuity.
- Assess the eye by first examining the area around the eye.
- Check the eyelid and the orbital rim before examining the eye itself.
- Check pupillary response and accommodation to light; document pupil size.
- Check for contact lenses and remove them if present.
- Keep the corneas moist.
- Prepare for a slit lamp exam or fluorescein exam, as needed, if a potential foreign body or sensation of foreign body exists.
- Check the eye pH if the possibility of chemical exposure is a concern (i.e., air bag deployment).

Box 17-1	**AIR BAG–RELATED EYE INJURIES**

Angle recession
Chemical keratitis
Corneal abrasions and edema
Eyelid contusion, abrasion, laceration
Globe rupture
Hyphema
Lens subluxation
Periorbital fractures
Retinal tear, detachment, or hemorrhage
Scleral rupture
Vitreous hemorrhage

DIAGNOSIS

- Clinical findings

THERAPEUTIC INTERVENTIONS

- Interventions depend on the specific findings.
- Perform eye irrigation, as needed, when any exposure to chemicals exists.
- An ophthalmologic consultation or referral may be needed for significant injuries.
- Patch the eye with a metal shield if suspicion of direct trauma or impeded foreign body exists.

Orbital Rim Injury

Orbital rim injuries occur as a result of blunt or penetrating trauma to the orbital rim area.

ASSESSMENT

- Inspect the eye for periorbital ecchymosis and edema.
- Palpate the eye for tenderness and deformity (step-off).
- Check visual acuity.
- Assess patient for visual disturbances such as diplopia.
- Check for extraocular motion for potential nerve entrapment.
- Thoroughly assess the patient for other associated injuries, especially to the globe of the eye.
- Assess patient for a fracture of the prominent supraorbital rim.
- Inspect patient for a cerebrospinal fluid leak.
- Check for subconjunctival hemorrhage.

DIAGNOSIS

- Clinical observation
- X-ray film or CT scan

THERAPEUTIC INTERVENTIONS

- Apply an ice pack.
- Elevate the head if spine clearance is assured to help reduce swelling.
- Administer tetanus prophylaxis and analgesia as needed.
- Treat for specific fractures.
- Provide aftercare instructions for head trauma.

Eyelid Trauma

With eyelid trauma there is usually a history of penetrating trauma or other associated major trauma to the face or body (Figure 17-9).

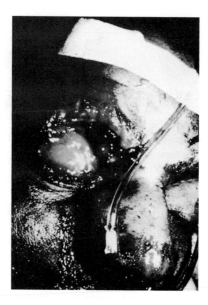

Figure 17–9. Avulsed eyelid. *(Courtesy Daniel Cheney.)*

ASSESSMENT

- Assess for visual acuity, if possible.
- Check for a foreign body.
- Check for eversion of the eyelid.
- Assess eye for a laceration of the lacrimal duct.
- Check for other associated trauma.

DIAGNOSIS

- Clinical observation

THERAPEUTIC INTERVENTIONS

- Irrigate the wound with normal saline solution.
- Early approximation of edges, before edema develops, usually is performed.
- A plastic surgery consultation may be needed if the patient has a major deformity, any tissue missing, or a duct injury.
- Administer tetanus prophylaxis and analgesia as needed.

Nonpenetrating Blunt Trauma to the Globe

Blunt trauma to the globe may cause aqueous humor to compress the iris and result in a hemorrhage or hyphema in the anterior chamber of the eye (Figure 17-10).

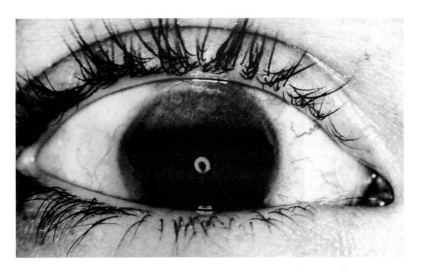

Figure 17-10. Traumatic hyphema that obscures the iris. The blood in the anterior chamber has not clotted but, during rest, forms a fluid meniscus. *(From Newell FW:* Ophthalmology: principles and concepts, *St Louis, 1996, Mosby.)*

ASSESSMENT

- Test visual acuity.
- Observe patient for hyphema in the anterior chamber of the eye.

DIAGNOSIS

- Clinical findings

THERAPEUTIC INTERVENTIONS

- Limit patient to quiet activity or bed rest with the head of the bed elevated 45 degrees.
- Consider the need for sedation in agitated or restless patients.
- Patch affected eye with a Fox shield.
- Obtain an ophthalmologic consultation.
- Monitor patient for increased intraocular pressure.

Blowout Fracture

A blowout fracture results from blunt trauma to the globe of the eye, causing increased intraocular pressure and a resultant fracture of the orbital floor.

ASSESSMENT

- Test visual acuity.
- Check the anterior chamber of the eye for the presence of leveling of blood (hyphema).
- Check the cornea for abrasion (with fluorescein if needed).
- Assess patient for periorbital hematoma.
- Monitor patient for subconjunctival hemorrhage.
- Assess patient for enophthalmos.
- Check for periorbital edema and/or any bony structure step-off.
- Monitor patient for complaints of diplopia.
- Check for limited extraocular movements (usually upward gaze) caused by trapping of the inferior rectus muscle or the inferior oblique muscle.

DIAGNOSIS

- Clinical findings
- X-ray film or CT scan

THERAPEUTIC INTERVENTIONS

- Apply a cold pack.
- Administer antibiotic prophylaxis as prescribed.
- Prepare the patient for surgery if appropriate.
- Patch the affected eye.
- Administer tetanus prophylaxis and analgesia as needed.

Penetrating Injuries to the Globe of the Eye

Perforation by a sharp object causes direct trauma and possible tissue evisceration to the globe of the eye (Figure 17-11).

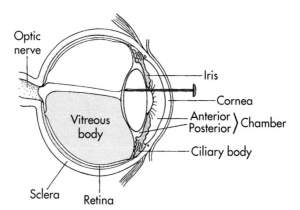

Figure 17–11. Do not remove the impaled object from the globe because this could result in the loss of humor from the anterior and posterior chambers.

ASSESSMENT

- Observation of the impaling object (do not remove; should be secured in place)
- Observation of the perforation

DIAGNOSIS

- Clinical observation
- Observation of the opaque object on x-ray film

THERAPEUTIC INTERVENTIONS

- Secure the impaled object.
- Patch the eyes bilaterally to minimize eye movement.
- Obtain an ophthalmologic consultation.
- Administer antibiotics intravenously as prescribed.
- Administer tetanus prophylaxis and analgesia as needed.

Ear Trauma

When caring for a patient with trauma to the ear, the goal is to repair current damage and prevent further damage. Circulation to the structures of the ear is poor, unlike the other structures of the head. Therefore much care should be taken to protect the injuries from possible necrosis or infection.

General guidelines for therapeutic intervention are as follows:

- If using lidocaine, use it *without* epinephrine.
- Splint the ear posteriorly with soft padding, and protect the inner areas from pressure and necrosis.
- If blood is draining from the inner ear, assume that it is mixed with cerebrospinal fluid and rule out a basilar skull fracture (do not pack). See Chapter 15 for more discussion of basilar skull fractures.

Simple Laceration

A simple laceration is the most common type of ear injury. The laceration usually is caused by a sharp penetrating object but also may result from blunt trauma to the ear.

ASSESSMENT

- Observe patient for bleeding from ear structures.
- Assess patient for any associated closed head injury symptoms.

DIAGNOSIS

- Clinical observation

THERAPEUTIC INTERVENTIONS

- Irrigate the wound with normal saline, cleanse it, and débride it.
- The physician will reanastomose the edges of the cartilage and suture the skin.
- Cover the wound with a thin layer of topical antibiotic ointment, and dress the wound with a protective dressing, being sure to pad the pinna.
- Administer tetanus prophylaxis and analgesia as needed.

Hematoma of the Pinna

Hematoma of the pinna results from impact to the pinna of the ear from a blunt object.

ASSESSMENT

- Visible hematoma

DIAGNOSIS

- Clinical observation

THERAPEUTIC INTERVENTIONS

- Prepare patient for the administration of local anesthesia.
- Assist with aspiration of the hematoma.
- Prepare for drain placement to facilitate drainage, if indicated.
- Apply a small pressure dressing on the local area of the injury only, if needed.

Traumatic Amputation of the Ear

Traumatic amputation of the structures of the outer ear (also known as auriculectomy) usually occurs as a result of a knife fight, a human bite, or of the person being ejected from a car through a windshield.

ASSESSMENT

- Observation of the amputation and the amputated segment

DIAGNOSIS

- Clinical observation

THERAPEUTIC INTERVENTIONS

- Ensure proper care of the amputated piece (see Chapter 14).

- Prepare the patient, if appropriate, for reanastomosis of cartilage and skin, which must be done with meticulous detail and usually is done in surgery.
- Administer antibiotics intravenously, if prescribed.
- Administer tetanus prophylaxis and analgesia as needed.

Nose Trauma

Injury to the nose may be associated with major trauma or may be caused by interpersonal violence, sports injuries, and falls. This type of injury frequently occurs with facial fractures and can be caused by blunt and penetrating trauma.

Epistaxis

Traumatic epistaxis (nosebleed) may occur as the result of blunt or penetrating trauma to the nose. Trauma usually results in anterior epistaxis, caused by disruption of the anterior and inferior turbinates at the area of Kiesselbach.

ASSESSMENT

- Assessment of the source of the bleeding anteriorly (most common) or posteriorly (ensure airway clearance)
- Observation of a deformity of the nose
- Other associated facial trauma
- Other associated trauma

DIAGNOSIS

- Clinical observation

THERAPEUTIC INTERVENTIONS

- Ensure the ABCs with particular attention to airway clearance.
- Reassure the patient.
- Begin volume replacement, if indicated.
- Check for anterior bleeding; apply direct pressure.
- Slightly hyperextend neck (after cervical spine injury has been ruled out).
- Suction clots from the nose.
- Identify bleeding sites.
- Apply a vasoconstrictor agent (such as phenylephrine [Neo-Synephrine]), if prescribed.
- Prepare the patient for procedures to manage the epistaxis as indicated: these include cauterization with silver nitrate, nasal packing, posterior packing for posterior bleeding, and/or angiography with selective embolization.

Nasal Fractures

A nasal fracture usually is caused by a blunt force to the front or side of the nose.

ASSESSMENT

- Observe nose for swelling and nares patency.
- Assess nose for anterior and posterior bleeding.
- Observe nose for a deformity.
- Palpate nose for crepitus.
- Palpate nose for a fracture.
- Assess nose for a septal hematoma.

DIAGNOSIS

- Clinical observation
- X-ray film (initial x-ray films may not be necessary if there is no evidence of malalignment and the nares are patent)

THERAPEUTIC INTERVENTIONS

- Apply a cold pack.
- Apply a splint if needed.
- Control bleeding with pressure.
- Administer a local anesthetic (usually topical and subcutaneous) as prescribed.
- As appropriate, prepare the patient for the fracture to be set, or explain that reduction may be performed at a later date.
- Prepare for draining of a septal hematoma, if needed.
- Pack the nose (bilaterally if the septum is fractured).
- Administer tetanus prophylaxis if needed.

Neck Trauma

Neck trauma may be caused by a blunt or penetrating mechanism and is considered a true emergency. The neck is unique because it contains many vital structures (airway, gastrointestional, vascular, and neurologic) in a small anatomic space.

Laryngotracheal Injuries

A fractured larynx and other laryngeotracheal injuries usually result from blunt trauma (Figure 17-12). These injuries most commonly occur by a victim's neck striking the steering wheel or dashboard during a vehicular crash. Other causes include sudden deceleration exerted by a rope or line, high-velocity impact such as with a hockey puck, and direct blows such as may be experienced with a karate chop.

ASSESSMENT

- Check the ABCs, ensuring spinal immobilization (special attention to airway for patency).
- Hoarseness
- Cough with hemoptysis
- Progressive respiratory stridor (airway loss may occur precipitously)

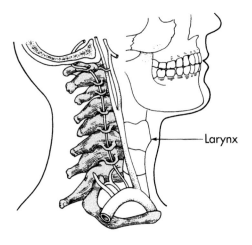

Figure 17–12. A laryngeal fracture usually results from blunt trauma to the neck.

Larynx

- Respiratory distress
- Subcutaneous emphysema
- Pain and/or tenderness
- Flattened-appearing larynx

DIAGNOSIS

- Clinical observation
- X-ray film or CT scan
- Direct observation with fiberoptic laryngoscopy may be the safest option in securing the airway to prevent catastrophic laryngeal detachment.

THERAPEUTIC INTERVENTIONS

- Closely check the ABCs (especially airway management).
- Prepare for endotracheal intubation (fiberoptic route preferred when available).
- Prepare for cricothyrotomy (always have a cricothyrotomy set at the bedside).
- Prepare for tracheostomy.

NOTE: The need to secure the airway must be balanced against the risk for further compromise in patients with altered anatomy. For stable or semistable patients, surgery may be the best plan. Endotracheal intubation should be avoided if possible, but if attempted, it must be performed gently. Cricothyrotomy is the next option; if the nature of the injury precludes this procedure, a formal tracheostomy is necessary.

- Administer high-flow humidified oxygen therapy.
- Administer broad-spectrum antibiotics, as prescribed.
- Prepare the patient for surgical repair.
- Have the patient rest the voice.
- Administer steroids if prescribed.
- Administer tetanus prophylaxis and analgesia as needed.

Penetrating Wounds

Penetrating objects, such as a bullet or a knife blade, easily can cause trauma to the structures of the neck. The patient's presentation will vary depending on the type of object that has penetrated, the angle and force of the penetrating object, and the structures involved with the injury.

Low injuries (zone I) may involve the major thoracic vessels, esophagus, thyroid gland, or trachea. High injuries (zone III) may affect the internal carotid and/or vertebral arteries, pharynx, spinal cord, and/or salivary glands. The main portion of the neck (zone II) is the most commonly injured, and any of the structures of the neck may be involved (Figure 17-13).

ASSESSMENT

- Obvious wound to neck
- Airway obstruction
- Signs and symptoms of hypovolemic shock
- Presence of expanding hematoma
- Potential associated spine or spinal cord injury
- Subcutaneous emphysema
- Presence of bruit

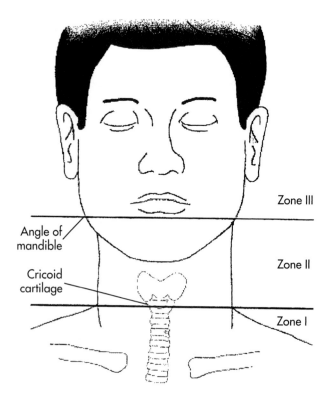

Figure 17-13. Zones of the neck. *(From Marx JA, Hockberger RS, Walls RM, editors:* Rosen's emergency medicine: concepts and clinical practice, *ed 6, St Louis, 2006, Mosby.)*

DIAGNOSIS

- Clinical observation
- Arteriography
- Possible exploratory surgery

THERAPEUTIC INTERVENTIONS

- Control the ABCs with spinal immobilization, if appropriate.
- Manage the airway.
- Manage breathing.
- Control bleeding with direct pressure.
- Secure impaled object in place: do not remove it.
- Establish intravenous lines of lactated Ringer's solution or normal saline solution.
- If appropriate, prepare the patient for emergency surgery.

Blunt Vascular Injuries

Blunt vascular injuries may have significant sequelae, including exsanguination, stroke, air embolism, and airway obstruction. Diagnosis is a challenge. Some patients have little external evidence of trauma, and the onset of symptoms may be delayed until thrombosis or emboli develop and stenose or occlude an artery. Blunt vascular injuries most commonly occur as a result of the victim being involved in a motor vehicle collision. Injury mechanisms involving severe cervical hyperextension, hyperrotation, or hyperflexion are suggestive of risk, as are basilar skull fractures involving the carotid canal or cervical spine fractures involving the foramen transversarium (through which the vertebral artery passes). The most common vessel injured is the internal carotid artery.

ASSESSMENT

- Soft tissue trauma
- Hematoma
- Bruit
- Thrill
- Diminished pulse
- Decreased level of consciousness
- Neurologic deficits resembling transient ischemic attack or stroke such as paresthesias, plegia, or paresis

DIAGNOSIS

- Initial CT scan may be normal
- Arteriography
- Magnetic resonance imaging/magnetic resonance angiography

THERAPEUTIC INTERVENTIONS

- Control the ABCs, especially airway management.
- Apply direct pressure to control bleeding.
- Administer an anticoagulant if possible and if prescribed.

- Prepare the patient for surgical revascularization or endovascular interventional therapy depending on the injury.

Esophageal Injuries

Esophageal injuries may result from blunt or penetrating trauma. These injuries are rare and often difficult to diagnose, and the clinician must have a high index of suspicion. In blunt trauma, isolated esophageal injury is uncommon; rather, it usually occurs in combination with laryngotracheal and/or spinal injuries.

ASSESSMENT

- Pain and/or tenderness
- Dysphagia
- Drooling
- Subcutaneous emphysema and/or crepitus
- Air in the mediastinal or fascial spaces

DIAGNOSIS

- Soft tissue neck x-ray films
- Continual airway observation for potential compromise
- Chest x-ray film that demonstrates air in the mediastinal space
- Contrast esophagography
- Rigid and flexible esophagoscopy

THERAPEUTIC INTERVENTIONS

- Prepare the patient for surgical repair.

Suggested Readings

Britt LD, Peyser MB: Penetrating and blunt neck trauma. In Mattox KL, Feliciano DV, Moore EE, editors: *Trauma,* ed 4, New York, 2000, McGraw-Hill.

Cantrill SV: Face. In Marx J, editor: *Rosen's emergency medicine: concepts and clinical practice,* vol 1, ed 5, St Louis, 2002, Mosby.

Emergency Nurses Association: *Trauma nursing core course,* ed 5, Park Ridge, Ill, 2000, The Association.

Frakes MA, Evans T: Evaluation and management of the patient with LeFort facial fractures, *J Trauma Nurs* 11(3):95-102, 2004.

Newton K: Neck. In Marx J, editor: *Rosen's emergency medicine: concepts and clinical practice,* vol 1, ed 5, St Louis, 2002, Mosby.

Watts DD, Kokiko J: Airbags and eye injuries: assessment and treatment for ED patients, *J Emerg Nurs* 25(6):572-574, 1999.

CHAPTER 18

CHEST TRAUMA

BENJAMIN E. HOLLINGSWORTH

Chest injuries can create some of the most urgent situations that the trauma team faces. Because of the significance of the organs enclosed in the thorax and the large area of the body that is involved, life-threatening situations can result from seemingly small mechanisms. Approximately 25% of all trauma deaths in the United States each year are related directly to chest trauma. Injuries to the chest are the most frequently missed injuries in the first hour of care, and the development of a thorough chest examination technique is essential to the emergency nurse. Many chest trauma patients die after reaching the hospital.

Most injuries to the chest occur from blunt trauma, primarily caused by impact of the chest with a relatively immobile object, such as an automobile steering wheel. Presence of a seat belt with shoulder harness and deployment of an air bag affects the degree of energy transferred during a crash and needs to be taken into consideration. An estimated 70% of motor vehicle crashes result in thoracic injuries.[1]

Most penetrating wounds to the chest are caused by bullets or knives. Clinical personnel must consider the effect of the mechanism of injury and the patient's preexisting cardiac or pulmonary disease on the potential severity of chest injuries so that diagnostic and therapeutic procedures can be administered before the patient's condition worsens.

GROSS ANATOMY OF THE CHEST

When assessing a patient and intervening for a possible injury to the chest, clinical personnel should be familiar with the gross anatomy of the chest. The thoracic cavity extends from the first rib to the diaphragm. The diaphragm may be anywhere from the fourth intercostal space on exhalation to the lower costal margin (about the tenth rib) on maximal inhalation (Figure 18-1). Any injury that occurs between these areas should be considered as thoracic and abdominal until each can be ruled out (Figure 18-2).

The thoracic cavity contains the heart, the great vessels (superior and inferior venae cavae and aorta), the lungs, and the lower airway (Figure 18-3). The thoracic cavity is surrounded by the ribs, the intercostal muscles, and the diaphragm. Movement of the thoracic cavity is assisted by the accessory muscles of respiration: the abdominal wall muscles, the pectoralis muscles, and the sternocleidomastoid muscles.

If the mechanism of injury suggests a chest injury, the chest injury should be considered severe until proven otherwise. Hypoxia, a major cause of death associated with chest trauma, may have four causes:

- Inadequate perfusion of unventilated lung
- Inadequate ventilation of unperfused lung
- Abnormal airway/lung relationship
- Hypovolemia

Figure 18–1. Level of diaphragm on inspiration and expiration.

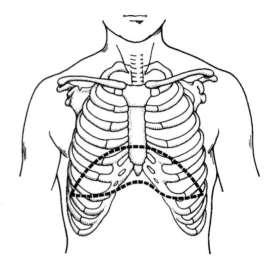

Figure 18–2. Injuries of the diaphragm are considered thoracic and abdominal.

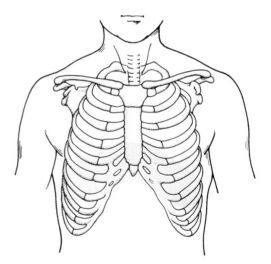

An injury database may be established to identify patterns of thoracic injury. This may include four areas of assessment, for example:

1. Type of incident: Was cause of injury a motor vehicle collision? Were seat belts worn? Was the patient the driver or a passenger? Were air bags deployed? Was injury penetrating?
2. What were the events of the incident? How fast was the vehicle traveling? What was the position in which the patient was found? Was the mechanism deceleration? If the injury was penetrating, what kind of weapon was used?
3. Mechanism of injury is of critical importance. Where on patients' chest was he or she struck? How far was the fall? What type of animal kicked the patient?
4. Were there any significant events during extrication or transport? Was there a prolonged extrication time? Did the patient have any airway or hemodynamic instability?

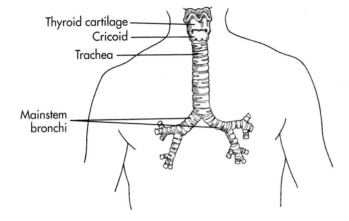

Figure 18-3. The lower airway is included with the thoracic cavity.

A database like this may help identify suspected injuries in an expeditious matter, leading to faster diagnosing and lifesaving measures.[2]

ASSESSMENT

In the patient with chest injuries, careful assessment of the airway, breathing, and circulation can affect the patient's survival.

- Check the patient's airway.
- Check air movement at nose and mouth.
- Be sure that airway is clear of obstruction(s).
- Check for breathing pattern.
- Auscultate breath sounds bilaterally.
- Check tidal volume using hands.
- Check for life-threatening injuries of the chest[3]:
    - Tension pneumothorax
    - Open pneumothorax
    - Massive hemothorax
    - Pericardial tamponade
    - Flail chest
- Check for injuries that are potentially life-threatening:
    - Pulmonary contusion
    - Tracheobronchial disruption
    - Esophageal disruption
    - Traumatic diaphragmatic hernia
    - Myocardial contusion
    - Aortic disruption
- Check for use of intercostal and accessory muscles.
- Check for epigastric and supraclavicular indrawing.
- Check for circulation. Check vital signs (auscultate blood pressure in both arms); skin color, turgor, temperature, and moisture; and other signs of hemodynamic status.

HIGH-FREQUENCY NURSING DIAGNOSES FOR PATIENTS WITH CHEST TRAUMA

- Ineffective breathing pattern
- Impaired gas exchange
- Fluid volume deficit
- Decreased cardiac output
- Ineffective tissue perfusion: cardiopulmonary, generalized
- Acute pain
- Risk for infection
- Fear
- Knowledge deficit: aftercare for injury

From NANDA International: *NANDA nursing diagnoses: definitions & classification, 2005-2006,* Philadelphia, 2006, The Association.

- Obtain a history of the event and mechanism of injury.
- Obtain an upright chest x-ray film (if spine stability has been established).
- Identify any entrance or exit wounds (describe appearance and location only; do not actually label "exit" or "entrance" because this is usually impossible to determine in the emergency department).
- Measure chest drainage.
- Measure urinary output.
- Monitor arterial oxygen saturation using pulse oximetry.
- Monitor arterial blood gases.
- Obtain 12-lead electrocardiogram.
- Monitor patient for dysrhythmias.

Nursing diagnoses relevant to the chest trauma patient are listed in the nursing diagnosis box.

DIAGNOSIS

- Mechanism of injury
- Clinical observations
- Chest x-ray film (preferably upright chest film)
- Evaluation of arterial oxygen saturation and/or arterial blood gases
- Observation of electrocardiogram

THERAPEUTIC INTERVENTIONS

Most patients with chest trauma require nonsurgical intervention to correct the hypoxic state, to improve circulation, or to remove a ventilatory obstruction.

- Ensure an open airway. Use airway adjuncts, as indicated.
- Ensure breathing. Administer oxygen at high flow.

- Initiate intravenous line(s) with large-bore cannulas and infuse crystalloid solutions or blood.
- Prepare for chest tube placement.
- Prepare for autotransfusion.
- Prepare for emergency thoracotomy.
- Provide interventions for specific chest injuries as indicated. (See Therapeutic Interventions sections for specific chest injuries.)

CHEST WALL INJURIES

Rib Fractures

Rib fractures are the most common chest injuries. They occur most frequently in the elderly and may cause subsequent problems because of inactivity and pain in this age group (Figure 18-4).[3] Another population that deserves special consideration when rib fractures occur is children. Because children's ribs are so elastic, they frequently do not fracture. However, when a child does suffer a rib fracture, clinical personnel should be highly suspicious of underlying thoracic injuries. Rib fractures may be caused by blunt or penetrating trauma to the chest wall. If there is a first rib fracture or if there are multiple ribs fractured, personnel should suspect major underlying trauma to the contents of the chest. Rib fractures may cause impaired ventilation, increased pulmonary secretions, atelectasis, and pneumonia.

ASSESSMENT

- Consider mechanism of injury.
- Patients will complain of pain upon inspiration or palpation.
- Patient will be splinting his or her chest.
- Chest wall ecchymosis will be apparent.
- Fracture is palpable.

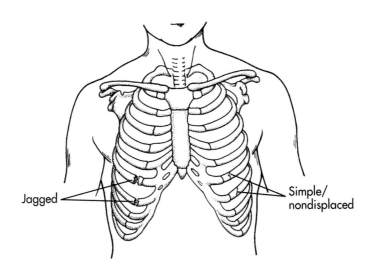

Figure 18–4. A rib fracture may be simple/nondisplaced or jagged.

DIAGNOSIS

- Chest x-ray film

THERAPEUTIC INTERVENTIONS

- Therapeutic interventions for various rib fractures are as follows:

Simple, Nondisplaced Fractures

- Administer analgesic agents. Regional anesthesia may be considered for pain control. Avoid systemic analgesics and constrictive devices.
- Consider hospital admission for close observation if the patient is elderly or has a history of underlying lung disease or if the fracture is jagged.

First, Second, or Third Rib Fracture

The patient must be hospitalized for fracture of the first, second, or third rib (Figure 18-5), and an arteriogram should be considered. It takes significant force to break these ribs; therefore, patients are at high risk for sudden death from central nervous system and tracheobronchial and vascular injuries.[4] The subclavian artery, vein, or aorta may be disrupted. A first rib fracture is difficult to visualize on an anteroposterior chest x-ray film.

Fourth to Twelfth Rib Fracture

The fourth to ninth ribs most often are injured in blunt trauma to the chest. In blunt trauma a bowing effect occurs, resulting in a middle shaft fracture. With fractures of these ribs, clinical personnel must consider intrathoracic injuries and intraabdominal injuries. Fractures of ribs 10 to 12 are associated with a high incidence of liver and spleen injuries.

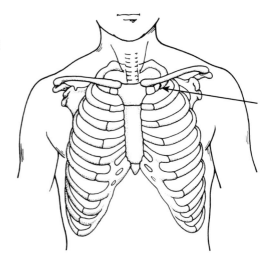

Figure 18–5. A first rib fracture *(arrow)* is significant because of subclavian artery and vein location and the amount of force required to fracture the first rib.

Flail Chest

A flail chest results from two or more consecutive ribs being fractured in two or more places. Flail chest also results from a detached sternum, which causes an incongruity of the chest wall that responds directly to intrathoracic pressure (Figure 18-6). When intercostal muscles contract and raise the rib cage, increased negative intrathoracic pressure causes the flail segment to draw inward. When the intercostal muscles relax, causing the rib cage to drop down, negative intrathoracic pressure decreases and the flail segment bulges outward. Because this motion is opposite that of the rest of the chest wall, it is known as *paradoxic motion.*

Flail chest usually is caused by a massive blunt force to the chest wall and results in rib fractures, as well as pulmonary contusion. Pain contributes to hypoventilation.[5] Although work of breathing is greatly increased, the main cause of hypoxemia is the underlying lung contusion.[6]

ASSESSMENT

- Mechanism of injury
- Dyspnea; poor air movement
- Chest wall pain
- Possible observation of movement of thorax as asymmetric and uncoordinated
- Palpation of subcutaneous emphysema

DIAGNOSIS

- Clinical observation
- Chest x-ray film
- Arterial blood gases; these values demonstrate hypoxia and should be carried out to evaluate increasing size of contusion

THERAPEUTIC INTERVENTIONS

Good ventilation is imperative in the treatment of a person with a flail chest.

- Perform selective endotracheal intubation.
- Administer supplemental, humidified oxygen.
- Control pain.
- Administer crystalloid intravenous solutions for volume replacement.

In absence of hypotension, be careful not to overload these patients with fluid. Injured lung tissue is sensitive to underresuscitation of shock and fluid overload.[3]

- Consider stabilizing the flail segment.
- Consider possible underlying injuries.
- Consider insertion of central venous pressure monitor to check fluid resuscitation.

Sternal Fracture

It takes a great force to fracture the sternum (Figure 18-7). Of prime concern should be underlying structural damage. One of the injuries most commonly associated with a sternal fracture

Figure 18-6. A, Flail chest: more than two ribs fractured in consecutive places *B* and *C*. Paradoxic motion. **B,** On exhalation the flail segment bulges outward. **C,** On inhalation the flail segment sucks inward.

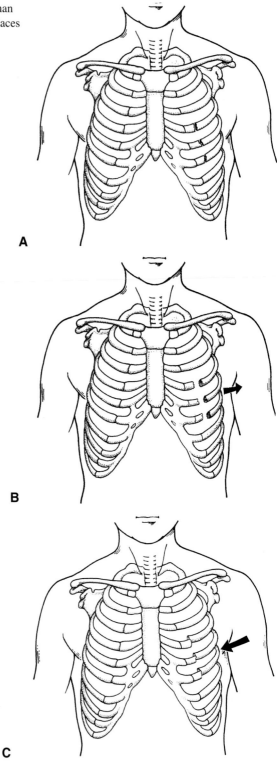

A

B

C

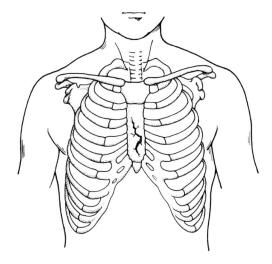

Figure 18-7. Sternal fracture.

is a myocardial contusion. Common causes are the chest hitting a steering wheel or use of gas-powered chest compressor or aggressive manual chest compression.

ASSESSMENT

- Mechanism of injury
- Chest wall contusion, ecchymosis
- Complaint of chest pain
- Dysrhythmias (especially premature ventricular contractions, atrial fibrillation, right bundle branch block, ST segment elevations)
- Pain upon inspiration
- Palpation of fracture
- Assessment for cervical spine injury

DIAGNOSIS

- Palpation of fracture
- Chest x-ray film

THERAPEUTIC INTERVENTIONS

- Observe patient.
- Monitor Pao_2.
- Administer analgesia.
- Treat dysrhythmias, as prescribed.
- Consider preparation for surgery for wiring if sternum is displaced.

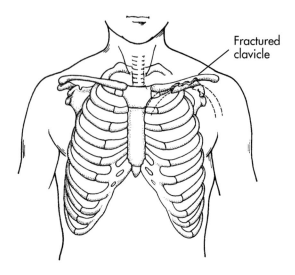

Fractured clavicle

Figure 18–8. A fractured clavicle may create concern because of the proximity of the subclavian artery and vein.

Clavicular Fracture

A clavicle fracture is usually not a serious injury, but a jagged edge of the fracture may perforate the subclavian artery or vein, causing disruption, hematoma, or clot formation (Figure 18-8). This injury usually is caused by blunt trauma directly to the clavicle or to the shoulder area laterally.

ASSESSMENT

- Mechanism of injury
- Pain on palpation
- Observation of deformity

DIAGNOSIS

- Clinical observation
- Chest x-ray film

THERAPEUTIC INTERVENTIONS

- Apply a figure-eight splint, sling, or sling and swathe as preferred by physician.
- Consider an arteriogram.
- Administer analgesic agents, as prescribed.

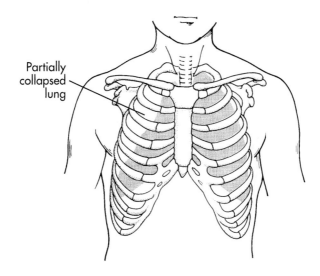

Figure 18–9. Simple pneumothorax. One lung partially collapsed; other structures unaffected.

LUNG INJURIES

Simple Pneumothorax

A simple pneumothorax causes a ventilation/perfusion defect (Figure 18-9). Blood is circulated to the nonventilated area and is not oxygenated. A loss of negative pressure in the intrapleural space causes a partial or total lung collapse. Pneumothorax may occur because of a tear in the lung tissue or from an opening in the chest wall. A simple pneumothorax usually results from blunt or penetrating trauma to the chest.

ASSESSMENT

- Mechanism of injury
- Complaint of sudden onset of chest pain
- Sudden onset of shortness of breath, tachypnea
- Absence of or diminished breath sounds on affected side
- Hyperresonance on percussion on affected side

DIAGNOSIS

- Clinical observation
- Chest x-ray film: upright, end-exhalation

THERAPEUTIC INTERVENTIONS

- Observe patient closely.
- Administer high-flow oxygen.

- Consider needle thoracostomy.
- Prepare for chest tube placement.
- Obtain chest x-ray film to confirm lung reexpansion.

Tension Pneumothorax

A tension pneumothorax is a life-threatening condition. The lung usually has good perfusion but poor ventilation, which eventually causes poor perfusion (Figure 18-10). A tension pneumothorax usually results from a penetrating injury but may be caused by blunt trauma. Tension pneumothorax may be caused by mechanical ventilation with positive end-expiratory pressure, a nonsealing puncture, rupture of an emphysematous bulla, or a parenchymal lung injury.

Figure 18–10. A, Right tension pneumothorax. **B,** Right tension pneumothorax as seen on x-ray film.

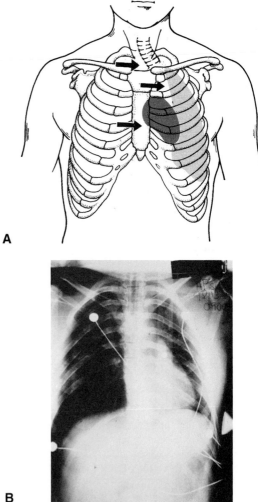

A

B

A tension pneumothorax forms when pressure enters the thoracic cavity during inspiration but cannot exit during exhalation. As this process continues, pressure not only collapses the affected lung but also pushes the mediastinum toward the unaffected side (mediastinal shift). This movement in turn causes a decreased blood flow to the right side of the heart and consequently a decrease in cardiac output. Tension pneumothorax also causes the unaffected lung to collapse.

ASSESSMENT

- Mechanism of injury
- Severe shortness of breath
- Deviated trachea (deviated toward unaffected side)
- Mediastinal shift, causing decreased venous return and impaired contralateral ventilation
- Distended jugular veins from impedance of blood return to right side of the heart
- Cyanosis
- Decreased blood pressure/hemodynamic deterioration
- Hyperresonance on percussion on affected side
- Unilateral absence of breath sounds

DIAGNOSIS

- Clinical observation
- Chest x-ray film

THERAPEUTIC INTERVENTIONS

- Administer oxygen.
- Perform a needle thoracostomy using a large-bore (at least 16-gauge) needle at the second intercostal space, midclavicular line.
- Prepare for chest tube placement. Be careful not to administer oxygen under positive pressure until after the chest tube is placed, because this may increase the tension.

NOTE: The results of a chest x-ray film are not necessary before providing therapeutic intervention if signs and symptoms of the tension pneumothorax are present.

Hemothorax

A hemothorax may be caused by blunt or penetrating trauma to the chest (Figure 18-11). If there is an injury to structures within the chest cavity (usually the lung or a vessel laceration) and bleeding occurs, this blood will collect in the intrapleural space, producing what is known as a hemothorax. The amount of collected blood varies depending on the extent of the bleeding. A collection of greater than 1500 mL of blood is considered a massive hemothorax. An initial drainage of 1000 mL of blood followed by a consistent drainage of more than 200 mL of blood for 4 hours or the initial loss of 1500 mL may be indicative of the need for emergency thoracotomy.[3]

Figure 18–11. Hemothorax.

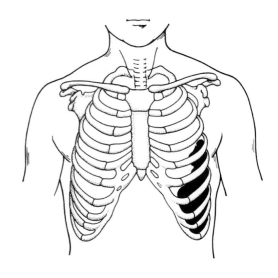

ASSESSMENT

- Mechanism of injury
- Signs of hypovolemic shock
- Restlessness to unconsciousness
- Cool, clammy skin
- Cool distal extremities
- Increased pulse
- Increased, shallow respirations
- Decreased blood pressure
- Decreased breath sounds on affected side
- Dullness to percussion on affected side

NOTE: Jugular veins may be distended or flat and are not useful in diagnosis.

DIAGNOSIS

- Clinical observation
- Chest x-ray film
- May be seen in combination with tension pneumothorax

THERAPEUTIC INTERVENTIONS

- Administer oxygen.
- Establish intravenous lines, and administer crystalloids or blood products.
- Prepare for placement of a large-bore chest tube (36°F).
- Consider autotransfusion.
- Consider preparation for emergency thoracotomy.

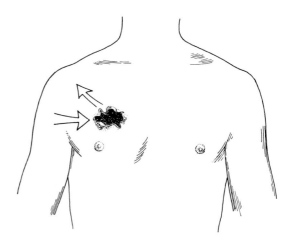

Figure 18–12. Sucking chest wound/open chest wound. Air preferentially enters and exits through the chest wall defect if the hole is greater than two thirds the diameter of the trachea. On expiration, air moves out of the defect. On inspiration, air preferentially enters the open wound.

Sucking Chest Wound/Open Pneumothorax

A sucking chest wound is caused by a penetrating force, especially that of a high-velocity missile (Figure 18-12). If the diameter of the hole in the chest wall is greater than two thirds the diameter of the trachea, there will be preferential flow of air through the chest wall defect, the path of least resistance. Loss of negative pressure in the chest from the defect will cause immediate equilibration between intrathoracic pressure and atmospheric pressure, thus causing a pneumothorax to form. If the defect produces a one-way valve, as air enters the thoracic cavity but cannot escape, a tension pneumothorax will form.

ASSESSMENT

- Mechanism of injury
- Sight of defect/audible sucking sound on inspiration
- Dyspnea
- Chest pain
- Signs of pneumothorax or tension pneumothorax

DIAGNOSIS

- Clinical findings

THERAPEUTIC INTERVENTIONS

- Administer oxygen.
- Seal the defect on three sides with a sterile, occlusive dressing. Leave one side open to act as a flutter valve to prevent the formation of a tension pneumothorax. Observe for the development of tension pneumothorax and remove the seal if this occurs. If the patient is intubated, this procedure is not necessary unless the wound is greater than the size of the trachea.

- Consider the placement of chest tubes, remote from area of injury.
- Consider autotransfusion.
- Consider surgery for repair.

Pulmonary Contusion

A pulmonary contusion is one of the most common types of chest injuries that occur in major trauma.[3] Pulmonary contusion often is seen with a flail chest or severe rib fractures (Figure 18-13). A pulmonary contusion usually is caused by severe blunt trauma to the chest. The contusion may be slow to develop, so close, on-going observation of patients with mechanisms of injury that would suggest a pulmonary contusion is imperative.

A contusion forms when an outside force against the chest wall is transmitted to the lung, rupturing tissues, small airways and alveoli. As this pressure releases, the chest wall springs back, pulling the lung with it and causing a resultant bruising injury sometimes accompanied by a pleural tear and laceration. This allows blood to extravasate into the parenchyma, causing the patient to become hypoxic.[2] Tracheal obstruction also may result. The contusion may be localized or massive.

ASSESSMENT

- Mechanism of injury
- Ineffective cough
- Hemoptysis or blood suctioned from endotracheal tube[4]
- Increasing hyperpnea
- Severe dyspnea
- Chest wall contusions or abrasions
- Additional severe injuries
- Hypoxemia on pulse oximetry or arterial blood gas

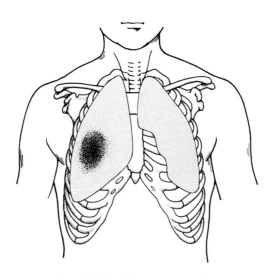

Figure 18-13. Pulmonary contusion.

DIAGNOSIS

- High index of suspicion
- Clinical observation
- Chest x-ray film

THERAPEUTIC INTERVENTIONS

- Maintain an adequate airway.
- Maintain adequate ventilation.
- Administer humidified oxygen, as prescribed.
- Selective endotracheal intubation may be necessary; consider the use of a ventilator.
- *Monitor the patient for acute respiratory distress syndrome.*
- In the absence of hypotension, limit intravenous fluids during the resuscitative and early intensive care phase.
- Use blood and colloids to maintain oncotic pressure and decrease pulmonary edema.
- Consider administering diuretics.
- Monitor pulse oximetry.
- Administer analgesics to keep the patient comfortable.
- Give morphine sulfate in 1- to 2-mg increments intravenously, not intramuscularly.
- Pay close attention to a decreased respiratory rate and increased hypoxia.[3]

Laceration of Lung Parenchyma

Laceration of lung tissue usually is caused by a jagged rib fracture or other penetrating injury (Figure 18-14).

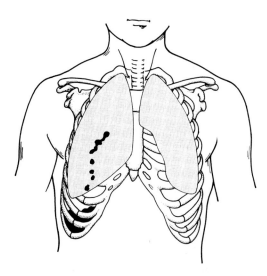

Figure 18-14. Laceration of the lung parenchyma.

ASSESSMENT

- Often a small hemothorax or pneumothorax
- Hemoptysis
- Subcutaneous emphysema

THERAPEUTIC INTERVENTIONS

- Usually no intervention is required because the process is usually self-limiting. If the injury is severe, surgical repair is necessary.

OTHER STRUCTURAL INJURIES

Tracheobronchial Injuries

Disruption of the tracheobronchial tree, most commonly near the bifurcation of the main stem bronchus 1 inch from the carina is where 79% of these injuries occur (39% in the right main stem bronchus and 40% in the left main stem bronchus)[7] and may be the result of blunt or penetrating trauma. Disruption may not be evidenced for up to 5 days after injury. If the disruption is below the carina, a chest x-ray film will show mediastinal air. Bronchoscopy is the most definitive diagnostic aid.

Bronchial injuries are subtle. Patients who arrive at the hospital with these types of injuries have a 30% mortality rate, often because of associated injuries.[3]

ASSESSMENT

- Mechanism of injury
- Observation for airway obstruction
- Noisy breathing
- Hemoptysis
- Cough
- Subcutaneous emphysema
- Progressive mediastinal emphysema
- Possible tension pneumothorax
- Air leak somewhere in chest

DIAGNOSIS

- Clinical findings
- Direct visualization on bronchoscopy
- Continuous air leak in chest tube drainage device

THERAPEUTIC INTERVENTIONS

- Maintain a patent airway.
- Administer high-flow oxygen.

- Prepare for chest tube placement.
- Prepare for surgery.

Diaphragmatic Rupture

Diaphragmatic rupture may be a life-threatening injury.[8] A diaphragmatic rupture is a disruption of the diaphragm, which is the main muscle of respiration, causing interference with the patient's ventilatory effort. Rupture may occur with any chest or abdominal injury from the level of the fourth intercostal space to the tenth rib. Diaphragmatic rupture may be caused by a stiff, forceful blow to the left side of the stomach or by an increase in intraabdominal pressure, as occurs with lap seat belts. If the trauma is blunt, the rupture usually results in large tears. If the trauma is penetrating, the rupture usually results in small perforations. Rupture usually is associated with other massive injuries.

ASSESSMENT

- Kehr's sign (epigastric pain radiating to the left shoulder)[7]; chest pain that may be referred to one shoulder
- Abdominal pain[5]
- Difficult breathing
- Decreased breath sounds
- Possible rhonchi (from the hemothorax)
- Bowel sounds auscultated in lower/middle chest[5]

DIAGNOSIS

- Supine x-ray film (look for presence of bowel that has herniated into the chest cavity and elevated the left hemidiaphragm) or the nasogastric tube in the thoracic cavity or loss of costophrenic angle on other side of injury[3]
- Contrast radiography (gastrointestinal series)
- Bowel sounds in chest

THERAPEUTIC INTERVENTIONS

- Administer high-flow oxygen.
- Position patient to facilitate breathing.
- Place a nasogastric tube.
- Prepare the patient for surgery.

Esophageal Rupture

Rupture of the esophagus is a rare injury, but mortality is high if diagnosis is missed. A rupture of the esophagus usually results from penetrating trauma or a severe epigastric blow. It may be seen in conjunction with a pneumothorax or hemothorax without evidence of fractures, or it may be an iatrogenic injury that occurs during esophagoscopy.

ASSESSMENT

- Mechanism of injury
- Substernal pleuritic pain radiating to neck and shoulders[5]
- Mediastinal emphysema
- Mediastinal crunch sound
- Particulate matter in chest tube drainage
- Shock without associated pain
- Elevated temperature

DIAGNOSIS

- Clinical observation
- Contrast radiography (upper gastrointestinal series)
- Endoscopy

THERAPEUTIC INTERVENTIONS

- Emergency surgery

CARDIAC AND GREAT VESSEL INJURIES

Myocardial Contusion

Establishing the mechanism of injury is important in suspecting the diagnosis of a myocardial contusion. One fourth of patients who have this injury have no sign of physical injury.[5] Myocardial contusion usually is caused by an impact of the myocardium on the chest wall, which causes a contusion to form. The contusion occurs as a result of a blunt trauma to the chest or a severe acceleration/deceleration force. Myocardial contusion also can occur following chest compression for cardiopulmonary resuscitation.

ASSESSMENT

- Mechanism of injury
- Complaints of severe chest pain, usually unaffected by vasodilatory drugs[8]
- Chest wall contusion/ecchymosis
- Dysrhythmias (usually within the first hour, but anywhere up to 24 hours), usually premature ventricular contractions, atrial fibrillation, right bundle branch block, or ST segment elevation in electrocardiogram; if there are premature ventricular contractions, there is possibility of ventricular injury

DIAGNOSIS

- High index of suspicion
- Mechanism of injury suggestive of severe blunt chest trauma (especially bent steering wheel)
- Possible signs of injury on 12-lead electrocardiogram (especially elevated ST segment in V_1, V_2, and V_3)

- Elevation of cardiac isoenzymes, similar to myocardial infarction
- Echocardiography

THERAPEUTIC INTERVENTIONS

- Assess and monitor the patient as if he or she were having a myocardial infarction.
- Administer oxygen.
- Administer an analgesia/narcotic for pain control.
- Administer the appropriate dysrhythmia therapy.
- Admit patient for observation and cardiac monitoring for at least 48 hours.

Pericardial Tamponade

A pericardial tamponade is caused by a bleeding myocardium, a ruptured coronary artery, or a lacerated pericardium. Blood from the wound is contained in the pericardial sac. This tamponade prevents the patient from hemorrhaging to death, but eventually it causes constriction of the heart, reducing cardiac output and causing hemodynamic deterioration. Pericardial tamponade most frequently is caused by a penetrating injury but may be caused by a severe blunt trauma to the chest. Clinical personnel should think about the possibility of a pericardial tamponade whenever an unexplained pump failure is not responsive to volume replacement.

ASSESSMENT

- Beck's triad
  - Increased central venous pressure, evidenced by distended neck veins
  - Decreased arterial blood pressure
  - Muffled heart sounds
- Cyanosis
- Pulsus paradoxus
- Pulseless electrical activity
- Patient unresponsive to resuscitation efforts

DIAGNOSIS

- High index of suspicion
- Clinical observation
- Chest x-ray film; widened mediastinum
- Pericardiocentesis
- Echocardiography

THERAPEUTIC INTERVENTIONS

- Administer oxygen.
- Initiate an IV.
- Prepare for pericardiocentesis or minithoracotomy (Figure 18-15).
- Monitor the patient.

Figure 18-15. Pericardiocentesis. *(From Budassi SA, Barber J:* Mosby's manual of emergency care, *ed 3, St Louis, 1990, Mosby.)*

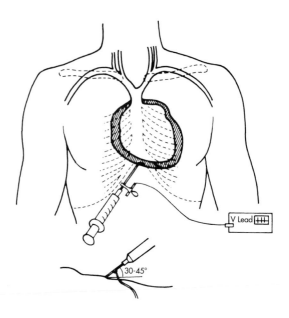

Aortic Trauma

In aortic trauma the aorta tears, usually as a result of a blunt force to the chest at the point where the aorta is attached or fixed. Tearing also may be caused by a penetrating force. Aortic trauma is associated most commonly with a motor vehicle collision (particularly lateral impact crashes) or a fall from a height where there is rapid deceleration.[9] The patient is critically injured and rarely survives long enough to reach the emergency department and definitive care. The mortality rate is 85% at the scene,[10] and one has only a 50% chance of surviving after arrival at the hospital.[4] The cause of death is exsanguination or massive pericardial tamponade.

The most common site for aortic rupture is at the ligamentum arteriosum (tethering point at junction between the aortic arch and the descending aorta). Two other common areas of aortic disruption are in the ascending aorta where it leaves the pericardial sac and in the descending aorta at the entry into the diaphragm.[2] The integrity of the aorta may be maintained for a brief period by an intact adventitia or collateral circulation.

ASSESSMENT

- Mechanism of injury
- Trauma arrest
- Chest wall bruise
- Presence of a first or second rib fracture
- Left parascapular murmur
- Presence of upper extremity discrepancy in blood pressure
- Decreased femoral pulses
- Sternal fracture
- Scapula or multiple rib fractures
- Paraplegia
- Tracheal deviation to the right

- Esophageal deviation (place nasogastric tube and observe deviation of tube)
- Lowered left main stem bronchus
- Elevated right main stem bronchus

DIAGNOSIS

Diagnosis of aortic trauma is made by a high index of suspicion because of the mechanism of injury.

- Visualized on x-ray film
  - Widened mediastinum, obliteration of aortic knob; and presence of pleural cap, hemothorax, or nasogastric deviation on x-ray film[3]
- Visualized on thoracic aortogram
- Visualized on chest computed tomography scan with contrast

THERAPEUTIC INTERVENTIONS

- If loss of vital signs, then administration of cardiopulmonary resuscitation (even though it may not be effective)
- Administration of intravenous solutions and blood products
- Preparation for emergency thoracotomy (Figure 18-16) and cardiothoracic surgery consultation to do the following:
  - Cross-clamp aorta.
  - Place patient on cardiopulmonary bypass.
  - Repair injury (resect and graft).
- Endovascular intervention
  - Delivered from remote access site, little vessel exposure and limited bleeding
  - Balloon expandable or self-expanding devices
  - Bare metal or covered grafts available; device selection based on injury type and location

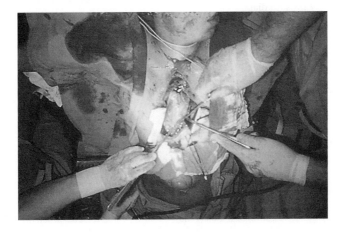

Figure 18-16. Thoracotomy. *(Courtesy Emanuel Hospital & Health Center, Portland, Ore.)*

- Applied on stable patients in controlled settings
- May be implemented in cases of blunt and penetrating injury[11]

Subclavian Artery Injury

Subclavian artery injury may result from blunt or penetrating force.

ASSESSMENT

- Mechanism of injury
- Observation of hematoma at base of neck
- Other signs of hemodynamic deterioration
- Difference in blood pressure between right and left arm[8]

DIAGNOSIS

- Clinical observation
- Arteriography

THERAPEUTIC INTERVENTIONS

- Administer oxygen.
- Administer intravenous fluids (place intravenous lines in lower extremities or on side opposite injury)
- Prepare patient for surgery.

SUMMARY

Any patient with an obvious chest injury or a mechanism of injury suggestive of a chest injury should be treated as if he or she has a critical injury until such an injury can be ruled out. With a high index of suspicion and aggressive appropriate therapeutic intervention, these patients may be saved from death or permanent disability.

References

1. Flynn MB, Bonini S: Blunt chest trauma: a case report, *Crit Care Nurse* 19(5):68-77, 1999.
2. McQuillan KA, Von Rueden KT, Hartsock RL et al, editors: *Trauma nursing: from resuscitation through rehabilitation,* ed 3, Philadelphia, 2002, WB Saunders.
3. Committee on Trauma, American College of Surgeons: *Advanced trauma life support instructor manual,* Chicago, 1993, The College.
4. Laskowski-Jones L: Meeting the challenge of chest trauma, *Am J Nurs* 95(9):22-29, 1995.
5. Jackimczyk K: Blunt chest trauma, *Emerg Med Clin North Am* 11:1, 1993.
6. Wilson R, Walt A: *Management of trauma: pitfalls and practice,* ed 2, Philadelphia, 1996, Williams & Wilkins.
7. Emergency Nurses Association: *Emergency nursing principles and practice,* ed 4, St Louis, 1998, Mosby.

8. Emergency Nurses Association: *Emergency nursing core curriculum,* ed 4, Philadelphia, 1994, Saunders.

9. Katyal D, McLellan BA, Brenneman FD et al: Lateral impact motor vehicle collisions: significant cause of blunt traumatic rupture of the thoracic aorta, *J Trauma* 42(5):769-772, 1997.

10. Emergency Nurses Association: *Trauma nursing core course instructors manual,* ed 4, Chicago, 1995, The Association.

11. Sheridan RL, editor: *The trauma handbook of the Massachusetts General Hospital,* Philadelphia, 2004, Lippincott Williams & Wilkins.

CHAPTER 19

ABDOMINAL, GENITOURINARY, AND PELVIC TRAUMA

ALICE A. GERVASINI

The abdominal cavity extends from the diaphragm to the pelvis and is highly susceptible to injury because of the lack of bony protection for underlying organs. The abdominal cavity is divided into three anatomic areas: the peritoneal space, the retroperitoneal space, and the pelvis. Free space in the abdomen can contain a large amount of shed blood before tamponade occurs, and exsanguination from abdominal injuries should be of utmost concern. Care of the patient with abdominal injuries on the surface appears simple yet may be complex.

Blunt trauma can cause severe injuries to abdominal contents as energy is diffused throughout the solid and hollow structures. Peritoneal injury and internal bleeding may not be recognizable immediately on arrival to the emergency department. Frequent reassessment and a high index of suspicion based on mechanism of injury, history, and signs and symptoms should guide the health care provider in identification of injury and management of the patient with abdominal trauma. Penetrating injury can result from any object that penetrates the abdominal wall. Underlying structures may or may not be affected, and diagnosis by clinical signs alone is unreliable. The patient demonstrating an altered mental status should always be evaluated for unknown injuries to the abdomen. An important factor in increasing survival from abdominal trauma is decreasing the time from the occurrence of the injury to definitive treatment. In the emergency setting it is more important to determine whether the patient requires urgent surgery than to determine which organs or viscera have been injured.

ANATOMY

The liver and spleen are located in the intrathoracic abdomen (high up in the abdomen; Figure 19-1). The small bowel, large bowel, bladder, and pelvic organs are located in what is known as the true abdomen. The retroperitoneal abdomen contains the kidneys, ureters, duodenum, and pancreas. These locations are important when considering the appropriate diagnostic examinations to use.

BLUNT TRAUMA

The most common mechanisms of blunt trauma are motor vehicle crashes, injury from contact sports, violence/abuse, and falls. The assessment and recommended diagnostic workup may be dictated by the inability to accurately evaluate the patient with blunt abdominal, genitourinary, and pelvic trauma. All trauma patients should have an abdominal exam and further diagnostic workup if the patient has altered mental status, inability to participate in the exam, or motor/sensory deficit including the thoracoabdominal area.

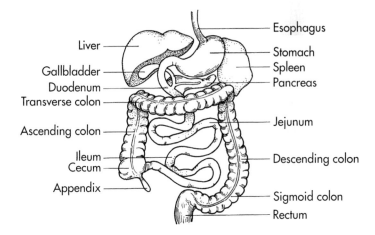

Figure 19–1. Anatomy of the abdomen.

PENETRATING TRAUMA

The extent of injury from penetrating trauma depends on the location of the penetrating object, its size and velocity, and the distance and angle of projection. Injury may range from minimal to severe and may not be confined to the direct path of the object. Therefore, penetrating injuries to the abdomen also should be considered penetrating trauma to the chest until proved otherwise. Clinical personnel should consider the mechanism of injury and observe carefully for hemodynamic compromise. If the mechanism of injury is suggestive of severe underlying trauma, if the wound was caused by a high-velocity missile, or if hemodynamic instability is present, exploratory surgery should be considered.

ASSESSMENT

An organized approach to assessment and reassessment of the abdomen and pelvis is critical to avoid delay in diagnosis:

- Perform primary and secondary surveys (see Chapter 11), and address all issues.
- Inspect the patient for areas of ecchymosis, abrasions, lacerations, or puncture wounds.
- Palpate the abdomen, flank, and perineum for tenderness or presence of masses.
- Observe for changes in abdominal size or distention.
- Auscultate for bowel sounds and bruits; lack of bowel sounds may indicate ileus; presence of bruit in the presence of penetrating injury may indicate major vascular disruption.
- Solicit for pain, tenderness, or guarding.
- Palpate for abdominal wall rigidity, masses, or crepitus.
- Perform rectal exam and assess for rectal tone and the position of the prostate gland (if appropriate), and determine the presence of blood; perform this before insertion of a Foley catheter.
- Inspect the urinary meatus for blood.
- Maintain a high index of suspicion in the presence of associated injuries, especially rib fractures, chest, and spinal cord injuries.
- Inspect the scrotum for edema, ecchymoses, hematomas, or testicular disruption.

HIGH-FREQUENCY NURSING DIAGNOSES FOR PATIENTS WITH ABDOMINAL, GENITOURINARY, OR PELVIC TRAUMA

- Fluid volume deficit
- Decreased cardiac output
- Ineffective tissue perfusion: gastrointestinal, renal, generalized
- Impaired urinary elimination
- Impaired physical mobility
- Acute pain
- Risk for infection

From NANDA International: *NANDA nursing diagnoses: definitions & classification, 2005-2006,* Philadelphia, 2006, The Association.

- Perform a vaginal exam (if appropriate) manually and with a speculum.
- Assess ability to void spontaneously.
- Do not remove impaled objects; stabilize them and prepare the patient for surgical removal.
- Nursing diagnoses commonly used with abdominal, genitourinary, and pelvic trauma are listed in the nursing diagnosis box.

DIAGNOSIS

Patients with blunt trauma to the abdomen are the most difficult to diagnose. The key to diagnosis is to obtain a complete history, including mechanism of injury, to assess and reassess the patient's physical/clinical signs and symptoms, and to conduct the appropriate diagnostic studies. Penetrating injury to the abdomen is also a challenge. Evidence of penetration does not equate to an immediate operation. As with blunt trauma, the history, assessment of physical findings, and hemodynamics play a major role in the diagnostic process.

Consider the following methods of assessment:

- Focused abdominal sonography for trauma performed in the emergency department, although operator dependent, can be helpful in early detection of free fluid in the abdomen; it can be used on pregnant women, does not interfere with resuscitation efforts, and plays a role in reassessment of the abdomen should hemodynamics change. It does not assess the retroperitoneal space.
- Pelvis, and chest x-ray films done in the resuscitation bay may be helpful in identification of pneumothorax, tube placements, and pelvic fractures (many trauma centers are forgoing these films with rapid access to computed tomography [CT])
- Abdominal CT (with intravenous contrast) assists with the identification of hemoperitoneum, pneumoperitoneum, retroperitoneal trauma, and solid organ injuries; and on advanced scanners, diaphragmatic, pancreatic, and hollow viscous injuries are better identified than in the past.
- CT cystogram identifies displacement of the bladder or leakage of urine.
- Use a guaiac test on any specimen from the rectum, bladder, or stomach to detect occult bleeding.
- Use a retrograde urethrogram to look for interruption of the urethra.

- Laboratory evaluation should include a complete blood count, liver enzymes, serum amylase, clotting factors, renal function studies, pregnancy test (if appropriate), urinalysis, and toxicology as indicated.
- Use diagnostic peritoneal aspiration and/or lavage to rule out blood and fecal contamination of the peritoneal fluid and possible intraabdominal injury. Current application is best seen in significant neurologic/head trauma in which the patient needs immediate operative intervention before CT scans of the abdomen, or in cases where the the patient's hemodynamics are such that the patient cannot be moved to the scanner.
- Laparoscopic exam is less invasive and can be used as the definitive procedure in diagnosing and treating the blunt or penetrating injury pattern.
- Exploratory surgery is also an option.

THERAPEUTIC INTERVENTIONS

- Administer oxygen, and initiate intravenous therapy with two large-bore catheters.
- Control external hemorrhage.
- Apply saline dressings to wounds or eviscerated tissue.
- Stabilize impaled objects.
- Insert a nasogastric/orogastric tube.
- If no contraindications are present (blood at meatus, high-rising prostate), insert a Foley catheter.
- Alert operating room staff of the potential need for urgent intervention.
- Stabilize the spinal column.

Organ-Specific Types of Injuries from Trauma

All intraperitoneal and retroperitoneal organs vary in injury patterns, from simple to complex, and functional disruption, from minimal to complete. The organ location and vulnerability affect the risk for injury and outcome. With blunt and penetrating injury, assessment and index of suspicion for potential hemodynamic instability are critical. Treatment strategies vary based on extent of injury and presence of active bleeding (Table 19-1; Figures 19-2 and 19-3).

Pelvic Fracture

Pelvic fractures usually result from a crush injury or rapid acceleration/deceleration injury that might occur in motor vehicle collisions or motorcycle crashes, penetrating trauma, falls from a significant height, or from a sudden contraction of muscle against resistance (Figure 19-4). Usually these injuries are associated with a high-energy impact, although in geriatric trauma patients, less energy is needed to result in a complex pelvic fracture. Classifications of pelvic fractures focus on the forces applied to the pelvis, including lateral compression forces, anterior-posterior compression forces, or a lateral shearing force. Each type of impact results in the disruption of the pelvis and potential for massive blood loss.

If a pelvic fracture is present (Figure 19-5), one should anticipate the potential for a massive amount of internal bleeding and prepare for blood volume replacement. The clinician should anticipate the loss of at least one unit of blood for each fracture pattern identified. Early involvement of an orthopedic surgeon for timely stabilization of the fractured pelvis is critical in helping to control bleeding. The use of pelvic binders or wrapping the pelvis in sheets helps stabilize the pelvis and potentially decreases ongoing bleeding. Concurrently, clinical personnel should search for other associated injuries while observing the patient carefully

Table 19-1   Abdominal/Pelvic Organs: Unique Features and Diagnosis and Treatment Options

Organ	Features and Diagnosis and Treatment Options
Spleen	Commonly injured dense organ; located in left upper quadrant under eighth to twelfth ribs; computed tomography (CT) confirms diagnosis; treatment choices include observation in the presence of hemodynamic stability, angiography/embolization of active bleeders, splenorrhaphy, and splenectomy
Liver	Commonly injured solid organ; located in right upper quadrant under anterior eighth to twelfth ribs; CT confirms diagnosis; treatment choices include observation in the presence of hemodynamic stability, angiography/embolization of active bleeders, and damage control laparotomy
Pancreas	Solid organ in retroperitoneal space, posterior midepigastrum; injured less frequently but most commonly missed injury; injury pattern not always evident on CT—often diagnosis is related to index of suspicion, increased abdominal pain, and signs of peritonitis; operative intervention includes débridement and drainage
Stomach	Hollow organ located in left upper quadrant; rarely injured in blunt forces, increased incidence in penetrating forces; CT may identify free air; operative intervention is required to repair injury
Intestines	Hollow organ at risk for blunt and penetrating injury; CT may identify free air, or the patient may demonstrate signs and symptoms of peritoneal irritation resulting from leak of gastrointestinal contents; laparotomy
Diaphragm	Should be considered as part of injury pattern for chest and abdominal trauma; more common injury on left versus right; small rents may go undetected for days to weeks until tear enlarges or abdominal contents move into the chest; CT identification via reformatted chest/abdominal images; controversial repair with laparoscopic or thoracoscopic procedure; laparotomy
Kidneys	Retroperitoneal organs at the level of T12-L3 (Figure 19-2); most frequently injured organ in the genitourinary system; at risk for injury from blunt and penetrating forces; increased suspicion with hematuria, but not necessary for diagnosis of injury; CT will confirm diagnosis; angiography/embolization is a potential option; often observation and bed rest the only interventions required; consider surgery in extreme cases
Ureters	Hollow structures, rarely injured with blunt forces; increased incidence with penetrating injuries to the lower abdomen or flank; delayed views from CT with contrast help identify the injury; usually operative repair is required
Bladder	Hollow organ at risk for injury from blunt forces or internal penetrating forces with associated pelvic fractures; CT cystogram; management strategies depend on location of injury and may require operative intervention
Urethra	More common in males and with associated pelvic fractures; suspect injury with obvious blood at the meatus; CT cystogram, retrograde urethrogram; repair varies—stenting with indwelling catheter and then potential for delayed closure

Table 19-1   Abdominal/Pelvic Organs: Unique Features and Diagnosis and Treatment Options—cont'd

Organ	Features and Diagnosis and Treatment Options
Penis/testis and scrotum	Injury can result from blunt or penetrating forces; treatment strategies for contusion includes cold pack and elevation; ultrasound to identify testicular injury; penile or testicular rupture requires immediate operative intervention; penile strangulation from external constricting objects requires immediate removal of objects and possible débridement of any necrotic tissue
Vascular	Major vessels include abdominal aorta, inferior vena cava, hepatic and mesenteric vessels (Figure 19-3); blunt and penetrating patterns result in disruption of the vessels; CT may demonstrate hematomas or active extravasation; angiography/embolization is a potential option, as is laparotomy

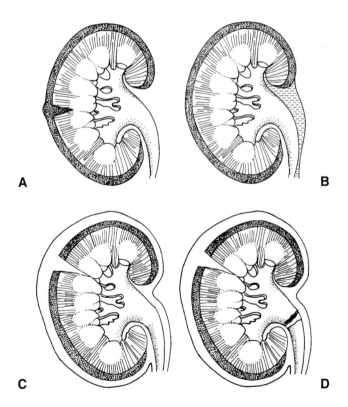

Figure 19-2. A, Lacerated kidney; bleeding contained in capsule. **B,** Fracture with extravasation of urine. **C,** Laceration through the capsule with blood extravasation. **D,** Fracture/laceration with extravasation of blood and urine.

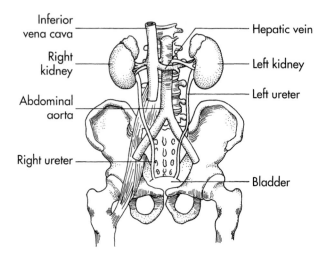

Figure 19–3. Location of the hepatic vein, inferior vena cava, and abdominal aorta.

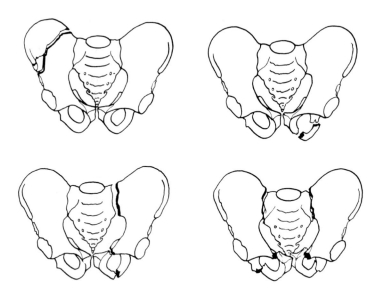

Figure 19–4. Types of pelvic fractures.

for hemodynamic compromise. Assume that there is major soft tissue abdominal injury as well, until proved otherwise, as a result of the tremendous amount of energy that is required to fracture the pelvis. Diagnosis is made on x-ray film with further delineation on CT with reformats. Therapeutic intervention ranges from bed rest to internal or external reduction and fixation and can be accomplished in planned, staged events. For patients in extremis from this injury, the concept of damage control for pelvic injuries includes a multidisciplinary approach with trauma and orthopedics to determine management strategies.

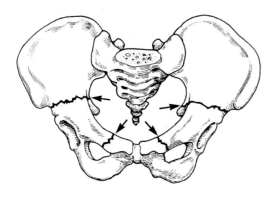

Figure 19–5. Fractured pelvis. Because of its ring formation, the pelvis usually fractures in two places. The common areas of fracture are indicated.

ASSESSMENT

- Perform primary and secondary survey (see Chapter 11), and address all issues.
- Perform ongoing assessment for hemodynamic instability.
- Palpate the pelvis for stability in lateral compression and anterior/posterior compression (this should be done just once in positive exams).
- Inspect soft tissue for ecchymosis, swelling, wounds, abrasions, and blood at the meatus of the penis.
- Perform rectal exam (assess for tone, prostate position, intactness of rectal wall, and guaiac for blood).
- Perform vaginal exam (if appropriate) to assess for blood and intactness of vaginal wall.
- Solicit patient for pain status with range of motion of lower extremities.
- Perform motor/sensory neurologic exam of lower extremities.
- Integrate abdominal exam and findings.

THERAPEUTIC INTERVENTIONS

- Administer oxygen, and initiate intravenous therapy with large-bore catheters.
- Control external hemorrhage.
- Treat hypovolemia.
- Consider early stabilization with pelvic binder or external fixation.
- Consider angiography and embolization of pelvic vascular structure.
- Monitor output; insert a Foley catheter if no contraindications or suprapubic cystotomy.
- Incorporate treatment strategies for abdominal injuries.

Complications from pelvic fractures include significant blood loss, coagulopathies, and associated injuries to the bladder, genitalia, and lumbosacral spine. Patients with abdominal and pelvic trauma are considered at high risk for poor outcomes and even death. A comprehensive approach to the management strategies along with an index of suspicion for the potential for hemodynamic instability is critical when caring for this patient population.

Suggested Readings

Brown CV, Velmahos G, Neville AL et al: Hemodynamically 'stable' patients with peritonitis after penetrating abdominal trauma, *Arch Surg* 140(8):767-772, 2005.

Clinical Policies Committee, American College of Emergency Physicians: Clinical policy: critical issues in the evaluation of adult patients presenting to the emergency department with acute blunt abdominal trauma, *Ann Emerg Med* 43(2):278-290, 2004.

Eckert KL: Penetrating and blunt abdominal trauma, *Crit Care Nurs Q* 28(1):41-59, 2005.

Montonye JM: Abdominal injuries. In McQuillan KA, Von Rueden KT, Hartsock RL et al, editors: *Trauma nursing from resuscitation through rehabilitation,* ed 3, Philadelphia, 2002, WB Saunders.

Morales CH, Villegas MI, Villavicencio R et al: Intra-abdominal infection in patients with abdominal trauma, *Arch Surg* 139(12):1278-1285, 2004.

Pape H, Pohlemann T, Gansslen A et al: Pelvic fractures in pregnant multiple trauma patients, *J Orthop Trauma* 14(4):238-244, 2000.

Teruy TH, Bianchi C, Abou-Zamzam AM et al: Endovascular treatment of a blunt traumatic abdominal aortic injury with a commercially available stent graft, *Ann Vasc Surg* 19(4):474-478, 2005.

Vrahas M, Joseph D: Orthopedic trauma 2: pelvic fractures. In Sheridan RL, editor: *The trauma handbook of the Massachusetts General Hospital,* Philadelphia, 2004, Lippincott, Williams & Wilkins.

Walker J, Criddle LM: Pathophysiology and management of abdominal compartment syndrome, *Am J Crit Care* 12(4):367-371, 2003.

CHAPTER 20

EXTREMITY AND VASCULAR TRAUMA

KATHLEEN J. BURNS

EXTREMITY TRAUMA

Injuries to arms and legs are more frequent and generally considered less life-threatening than injuries to the torso. When the patient has suffered multiple injuries, it is important to recall the principles of the trauma assessment and first identify and focus on life-threatening injuries and not be distracted by the deformities that frequently accompany extremity injuries. However, a great number of the disabilities and days of missed work that are suffered every year are the direct result of limb trauma. Prompt and appropriate management not only may be lifesaving and limb saving but also may prevent subsequent disabilities and reduce the costs of those disabilities to individuals and society.

EMERGENCY MANAGEMENT

After identifying life-threatening injuries, it is important to assess and stabilize all limb injuries. Obtain a brief history, and review the mechanism of injury. Consider patterns of injury to assist with diagnosis. For instance, a fractured right humerus and a fractured left femur in a patient who was struck by debris in an explosion would suggest that the plane of injury also may include the chest, abdomen, and pelvis, the structures that lie between the two obviously injured parts. Early treatment includes the following:

- ABCs (airway, breathing, and circulation)
- Quick assessment for other major trauma (head, cervical spine, chest, and abdomen)
- Protection of head and cervical spine
- Immobilization of traumatized limb to include joints above and below the trauma site
- Evaluation of neurologic/vascular status of limb distal to injury before and after immobilization:
  - Pulses distal to trauma
  - Color
  - Temperature
  - Capillary refill
  - Voluntary movement
  - Sensation
- Reduction of the fracture *only* if vascular status is compromised
- Elevation and support of limb, if possible
- Application of cold pack to area
- Transportation to hospital

Immobilization is accomplished before movement or transport to prevent further damage and to reduce the amount of pain and avoid further discomfort. Clinical personnel should note any swelling, discoloration, contusions, abrasions, or obvious deformities. If the injury includes an open fracture, perform the following:

- Irrigate the wound site with normal saline.
- Apply a sterile, normal saline dressing; cover it with a dry sterile dressing.
- Apply a slight compression dressing to control hemorrhage.
- Splint the limb.
- Do not attempt to reduce a fracture in the field.
- Assess the need for a tetanus shot; administer booster, if needed.

A tourniquet should be used only as a lifesaving measure. The limb may have to be amputated if all circulation ceases for an extended time.

When the patient arrives in the emergency department, he or she should be undressed to avoid missing any injuries. The patient should be turned to examine the front and back, stabilizing the injured limb throughout the maneuver. See Chapter 11 for initial assessment.

SOFT TISSUE INJURIES

Strains/Sprains

A strain is a weakening or stretching of a muscle at the tendon attachment. A strain may result from any trauma that stresses the attachment or injures the muscle in that area. Generally, strains have local point tenderness and mild swelling. Management strategy for strains includes resting the affected area, elevating it, and applying ice intermittently for up to 48 hours.

A sprain is a ligament that has been stretched or torn. The mechanism of injury may be the same as for a strain, but usually one with exaggerated force. Joint motion exceeds its normal limits. Most common sprains are in the shoulders, knees, wrists, and ankles. Sprains range from mild to severe and generally have pain and swelling, ecchymosis, and depending on the degree of injury, varying functional incapacity. Management strategy for sprains includes rest, elevation, intermittent ice application for up to 48 hours, and depending on the joint involved and the degree of injury, splinting and decreased function or weight-bearing status. Persistent pain or dysfunction should trigger an orthopedic consult.

Achilles Tendon Rupture

An Achilles tendon rupture occurs most often in athletes over 30 years old. The injury usually occurs in stop-and-start sports (such as tennis or racquetball) in which one steps off abruptly on the forefoot with the knee forced in extension. The patient usually describes a "snap" or "pop" noise and little or no pain at the time of injury. Many athletes who suffer this injury do not seek immediate care because of the lack of pain. Generally, these patients have the inability to extend their foot on the affected side, along with a deformity and a palpable gap in the tendon, and a positive Thomson's sign (with the leg extended and the foot over the end of the stretcher, squeeze the calf muscle, and no heel pull or upward movement will be observed). Once diagnosed, these patients require rest, elevation, and ice to the affected area. The limb should be immobilized in a toe-to-knee splint, and the patient should be instructed not to bear weight on that leg. Ambulation assist devices are necessary, and an orthopedic consult is necessary.

Table 20-1   Modes for Assessing Common Peripheral Nerve Injuries

Nerve	Frequently Associated Injuries	Assessment Technique*
Radial	Fracture of humerus, especially middle and distal third	Inability to extend thumb in hitchhiker's sign
Ulnar	Fracture of medial humeral epicondyle	Loss of pain perception in tip of little finger
Median	Elbow dislocation or wrist or forearm injury	Loss of pain perception in tip of index finger
Peroneal	Tibia or fibula fracture, dislocation of knee	Inability to extend great toe or foot; also may be associated with sciatic nerve injury
Sciatic and tibial	Sciatic nerve injuries should be considered in patients with hip fractures or dislocations; tibial nerve injuries are associated with knee injuries	Loss of pain perception in sole of foot

*Test is invalid if extension tendons are severed or if severe muscle damage is present.

PERIPHERAL NERVE INJURIES

Peripheral nerve injuries caused by trauma usually are associated with lacerations, fractures, dislocations, and penetrating wounds. Accurate assessment requires an understanding of the distribution of nerves, the origin of motor branches, and the muscles they supply (Table 20-1).

The clinician should recognize that motor loss tests are accurate only if he or she can palpate or visualize the tendon or muscle belly under consideration. Diagnostic tests such as electromyography, nerve conduction tests, and electrical stimulation are of little or no value in the emergency evaluation of peripheral nerve injury.

Repair of peripheral nerves should not be undertaken as an emergency department surgical intervention.

FRACTURES

Fractures are divided into two general categories:

- *Closed* (simple): The skin is not disrupted.
- *Open* (compound): The skin is disrupted by bone puncturing from inside out or an object puncturing from outside in, with resultant fracture.

The many different types of fractures are the following (Figure 20-1):

- *Transverse:* Results from angulation force or direct trauma
- *Oblique:* Results from twisting force
- *Spiral:* Results from twisting force with firmly planted foot
- *Comminuted:* Results from severe direct trauma; has more than two fragments

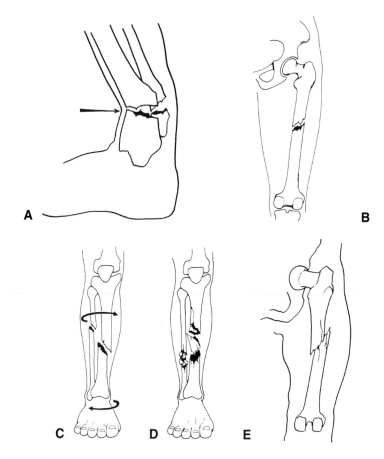

Figure 20-1. Types of fractures. **A,** Transverse. **B,** Oblique. **C,** Spiral. **D,** Comminuted. **E,** Impacted.

- *Impacted:* Results from severe trauma causing fracture ends to jam together
- *Compressed:* Results from severe force to top of head or os calcis or from acceleration-deceleration injury
- *Greenstick:* Results from compression force; usually occurs in children under 10 years of age and middle school or high school athletes
- *Avulsion:* Results from muscle mass contracting forcefully, causing bone fragment to tear off at insertion
- *Depression:* Results from blunt trauma to flat bone; usually involves much soft tissue damage

ASSESSMENT

When treating a patient with a suspected limb fracture, one should always assess for the *five P*'s:

- Pain and point tenderness
- Pulse (distal to fracture site)
- Pallor

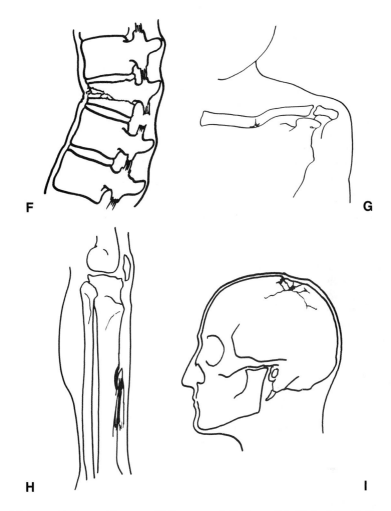

Figure 20–I, cont'd. Types of fractures. **F,** Compressed. **G,** Greenstick. **H,** Avulsion. **I,** Depression.

- Paresthesia (distal to fracture site)
- Paralysis (distal to fracture site)

The following factors also should be included in the assessment:

- Mechanism of injury
- Deformity
- Swelling
- Crepitus
- Discoloration
- Open wounds
- Other injuries

Clinical personnel should always suspect a fracture in limb trauma until proved otherwise. The patient's inability to move the limb or the presence of pain on movement should make the examiner suspicious of fracture. Radiographic examination is the most definitive way of detecting a fracture. The film should include the joints above and below the suspected fracture and should be taken in anteroposterior and lateral views.

THERAPEUTIC INTERVENTIONS

- Check the ABCs.
- Immobilize the limb (above and below fracture site).
- Reassess neurovascular status.
- Apply traction if circulatory compromise is present.
- Elevate injured limb, if possible (to decrease swelling and hemorrhage).
- Apply cold pack (to cause vasoconstriction and reduce swelling, spasm, and pain).

Complications of fractures include the following:

- Blood loss causing hypovolemia and shock (Chapter 12)
- Injury to vital organs
- Neurologic and/or vascular damage
- Infection (in open fractures)
- Fat embolism
- Deep vein thrombosis
- Rhabdomyolysis
- Compartment syndrome

Fat Embolism

Fat embolism may occur 24 to 48 hours after trauma and usually comes from a pelvic, tibial, or femoral fracture, but it may come from any other fracture site. Fat embolism has a high mortality rate and is a life-threatening situation.

ASSESSMENT

- Elevated temperature
- Rapid pulse
- Decreasing level of consciousness
- Inefficient respirations, leading to respiratory failure
- Cough
- Dyspnea
- Cyanosis
- Pulmonary edema
- Petechiae

THERAPEUTIC INTERVENTIONS

- Oxygen at high flow
- Close observation and monitoring
- Supportive therapy

Crush Injuries

Crush injuries frequently occur in industrial settings when limbs get caught in equipment or between equipment, motor vehicle/motorcycle collisions in which extremities get pinned, or from being down in one position for a prolonged time. The clinician must know the mechanism of injury because the patient may have few symptoms initially. Crush injuries often cause damage to skin, muscle, bone, nerve, and vascular structures. Tissue necrosis can occur within a few hours, resulting in the development of compartment syndrome, rhabdomyolysis, and shock.

Compartment Syndrome

Compartment syndrome should be suspected in patients with severe fractures or crush injuries. This syndrome develops from an increase in the pressure of the compartment from edema or bleeding, resulting in a decrease blood supply to the muscles and nerves. Patients will develop ischemia and necrosis if the pressures are not reduced. Compartment syndrome usually occurs within 6 to 8 hours of injury. It may occur in any soft tissue compartment but is seen most commonly in the forearm and lower extremities. Suspected extremities require timely reassessment and measurement of the compartment pressures.

ASSESSMENT

- Throbbing pain out of proportion to injury that is not relieved by analgesia
- Increased pain with passive stretching
- Firmness/edema over compartment; compare with uninjured extremity

THERAPEUTIC INTERVENTION

- Ongoing assessment of compartment for pain and firmness
- Compartment pressures checked by orthopedist
- Fasciotomies to relieve elevated pressures and prevent further damage

Rhabdomyolysis

Rhabdomyolysis is a syndrome seen with fractures and crush injuries when there is major muscle destruction along with ischemia and edema, causing the release of potassium and myoglobin. Potassium and creatine kinase levels need to be monitored. The myoglobin often affects kidney function because the large particles obstruct filtration, resulting in tubular necrosis. Treatment strategies include high-volume intravenous fluids, use of osmotic diuretics, and bicarbonate in the intravenous fluids. Complications of rhabdomyolysis include hemodynamic and metabolic disturbances, compartment syndrome, and acute renal failure. Rapid identification of the problem and treatment helps minimize the complications.

VASCULAR TRAUMA

A person who sustains trauma to the vascular system is at risk of losing an extremity or his or her life. Vascular trauma is often the consequence of blunt or penetrating injury. Vascular trauma may be seen with fractures, deceleration injuries, or crush injuries. Injuries may involve veins, arteries, or both. Usually, when penetrating trauma such as a gunshot wound, stab wound, or blast injury occurs, the resulting vascular trauma is a laceration or transection. Blunt trauma, such as occurs with deceleration injuries, crush injuries, and joint disruptions, may cause dissections, hematomas, or disruptions. Vascular injuries may be subtle, resulting in internal hemorrhage, or obvious, as demonstrated by an external hemorrhage.

Arterial injuries may cause the following:

- Pain
- Pallor
- Pulselessness
- Paresthesias
- Paralysis (neurologic deficit)
- Cold distal extremity
- Pale distal extremity

When a trauma patient arrives at the emergency department, clinical personnel should think about the mechanism of injury, the location of the injury, and the proximity of the injury to arterial structures while they are completing a primary and secondary survey.

During the secondary survey, clinical personnel should check the affected limb for the following:

- Pulses (to be described as normal, diminished, absent, or Doppler)
- Capillary refill
- External blood loss
- Skin color, temperature, and moisture
- Type of wound
- Neurovascular status
- Hematoma (may be pulsatile)
- Bruits
- Differences in extremities

Definitive diagnosis of arterial injury can be made by the following:

- Pulselessness
- Angiography
- Computed tomography scan

SPECIFIC FRACTURES AND ASSOCIATED VASCULAR INJURIES

Assessment and management strategy of fracture patterns and associated vascular injuries as previously described is essentially the same for upper and lower extremities. A high index of suspicion based on the mechanism of injury and the pattern of trauma should help the clinician with timely identification of injuries. Table 20-2 outlines specific patterns or associations (Figures 20-2 to 20-8).

DISLOCATION

Dislocation occurs when a joint exceeds its range of motion and the joint surfaces are no longer intact. This type of injury generally is accompanied by a large amount of soft tissue injury in the joint capsule and surrounding ligaments; much swelling; and possible vein, artery, and nerve damage. When obtaining a history, clinical personnel should determine the force that

Table 20-2   Fracture Sites and Associated Neurologic/Vascular Concerns

Fracture Site	Associated Neurologic/Vascular Concerns
Clavicle	Subclavian artery/vein; observe for expanding hematoma that can cause airway compromise
Shoulder: glenoid, humeral head, humeral neck	Increased incidence in elders; may have associated axillary nerve injury; requires rapid determination if dislocation exits
Scapula	High-energy injury; timely rule out of associated intrathoracic injury
Humeral shaft	Brachial artery; radial nerve
Elbow (Figure 20-2)	Brachial artery; median or radial nerve damage; Volkmann's contracture*
Forearm (radius/ulna; Figure 20-3); wrist (Figure 20-4)	Common injury after fall with outstretched hand; median nerve at risk; timely reduction of fracture pattern
Hand/fingers	Injury pattern associated with dislocations and fractures; increase incidence of industrial injuries resulting in amputations/mangled soft tissues
Hip (Figure 20-5)	Common injury in elders with minimal energy transfer; generally requires high-energy transfer in younger patients
Femur (Figure 20-6)	Femoral artery; potential for significant blood loss into the surrounding soft tissue
Knee (supracondylar femur, intraarticular fracture of femur or tibia; Figure 20-7)	Popliteal artery; peroneal and posterior tibial nerve; can be complex/limb-threatening injury
Patellar	Usually associated with direct impact (fall) or indirect trauma (severe muscle pull)
Tibial shaft and/or fibular shaft (Figure 20-8)	If the result of twisting motion, be sure to assess knee and ankle for associated injuries; high incidence of associated compartment syndrome
Ankle	Torsion/twisting a common mechanism for injury
Heel (os calcis)	Usually associated with direct axial loading (fall, jump from a height landing on feet); always assess for associated injuries (compression spinal fractures)

*In Volkmann's contracture, degeneration and contraction of muscles occur because of ischemia caused by decreased arterial blood flow.

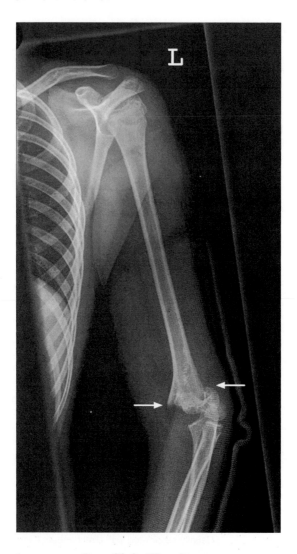

Figure 20–2. Elbow fracture.

caused the injury to project a diagnosis. For all joint injuries the assessment and general therapeutic interventions are similar. Table 20-3 lists specific patterns and associations.

ASSESSMENT

- Severe pain
- Joint deformity
- Inability to move joint
- Swelling
- Point tenderness

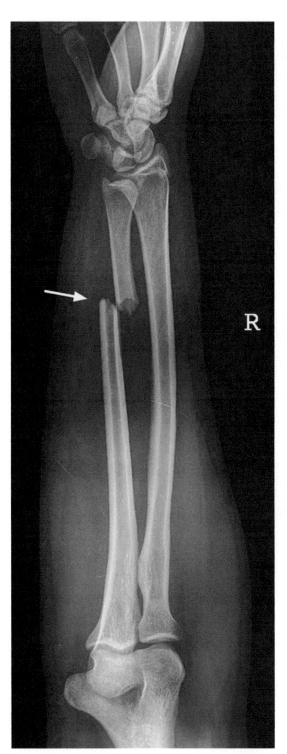

Figure 20–3. Forearm fracture.

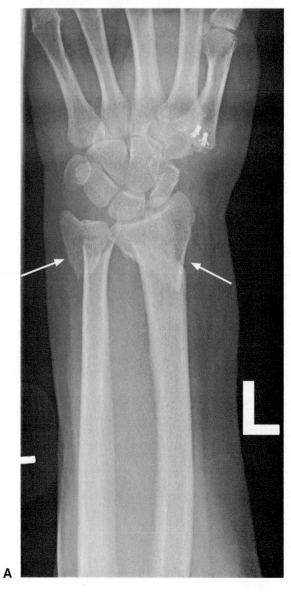

Figure 20–4. Wrist fractures. **A,** Anteroposterior view.

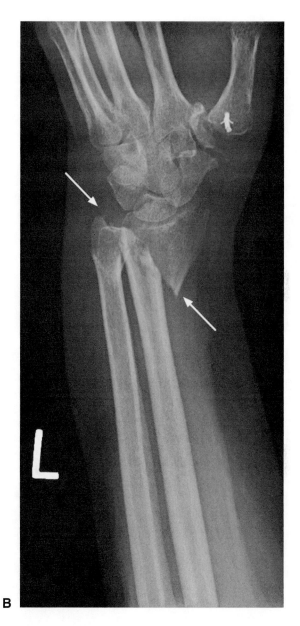

Figure 20–4, cont'd. Wrist fractures. **B,** Lateral view.

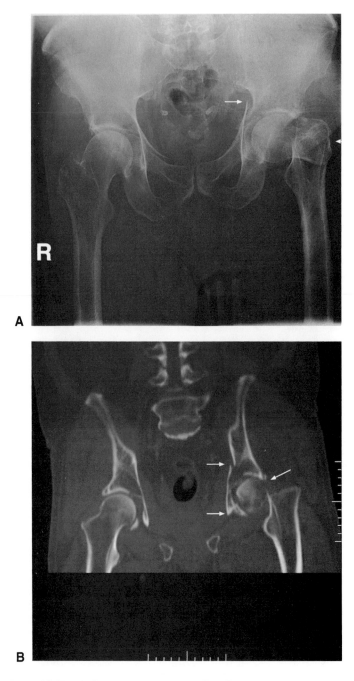

Figure 20–5. Hip fractures. **A,** Plain x-ray film. **B,** Computed tomography scan.

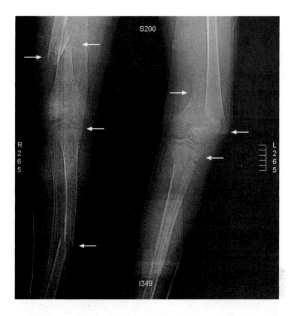

Figure 20-6. Femur fracture.

Table 20-3 Dislocation Sites and Associated Concerns

Dislocation Site	Associated Concerns
Acromioclavicular separation	Common athletic injury, inability to raise affected arm or bring arm across chest, point tenderness with or without step-off
Shoulder	Anterior dislocation associated with fall on an extended arm that is abducted and externally rotated, resulting in the head of the humerus locating anterior to the shoulder joint; posterior dislocation is rare, associated with extended arm that is abducted and internally rotated or from a direct blow; high incidence of recurrent dislocation
Elbow	Prominent olecranon with more common posterior dislocation; Generally results from fall on to extended arm; in young children can result from lifting the child by a single arm causing displacement of the ulna (nursemaid's elbow)
Hip	Generally associated with high-energy transfer (with extended leg and foot on brake pedal before impact or with knee hitting dashboard); more common posterior dislocation, always assess knee and ipsilateral hip
Knee	Usually high-energy transfer and grossly unstable; detailed neurologic/vascular assessment with ongoing reassessment until definitive care is complete
Patella	Usually from a direct blow; always assess hips for associated injury
Ankle	Soft tissue at great risk; timely reduction and support.

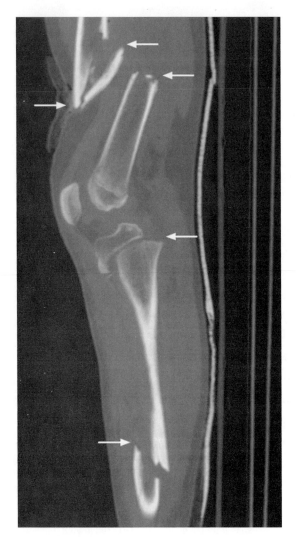

Figure 20–7. Knee fracture (supracondylar femur and tibia).

THERAPEUTIC INTERVENTIONS

- Palpate the joint area carefully.
- Splint the joint "as it lies."
- Do *not* reduce a dislocation in the field.
- Early reduction with adequate anesthesia is required in the emergency department, but only after x-ray examination to rule out accompanying fracture.
- Compare injured side to other side for symmetry, droop, edema, and deformity.
- Obtain an orthopedic consult.

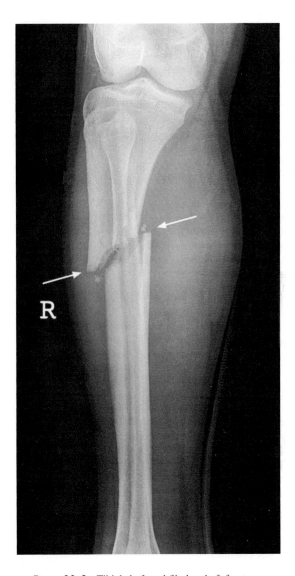

Figure 20-8. Tibial shaft and fibular shaft fracture.

PEDIATRIC LIMB TRAUMA

Special attention should be paid to pediatric limb trauma when fractures occur at the epiphysis, or growth center. A fracture at the epiphysis may cause an early closure of the plate, which results in a short extremity as the child grows, or it may stimulate long-bone growth, resulting in unequal limb length. If the fracture is a partial fracture, an angular deformity may result. A child with such a fracture should be followed by an orthopedic surgeon for several months because it is difficult to predict the outcome at the time of injury.

TRAUMATIC AMPUTATIONS

Traumatic amputations are common to farm workers, factory workers, and motorcyclists. They occur under many different circumstances. The affected part can be amputated completely or partially or demonstrate extensive damage in the form of a mangled extremity where the appendage is at significant risk for viability. All body parts are at risk for these type of injuries: upper and lower extremities at any point along the extremity, along with ears, nose, face, or penis.

THERAPEUTIC INTERVENTIONS

- Ensure the ABCs.
- Control bleeding.
- Support affected part in position of function.
- Initiate fluid replacement with two large-bore intravenous lines.
- Type and crossmatch for possible blood replacement.
- Administer high-flow oxygen.
- Transport patient to hospital.
- Prepare patient for surgery.

Preservation of Amputated Part

Perform the following to preserve the amputated extremity:

- Use hypothermia; do not freeze the amputated part.
- Soak or dress the part in sterile normal saline or lactated Ringer's solution.
- Place part in dry container; then place the container—but *not* the part—on ice.
- Maintain correct anatomic position of severed limb, if limb is partially attached.

Care of Stump

Care for the stump as follows:

- Treat patient for shock.
- Apply direct pressure to reduce blood loss.
- Apply ice and elevate extremity.
- Consider débridement, if wound is contaminated.

Limiting Factors in Replantation

The following factors limit the possibility of replantation:

- Availability of replantation team
- Severity of damage to amputated part *(including damage during preservation technique)*
- Amount of time since incident occurred
- Physical status of patient

Upper extremity replantations have been more successful than lower extremity replantations.

SPLINTING

Splinting prevents further damage to soft tissues, arteries, and veins; decreases pain; and minimizes muscle spasm. Clinical personnel should always splint above and below the injury site. For example, if the ankle is injured, also splint the foot and knee. If the knee is injured, also splint the lower leg and the trunk on the injured side.

Splints are divided into four basic types:

- Soft splint: soft, not rigid, such as a pillow
- Hard splint: firm surface; rigid, such as a board
- Air splint: inflatable; provides rigidity without being hard (do not use if patient to be transferred by air)
- Traction splint: provides support, decreased angulation, and traction

A variety of splint materials are used:
- Thomas*
- Reel*
- Hare*
- Sagar*
- Backboard
    - Short board (or Kendrick extrication device)
    - Long board
- Aluminum long-leg

General Principles of Splint Application

Consider the following principles of splint application:

- Immobilize the injured part, including joint above and below injury and proximal and distal to injury.
- Correct severe angulation only if it is impossible to splint or if vascular compromise is present.
- Use at least two persons for splinting: one to maintain manual alignment and one to apply the splinting apparatus.
- Secure the injured part to the splint (do *not* use elastic bandage).
- Monitor the extremity for swelling.
- Perform a neurovascular exam: check the color, sensitivity, and motion before and after splint application to ensure the splint does not impede neurovascular status

SUMMARY

When a patient has limb trauma, the caregiver needs to do a thorough assessment. Clinical personnel must assess for potential fractures and must think about the underlying vascular supply. Keeping the fracture and underlying structures in mind will help the caregiver anticipate the diagnostic signs and symptoms particular to that limb. When these signs and symptoms are detected early, the caregiver can provide appropriate, timely interventions and can optimize the patient's care.

---

*Use for femoral shaft fractures or fractures of the upper third of the tibia; these splints should not be used on fractures of the hip, lower tibia, fibula, or ankle.

Suggested Readings

Dolan B: *Accident and emergency: theory into practice,* Edinburgh, 2000, Balliere Tindell.

Khatod M, Botte MJ, Hoyt DB et al: Outcomes in open tibia fractures: relationships between delay in treatment and infection, *J Trauma* 55(5):949-954, 2003.

Klineberg EO, Crites BM, Flinn WR et al: The role of arteriography in assessing popliteal artery injury in knee dislocations, *J Trauma* 56(4):786-790, 2004.

Newberry L, editor: *Sheehy's emergency nursing: principles and practice,* ed 4, St Louis, 1998, Mosby.

Rios A, Villa A, Fahandezh H et al: Results after treatment of traumatic knee dislocations: a report of 26 cases, *J Trauma* 55(3):489-494, 2003.

Rozycki GS, Tremblay LN, Feliciano DV et al: Blunt vascular trauma in the extremity: diagnosis, management, and outcome, *J Trauma* 55(5):814-824, 2003.

Sahin V, Karakas ES, Aksu S et al: Traumatic dislocations and fracture-dislocation of the hip: a long-term follow-up study, *J Trauma* 54(3):520-529, 2003.

Sheridan RL, editor: *The trauma handbook of the Massachusetts General Hospital,* Philadelphia, 2004, Lippincott, William & Wilkins.

Smith J, Greaves I: Crush injury and crush syndrome: a review, *J Trauma* 54(5):50-529, 2003.

UNIQUE POPULATIONS

CHAPTER 21

TRAUMA IN PREGNANCY

MARY LOU LYONS AND ALICE A. GERVASINI

Trauma is the leading cause of death in women during the reproductive ages of 15 to 44. Physical injury affects approximately 7% of all pregnancies. The most common cause of trauma in pregnant women is motor vehicle crashes, followed by falls, penetrating injuries/domestic violence, and burns/smoke inhalation.

When a woman of childbearing age arrives as a victim of trauma, a pregnancy test should be done with the initial trauma lab tests, for early signs of pregnancy may not be readily visible or assessible. If the woman is pregnant, the gestational age of the fetus should be established. When a pregnant woman has been injured, the mother and the fetus need to be taken into consideration, although the health of the mother always takes precedence over the fetus. Decisions regarding management strategy for the pregnant trauma patient should reflect the mother's viability and gestational age of the fetus. Considerations for the fetus less than 23 to 24 weeks' gestational age focus on radiation and medication exposure. In general, fetal viability is at the 23- to 24-week mark, and assessing the height of the uterine fundus can approximate this. Generally, the fundus height is approximately 1 cm per week of gestation and therefore is between the umbilicus and the xiphoid at the 23- to 24-week point. The physiologic changes that occur in pregnancy must be considered when the patient has been traumatized. The more severely injured the mother is, with associated hypotension and hypovolemia, the greater the incidence of fetal complications and death.

Also important to remember is that the initial assessment and interventions remain the same: airway, breathing, and circulation. Clinical personnel should perform a primary and secondary survey, just as on any other trauma patient (Chapter 11). The obstetric team should participate

---

HIGH-FREQUENCY NURSING DIAGNOSES FOR PREGNANT TRAUMA PATIENTS

- Impaired gas exchange
- Decreased cardiac output
- Ineffective tissue perfusion: maternal-fetal unit
- Acute pain
- Fear
- Anticipatory grieving
- *Nursing diagnoses specific to injury*

From NANDA International: *NANDA nursing diagnoses: definitions & classification, 2005-2006*, Philadelphia, 2006, The Association.

in the evaluation of the patient and assist with care. High-frequency nursing diagnoses for the pregnant trauma patient are listed in the nursing diagnosis box. An understanding of the normal anatomic and physiologic changes in the pregnant patient needs to be incorporated into the trauma team's management strategy (Table 21-1).

Table 21-1 Normal Anatomic and Physiologic Changes of Pregnancy

System	Normal Changes	Implications
Cardiovascular	Increased heart rate: 10-15 beats/min above baseline Cardiac output increases by 30%-50% and plateaus at the end of the second trimester Decrease in systemic vascular resistance Decrease in pulmonary vascular resistance Supine hypotension increases as gestational age increases and can result in decreased preload 95% of women develop systolic murmur at 22 weeks Vasodilation such that skin color remains good even in the presence of shock Left axis shift of 15 degrees of the heart by the third trimester Physiologic anemia resulting from 40%-50% increase in plasma with a smaller increase in red blood cells Increase in clotting factors	Acute blood loss of 10%-20% may not result in vital sign changes and may lead to false sense of hemodynamic stability Position patient to remove uterus from compressing inferior vena cava; less than 24 weeks' gestation, lateral displacement of the uterus toward the maternal left side; greater than 24 weeks, a 30-degree left lateral tilt should be considered; if positioning changes are not feasible, the uterus should be displaced manually Potential electrocardiogram changes including T wave flattening or inversion in lead III, Q waves in lead III, and augmented V leads Lower hematocrit Hypercoagulation state—rapidly decreases in the presence of bleeding
Respiratory	Elevated diaphragm (gestational age specific) Elevated oxygen consumption by 15%-20% Increased tidal volume and vital capacity Decreased functional residual capacity Respiratory alkalosis because of hyperventilation leading to slight alkalemia Decreased oxygen reserve and buffering capacity	Hypoxemia occurs earlier in pregnant women; monitor rate, depth, and pattern because subtle changes are significant—poor compensation Early use of oxygen therapy Gestational age directly affects all parameters of respiratory function
Gastrointestinal	Decreased gastric emptying Decreased gastric tone Increased gastric acid production	Increased potential for aspiration

Continued

Table 21-1   Normal Anatomic and Physiologic Changes of Pregnancy—cont'd

System	Normal Changes	Implications
Genitourinary	Increased urinary frequency Displaced bladder anteriorly and superiorly Dilation of the renal pelvis and ureters	Bladder repositioned intraabdominally and more susceptible to injury Blood urea nitrogen/creatinine will decrease to 50% of normal adult values
Musculoskeletal	Widened symphysis pubis Joint laxity Altered center of gravity	Alteration in gait and balance Potential to misread x-ray films
Vital signs	Pulse: increased by 15-20 beats/min by the middle of the second trimester; normal pulse is 90-100 beats/min Respirations: increased because of progesterone stimulation of the medullary respiratory center Temperature: not affected by pregnancy Blood pressure normally slightly elevated	Maternal hypovolemia can result in a 20% reduction in uterine blood flow without changes in her blood pressure

GENERAL THERAPEUTIC INTERVENTIONS FOR THE TRAUMATIZED PREGNANT WOMAN

Perform the following interventions for the pregnant woman with trauma:

- Perform standard trauma care (airway, breathing, circulation).
- Administer high-flow oxygen.
- Depending on gestational age, while the patient is flat, displace the uterus off the retroperitoneal vasculature.
- If fluids are required, give blood products early. Avoid large volumes of crystalloid solutions. Type and crossmatch blood.
- Check the patient's Rh status, and determine the need for $Rh_0(D)$ immune globulin (RhoGAM).
- Ensure current tetanus prophylaxis.
- Focused abdominal sonogram of trauma has been shown to be beneficial.
- Shield the abdomen during radiologic procedures whenever possible.
- Insert a gastric tube because gastric emptying is prolonged.
- Once fetal viability (approximately 23 to 24 weeks) has been estimated, provide continuous fetal/uterine monitoring.

SPECIFIC INJURIES AND INDICATIONS IN PREGNANCY

In addition to standard therapeutic interventions for trauma to any patient, caregivers should be particularly cognizant of the following in the injured pregnant patient.

Head Trauma

Following minor or major trauma, there is a significant potential for head and neck injury. A complete neurologic exam with radiographic diagnostic tests should be included in the plan of care.

Chest Trauma

Pulmonary volume may be decreased as a result of anatomic changes in the second and third trimesters. The diaphragm is elevated, and vital capacity is decreased. Chest tube placement may require insertion one or two intercostal spaces higher than in the nonpregnant patient. Chest trauma that causes even small changes in lung volumes and expansion may be lethal.

Gastrointestinal Trauma

Trauma to the gastrointestinal system requires the following considerations:

- Caregivers should assume that the patient has a full stomach and therefore is at risk for aspiration. Bowel sounds may be absent.
- Lower abdominal injuries may not cause intestinal trauma because the intestines are relocated high anatomically.
- An aberration in referred pain may result from relocation of the abdominal contents.
- A 5% to 10% incidence of disseminated intravascular coagulation occurs with significant blunt abdominal trauma.
- With lower abdominal blunt forces, the risk for significant pelvic fractures, uterine injury, and abruptio placentae is high. The uterus is more elastic than the placenta, which may result in a lower injury pattern to the uterus but still significant placental disruption. All of these injury patterns are associated with significant bleeding and the potential for preterm labor.

Genitourinary Trauma

Trauma to the genitourinary system requires the following considerations:

- The bladder is pushed out of the pelvic ring and is less protected in late pregnancy.
- Blood urea nitrogen and creatinine will decrease to 50% of normal adult values, and urine glucose will increase.
- Any blood found in the urine—gross or microscopic—is not normal, and further investigation should occur to determine its cause.

Vaginal/Fetal Trauma

Consider the following interventions for vaginal and fetal trauma:

- Ultrasound procedures may be advantageous in this situation because they can help determine fetal well-being, gestational age, and placental and uterine injuries.
- Pelvic examination should be performed by a person who understands obstetric findings in trauma.
- Contractions may occur prematurely. Uterine activity must be monitored carefully.
- Any fluid coming from the vaginal vault should be tested to determine whether it is amniotic fluid. The pH of amniotic fluid is 7 to 7.5. If the fluid has been determined to be amniotic fluid, a stat obstetric/gynecologic consult should be obtained.

- Check for frank blood or hemorrhage. This may be indicative of abruptio placentae or fetal injury. Signs and symptoms of abruptio placentae include premature labor, abdominal pain, fetal distress, uterine tenderness, or maternal shock. Obvious vaginal bleeding may or may not be present. Stat cesarean section should be considered.
- Fetal trauma during the first and second trimester is not common (except in massive blunt abdominal trauma or penetrating abdominal trauma) because of the cushioning effect of amniotic fluid. During the third trimester, the ratio of amniotic fluid to fetus is reversed, and the cushion effect is decreased, potentially resulting in fetal trauma.
- The fetal skull may be damaged from an acceleration/deceleration motion (when the mother is wearing only a lap seat belt).

Burns/Smoke Inhalation

Consider the following interventions for burns and smoke inhalation:

- The patient with a burn injury has increased fluid needs.
- The rule of nines may not apply to the pregnant patient when measuring body surface area because of the great increase in body surface area during pregnancy. One may use the area of the palm of the patient's hand to estimate the amount of body surface area burned (palmer surface of the patient's hand is approximately 1% of total body surface area).
- There is an increased risk of preterm labor in the patient who has sustained a large thermal burn.
- If smoke inhalation has occurred, it is essential to administer high-flow oxygen and obtain an oxygen saturation measurement and arterial blood gases.

Fetal Assessment

Fetal assessment requires the following considerations:

- Estimate gestational age by using a measurement of the height of the fundus and, if available, the date of the patient's last menstrual period.
- Fetal monitoring should be continual for those patients with fetuses of a gestational age of at least 23 to 24 weeks. Fetal heart tones normally should be between 110 and 160 beats/min.
- If fetal heart rate is nonreassuring, stat cesarean section may be appropriate depending on the condition of the mother, the nature of the injuries, and the gestational age of the fetus (at least 23 to 24 weeks).
- If the pregnant mother is moribund and there is a possibility that the fetus may be viable, consider preparation for a stat cesarean section, possibly to be done in the emergency department. This also may be considered if the mother is recently (minutes) deceased.
- In the event of fetal death, appropriate support personnel should be available to the mother, the family, and significant others to support them through the grieving process.

SUMMARY

The traumatized pregnant patient represents approximately 7% of all pregnancies. Although fairly rare, the clinical management challenge for the trauma nurse is significant and requires a comprehensive approach by the trauma service and the obstetric service to ensure optimal outcomes.

Suggested Readings

D'Amico CJ: Trauma in pregnancy, *Top Emerg Med* 24(4):26-39, 2002.

Grossman NB: Blunt trauma in pregnancy, *Am Fam Physician* 70(7):1303-1310, 2004.

Mattox KL, Goetzl L: Trauma in pregnancy, *Crit Care Med* 33(10):S385-S389, 2005.

Pape H, Pohlemann T, Gansslen A et al: Pelvic fractures in pregnant multiple trauma patients, *J Orthop Trauma* 14(4):238-244, 2000.

Rand L, Dennehy K: Considerations in the pregnant women. In Sheridan RL, editor: *The trauma handbook of the Massachusetts General Hospital,* Philadelphia, 2004, Lippincott, Williams & Wilkins.

Shah AJ, Kilcline BA: Trauma in pregnancy, *Emerg Med Clin North Am* 21:615-629, 2003.

Smith LG: Assessment and initial management of the pregnant trauma patient, *J Trauma Nurs* 1:8-20, 1994.

Smith LG: The pregnant trauma patient. In McQuillan KA, Von Rueden KT, Hartsock RL et al, editor: *Trauma nursing: from resuscitation through rehabilitation,* ed 3, Philadelphia, 2002, WB Saunders.

Stone IK: Trauma in the obstetric patient, *Obstet Gynecol Clin North Am* 26(3):459-467, 1999.

PEDIATRIC TRAUMA

CAROLE C. ATKINSON

Trauma remains the leading cause of death in children, and each year a significant number of children suffer permanent disability. The impact affects not only the child but the family and community at large. The pathophysiologic mechanism of traumatic injury in children is similar to that of the adult, although there are unique characteristics that need to be explored.

EPIDEMIOLOGY

Unintentional injury continues as the number one cause of death in the 1- to 24-year-old age group. Table 22-1 outlines the leading causes of injury death in children by age group. Thousands of children are estimated to be hospitalized each year, and millions more are treated in emergency departments and physician's offices for unintentional injury. Table 22-2 outlines the leading causes of nonfatal injuries treated in hospital emergency departments by age group.

T a b l e 22–I   Leading Causes of Injury/Death in Children by Age Group

	Age in Years			
Rank	**<1**	**1-4**	**5-9**	**10-14**
1	Unintentional suffocation	Motor vehicle (MV) traffic	MV traffic	MV traffic
2	MV traffic	Drowning	Drowning	Drowning
3	Homicide	Fire/burn	Fire/burn	Suicide/suffocation
4	Homicide/ unspecified	Homicide/ unspecified	Homicide/firearm	Homicide/firearm
5	Drowning	Unintentional suffocation	Other land transport	Suicide/firearm
6	Fire/burn	Pedestrian	Unintentional suffocation	Fire/burn
7	Undetermined suffocation	Homicide	Fall	Other land transport
8	Homicide suffocation	Homicide firearm	Pedestrian	Unintentional suffocation
9	Adverse effects	Homicide	Struck by/against	Firearm
10	Fall	Natural/environment	Other transport	Pedestrian

Adapted from National Center for Health Statistics, Vital Statistics Systems, and National Center for Injury Prevention and Control, 2001.

Table 22-2   Leading Causes of Nonfatal Injuries Treated in Hospital Emergency Departments by Age Group

	Age in Years			
Rank	<1	1-4	5-9	10-14
1	Fall	Fall	Fall	Fall
2	Struck by/against	Struck by/against	Struck by/against	Struck by/against
3	Fire/burn	Bite/sting	Cut/pierce	Overexertion
4	Bite/sting	Foreign body	Pedal cyclist	Cut/pierce
5	Motor vehicle (MV) collision: occupant	Cut/pierce	Bite/sting	Pedal cyclist
6	Unintentional poisoning	Unintentional poisoning	MV collision: occupant	Unspecified
7	Foreign body	Overexertion	Overexertion	MV collision: occupant
8	Unspecified	Fire/burn	Foreign body	Assault
9	Inhalation/ suffocation	MV collision: occupant	Dog bite	Other transport
10	Overexertion	Unspecified	Unspecified	Bite/sting

Modified from chart developed by the National Center for Injury Prevention and Control, Centers for Disease Control and Prevention, 2002.
Data source: National Electronic Injury Surveillance System operated by the Consumer Product Safety Commission.

ASSESSMENT

Although the management priorities for children are the same as for the adult trauma patient, consideration must be given to their significant anatomic, physiologic, and developmental differences. Table 22-3 outlines these differences by system. The nursing diagnosis box lists nursing diagnoses common to pediatric trauma patients.

HIGH-FREQUENCY NURSING DIAGNOSES FOR PEDIATRIC TRAUMA PATIENTS

- Risk for aspiration
- Impaired gas exchange
- Decreased cardiac output
- Hypothermia
- Acute pain
- Fear
- Post-trauma syndrome
- Impaired parenting
- *Nursing diagnoses specific to injury*

From NANDA International: *NANDA nursing diagnoses: definitions & classification, 2005-2006,* Philadelphia, 2006, The Association.

Table 22-3   Some Unique Anatomic and Physiologic Characteristics of Infants and Children

System	Anatomic Uniqueness	Physiologic Consideration
Respiratory		
Airway	Small oral cavity Narrowest section is cricoid cartilage Large epiglottis, tonsils, and adenoid tissue	Tongue can occlude oropharnyx Secure endotracheal tube and prevent aspiration Protect the lower airway
Breathing	Infants are obligate nose breathers Infants have a thin, pliable chest wall The diaphragm is used for respiration because intercostal muscles are underdeveloped	Nasal obstruction increases work of breathing Blunt forces are transmitted to internal structures Faster breathing results in higher rate of oxygen consumption and rapid hypoxemia
Cervical spine immobilization	Prominent occiput results in hyperflexion of the short neck	Airway occlusion with neck flexed and endotracheal tube dislodges with neck motion
Cardiovascular		
Circulation	Circulatory blood volume is 80 mL/kg	When blood volume decreases, the cardiac output increases and the heart rate increases; blood pressure can remain unchanged because of compensatory mechanisms
Neurologic		
Disability	Large head size and lax neck muscles, so child more susceptible to head injury; blunt head injury is the major cause of morbidity and mortality of children	External and internal hemorrhage may result in shock; hypoxia and severe head trauma can result in cerebral edema that is difficult to control
Gastrointestinal	Small amount of protective subcutaneous fat around organs and undeveloped supportive musculature; liver and spleen most susceptible to injury	Intraabdominal hemorrhage and shock
Genitourinary	The kidneys take up a larger space in abdominal cavity, sit lower, and have less protective fat Pliable ribs do not protect Renal capsule and vascular pedicle are less developed and susceptible to injury	Intraperitoneal bleeding and shock

Table 22-3   Some Unique Anatomic and Physiologic Characteristics of Infants and Children—cont'd

System	Anatomic Uniqueness	Physiologic Consideration
	Bladder is an abdominal organ in children	
Musculoskeletal	Growth plates not fused Bone ossification incomplete; ligamentous injury	Bone growth arrest Unstable injuries with management challenges
Psychosocial	Chronologic age and physical or psychological development do not always coincide; age-appropriate pain measurement scales must be used for accurate assessment Consideration must be given to suspected child abuse if the history does not correlate with the injury pattern	

PEDIATRIC-SPECIFIC INTERVENTIONS AND TREATMENT

A multidisciplinary team approach is essential for comprehensive care of the trauma patient—adult or pediatric. For a detailed review of the initial assessment of the trauma patient with a focus on primary and secondary survey and interventions, see Chapter 11. Incorporating the distinctive anatomic features and physiologic responses for the pediatric trauma patient is critical to the successful management of this patient population.

Primary Survey

Airway

Perform the following interventions for airway management:

- Use the jaw thrust maneuver to open the airway in an unconscious child.
- Suction any obstructing matter such as blood, emesis, or secretions from the airway; do not use the blind finger sweep method to clear the oral cavity.
- Oral airways, when required, are inserted using a forward motion with the tongue depressed outward. Rotation of the airway is contraindicated because it may cause trauma to the soft tissues of the palate and hypopharynx.
- Nasopharyngeal airways are tolerated better by the conscious child and are to be used only in the absence of maxillofacial injuries or suspected basilar skull fractures.
- Intubation is recommended when respiratory distress or poor ventilation persist or when the child has a Glasgow Coma Scale score of 8 or less (Table 22-4). Use an uncuffed tube for children less than 8 years old to avoid vocal cord trauma, subglottic edema, and pressure necrosis.
- Use a length-based equipment tool such as a Broselow tape to expedite equipment setup.

Table 22-4   Glasgow Coma Scale

Infant/Toddler	Child/Adult
Eye Opening	*Eye Opening*
Spontaneous 4	Spontaneous 4
To voice 3	To voice 3
To pain 2	To pain 2
None 1	None 1
Best Verbal Response	*Best Verbal Response*
Smiles, interacts 5	Oriented 5
Consolable 4	Confused 4
Cries to pain 3	Inappropriate words 3
Moans to pain 2	Incomprehensible words . . .2
None 1	None 1
Best Motor Response	*Best Motor Response*
Normal spontaneous. 6	Obeys commands 6
Localizes pain 5	Localizes pain 6
Withdraws to pain 4	Withdraws to pain 5
Abnormal flexion 3	Abnormal flexion 4
Abnormal extension 2	Abnormal extension 2
None 1	None 1

From Teasdale G, Jennett B: Assessment of coma and impaired consciousness, *Lancet* 2:81-84, 1974.

Breathing

Perform the following interventions for breathing management:

- Administer 100% oxygen by non-rebreather mask to all children.
- Monitor oxygen saturation, via pulse oximetry, noting that readings are unreliable in children with poor peripheral perfusion.

Circulation

Perform the following interventions for circulation management:

- *If the child is pulseless,* initiate cardiopulmonary resuscitation, and follow pediatric advanced life support protocols.
- If a pulse is present but ineffective, obtain vascular access using two large-bore intravenous catheters (or obtain intraosseous access) and administer a 20 mL/kg bolus of warmed normal saline or lactated Ringer's solution. If response is unsatisfactory, repeat the bolus, follow by administration of 10 mL/kg of packed red blood cells, type specific or O negative.

Disability

Perform the following interventions for disability management:

- Consider pharmacologic intervention such as naloxone or D_{25} to improve mental status.
- Calculate the Glasgow Coma Scale score using the infant/toddler scale for preverbal children.

Secondary Survey

Perform the following assessments during the secondary survey:

- *Expose* the child by removing all clothing so that a complete assessment can be performed. Remember that the ratio of surface area to body mass in the child is greater than in the adult; therefore, the child's body temperature will drop quicker. Initiate warming interventions such as blankets, radiant warmers, and warmed intravenous fluids.
- *Get a full set of vital signs,* including a blood pressure, rectal temperature, oxygen saturation, and end-tidal carbon dioxide measurement, as well as a pain assessment.
- *Head-to-toe assessment* is performed in detail, including the anterior and posterior body surfaces.
- *History* should be obtained from the caregiver and emergency medical services personnel. The history should include mechanism of injury, treatment before arrival in the emergency department, medical history, allergies, medications, immunization status, and last food/fluid intake.

Interventions

Perform the following interventions during the secondary survey:

- Trauma lab tests:
  - Complete blood count, urinalysis, and blood bank sample are usually sufficient.
  - Prothrombin time and partial thromboplastin time are indicated with severe brain injury and/or shock.
  - Accuracy of lab results depends on appropriate technique; use of existing peripheral intravenous lines may result in diluted or hemolyzed samples and inaccurate results.
  - Obtain urine or serum human chorionic gonadotropin in females less than 12 years old and younger if menstruating.
  - Toxin screen is indicated if clinical assessment does not correlate and/or further interventions may be affected adversely by illicit substances.
- Radiographs:
  - Obtain radiographs based on clinical indication.
  - Obtain plain cervical spine radiographs: two views if less than 5 years old; three views if more than 5 years old.
  - Panoramic scanning should be avoided for two reasons: the adverse radiation dosage effect and the lack of relevant clinical data gathered.
  - An abdominal/pelvic computed tomography scan with intravenous contrast is the gold standard for evaluation of acute intraabdominal injuries; in the acute trauma patient, oral administration of contrast medium should be avoided because it frequently is vomited and/or does not pass into the bowel effectively.
  - Comparison views of uninjured extremities may be required to determine injury versus normal variants; x-ray films of the joint above and below a subtle or suspected injury may be necessary.

- Expeditious removal of the backboard, Kendrick extrication device, cervical collar, and prehospital splinting equipment such as HARE traction devices is recommended to avoid pressure at sensitive areas.
- Place a urinary catheter and/or nasogastric/orogastric tube if indicated.
- Pharmacologic agents: Safe and effective administration of medications to children includes familiarity with drug dosage recommendations and adverse effects.
- Use a length-based drug dosage tool such as a Broselow tape.
- Rapid sequence intubation:
  - *Lidocaine* administered before intubation in the head-injured child is recommended to protect against increasing the intracranial pressure.
  - *Opioids* and *benzodiazepines* may cause respiratory depression, especially if given simultaneously.
  - *Fentanyl* can result in chest wall rigidity in young children if given rapidly.
  - *Succinylcholine* should be avoided in children with spinal cord injury, burn, or crush injury because of associated hyperkalemia.
  - Topical anesthetics such as EMLA (lidocaine and prilocaine) and LET (lidocaine, epinephrine, and tetracaine) have been safe and effective.
  - *Procedural sedation* should be undertaken with age-appropriate monitoring capabilities, including capnography.
- Current trends:
  - Focused abdominal sonogram of trauma exam for pediatric abdominal trauma evaluation is not widely used.
  - Embolization of liver, spleen, kidney, and pelvic vascular injuries is a treatment option.
  - Routine closed reduction and internal fixation of long-bone fractures without casting is used.
  - Prophylactic use of anticonvulsants for most head injuries is not recommended.
  - High-dose steroid administration after spinal cord injury has more adverse effects.
  - A short hospital stay and observation status are recommended.

Suggested Readings

Eichelberger MR: *Pediatric trauma: prevention, acute care, rehabilitation,* St Louis, 1993, Mosby-Year Book.

Infosino A: Pediatric upper airway and congenital anomalies, *Anesthesiol Clin North Am* 20:747-766, 2002.

Isaacs RS, Sykes JM: Anatomy and physiology of the upper airway, *Anesthesiol Clin North Am* 20:733-745, 2002.

Moloney-Harmon PA, Czerwinski SJ: *Nursing care of the pediatric trauma patient,* Philadelphia, 2003, Saunders.

O'Carroll BM: *Principles of basic trauma nursing,* Easton, Mass, 2000, Western Schools.

Sheehy SB, Blansfield JS, Danis DM et al: *Manual of clinical trauma care: the first hour,* ed 3, St Louis, 1999, Mosby.

Sullivan KJ, Kissoon N: Securing the child's airway in the emergency department, *Pediatr Emerg Care* 18(2):108-120, 2002.

Walls RW: *Manual of emergency airway management,* Philadelphia, 2000, Lippincott Williams & Wilkins.

Chapter 23

Intimate Partner Violence

Deborah A. D'Avolio

Intimate partner violence has grave consequences for women's health. The statistics on the prevalence of intimate partner abuse and trauma are staggering. Given these figures, it is likely that health care professionals will treat patients who have been abused or are at risk of abuse. Findings from the National Violence against Women survey revealed that 25% of women seen in health care settings have experienced intimate partner violence. The health care community has treated an estimated 4.8 million intimate partner rapes and physical assaults annually.[1] Patients experiencing abuse present at a variety of health care settings. A prevalence of intimate partner violence of 18% has been found among patients admitted to trauma centers.[2] Women who have been abused also experience multiple nonspecific symptoms and risky behaviors: smoking cigarettes, binge drinking, and poor nutritional habits.[3] Abused women have been found to have a 50% to 70% increase in gynecologic, central nervous system, and stress-related difficulties.[4]

The cost of intimate partner violence, rape, and stalking is greater than $5.8 billion each year, with close to $4.1 billion for direct medical and mental health services. The cost of intimate partner violence also includes almost $0.9 billion in lost productivity from paid work and household chores for victims of nonfatal violence and $0.9 billion in lifetime earnings lost by victims of intimate partner violence homicide.[5]

Pregnant women can be at increased risk for domestic violence. Homicide was revealed as a leading cause of death in pregnant or recently pregnant women.[6] Pregnancy is often a positive time in a woman's life. A controlling, manipulative abuser can feel threatened with this positive focus, and the abuse may increase. Studies point to violence as the cause of miscarriages and multiple abortions. Abused women are twice as likely to delay prenatal care until the third trimester of pregnancy.[7] Intimate partner violence has been shown to increase the risk of negative health effects for low-income and high-income pregnant women.[8] Screening for abuse and provision of intervention is indicated for all pregnant women during health care and prenatal visits.

Health care providers have identified multiple and complex obstacles to intimate partner screening, including concern about what to do, lack of organizational support, and pressure to see more patients quickly during their practice sessions. Training clinicians to screen and intervene and to provide on-site resources can improve screening rates and the care of victims of violence.[9] In response to the need for improved health care response, the Joint Commission on Accreditation of Healthcare Organizations has established requirements for intimate partner violence care. Health care organizations are required to have polices and procedures and to provide education to staff on the care of victims of intimate partner violence.[10] Health care providers should become familiar with the systems in their health care institutions that provide the necessary support and intervention for victims of violence. Intimate partner violence has been underrecognized by society and in the past has been given low priority. Agencies such as the World Health Organization are working on an international level to examine the impact of violence on society.[11]

Intimate partner violence, or domestic violence, has been defined in many ways; there are also differing legal definitions. Most of the victims of intimate partner violence are women; therefore, in this chapter the patient will be referred to as a woman. Intimate partner violence occurs in all intimate partner relationships including same-sex relationships. Partners may be married or not married; heterosexual, gay, or lesbian; or living together, separated, or dating. Women of all cultures, educational levels, races, incomes, and ages are battered by husbands, boyfriends, lovers, and partners. Violence can happen frequently or occasionally. Women who leave a violent relationship are also at risk of continued abuse. Ending the relationship with a violent partner sometimes can escalate the violence.

Intimate partner violence includes partner abuse, teen dating violence, and spouse abuse. Violence in adolescent dating relationships often is unrecognized because of lack of awareness. Intimate partner violence is a pattern of behaviors that includes physical and psychological abuse.

Examples of intimate partner violence include the following:

- Withholding of economic resources, which is used to intimidate and coerce the victim
- Physical assault
- The threat of harm
- Isolation from family and friends
- Controlling or degrading behaviors
- Name calling
- Stalking
- Intimidation
- Sexual assault

At times, the abuser may threaten to abuse the victim's children or commit abusive acts against the children as a form of power and control over the victim. Intimidation and attacks against pets or property are forms of control that inflict fear on the victim.

In some states the threat of harm and acts of intimidation are considered intimate partner violence or domestic violence. Each state has different definitions and legal remedies. Several states have mandated reporting laws for domestic violence and may require health care providers to report domestic violence to law enforcement authorities. Health care providers must be familiar with the laws of the state in which they practice.

SPECIAL POPULATIONS

A knowledge base of special populations that are at risk of intimate partner violence is essential for all health care providers. These special populations are the elderly, the disabled, and children. Health care organizations usually have policies, procedures, guidelines, and training and education for responding to different types of intimate partner violence. Training and education to provide support to these special populations are essential for health care providers.

With our aging society, maltreatment of the elderly now is recognized as a significant problem. In the 1981 the U.S. Select Committee on Aging suggested that there is an annual occurrence of 500,000 to 1.5 million cases of elder abuse in the United States. Health care providers in all settings are in an ideal position to detect abuse and neglect of the elderly.

The following are several types of elder abuse:

- Physical abuse
- Physical neglect

- Psychological abuse or neglect
- Financial or material abuse
- Violation of personal rights or exploitation

Health care providers must know about the adult protective service systems and the reporting laws in their state. Elder abuse laws vary from state to state. Health care providers must know necessary information related to the reporting law in their practice state, including the following:

- The patient's age
- Which events are reportable
- The required timeliness of filing a report
- The necessary forms
- When an investigation should begin
- The penalty for failure to report

The disabled are another population at risk for maltreatment. Usually the disabled patient depends on another adult, and the victim and the perpetrator generally live together. Again, clinical personnel must know about the reporting law in the state in which they practice.

SCREENING AND INTERVENTION

If health care providers wait for a "classic presentation" before assessing for intimate partner violence, they will lose many opportunities to offer support. The injuries can range from simple soft tissue contusions to gunshot wounds. Recent research has shown that often chronic presentations without evidence of pathologic condition—headaches, abdominal pain, pelvic pain, and back pain—can be attributed to interpersonal violence. Vague, nonspecific complaints can be manifestations of battering. Abused patients may have a history of multiple medical visits for depression or anxiety, drug use, or suicide attempts. A number of signs of abuse are possible; however, the patient assessment should include questions about abuse. Support for abused patients can be life-changing and at times lifesaving. Almost any type of injury or trauma can be a result of domestic violence.

Victims of violence may come to any clinical setting, including emergency departments, trauma centers, health maintenance organizations, clinics, and private medical offices, and they may remain silent about their abuse even when providers perform a screening. The health care visit is an opportunity to establish a relationship of respect and trust to facilitate disclosure about abuse. Health care providers should include screening questions about abuse in routine triage and exams. An essential part of a triage assessment is a violence assessment. Health care providers must be familiar with organizational and local resources for domestic violence. Organizations often have trained social workers or victim advocates who are expert at providing assistance to help victims of intimate partner violence. Nursing diagnoses common to interpersonal violence are listed in the nursing diagnosis box.

Patients are assessed for abuse during their health care visit by asking a few key questions. Examples of questions are the following:

- Are you concerned about your relationship?
- Are you ever afraid of your partner?
- Does anyone try to control you?
- Does anyone make you feel afraid?
- Has anyone threatened you?
- Is someone you know hurting you?

HIGH-FREQUENCY NURSING DIAGNOSES FOR VICTIMS OF INTERPERSONAL VIOLENCE

- Fear
- Rape-trauma syndrome
- Post-trauma syndrome
- Powerlessness
- Impaired parenting
- Caregiver role strain
- Risk for violence: other directed
- *Nursing diagnoses specific to injury*

From NANDA International: *NANDA nursing diagnoses: definitions & classification, 2005-2006,* Philadelphia, 2006, The Association.

- Are you afraid of the person you have a relationship with?
- Some of the women for whom I care have injuries similar to yours, and they have been hurt by someone they care about. Did someone hurt you?

Assessment for intimate partner violence is conducted in privacy. A few minutes alone with the patient are part of normal practice in the health care setting. Family members or significant others can remain in the waiting area during the initial patient evaluation. An environment of safety is essential for patient disclosure of abuse. The interview is held in a quiet and secure area where patient confidentiality can be ensured. The question of abuse can be incorporated into routine health screening (medical history, medications, and allergies). Health care settings also may have specific screening tools or questions to ask all patients.

The screening questions are concluded with a supportive statement, which lets the patient know that there are persons who can help and places that offer help. The patient then is reassured that she is not alone, it is not her fault, no one deserves to be hurt, and it is not an uncommon occurrence.

Disclosure of abuse at times can put the patient at increased risk for violence, and this may be a reason why the patient may decline intervention or services. If a patient discloses abuse and declines intervention, seize the opportunity to provide essential resource and referral information, which the patient may use in the future. A therapeutic relationship of trust can be established. Women have returned to the health care setting uninjured to access the services that were offered during the initial screening.

Also important is to let the patient know that confidentiality will be maintained within the limits of state law. If your state law requires health care providers to report suspected intimate partner violence, then you should discuss this with the patient. Inform the patient that the health care provider is a mandated reporter and that state services will be provided to help keep her and the children safe.

PHYSICAL EXAMINATION AND DOCUMENTATION

A thorough physical examination is conducted during an abuse disclosure visit. Injuries are evaluated and documented in the chart. Many hospitals provide a body map that is helpful to describe and document the injuries. A careful evaluation and description of the injury should include the type, number, size, and location of the injury. Hospitals often provide education on the use of photographs as a tool for documentation. Documentation includes the internal and external services and/or resources that were offered to the patient.

Screening and assessment for other injuries, such as sexual assault, is indicated during the visit. If the patient has been raped, then follow the sexual assault procedures of the health care facility.

In some cases in which intimate partner violence is suspected, the patient may decide not to disclose a history of abuse. Health care providers then should document that intimate violence screening was conducted. Also, if indicated, document any inconsistencies between the pattern of injury and the history of the injury the patient provides. The patient's decision not to disclose abuse should be respected. As with all patients, provide a comfortable, trusting environment to which the person feels comfortable returning in the future. If trust is established, the patient may disclose abuse during a future visit.

It is essential to ensure the safety of the patient and the staff members at all times. If an abused patient feels at risk of further injury in the health care setting, discuss with the patient the importance of notifying security of the potential risk.

Once disclosure of abuse has occurred, then assess the patient's needs:

- Does she want clinical personnel to notify the police?
- Is she safe to return home?
- Does she want to go to a shelter?

All victims of violence should be assessed for risk of homicide or serious injury. One should consider several risk factors when assessing for the risk of serious injury. Questions to consider are the following:

- Have threats been made to kill the victim, the children, or other family members?
- Does the abuser have a history of drug and/or alcohol abuse?
- Has the abuser been arrested before?
- Is the abuser stalking the victim?
- Has the abuser been involved in violent relationships in the past?
- Does the abuser own a gun or a knife? (The possession of a gun or a knife is a serious risk.)
- Is the victim afraid that she will be killed?

Clinical personnel should review with the patient their concerns about the patient's safety and risk for further injury. Discussion of abuse may help the patient realize the seriousness of the violent relationship. Health care providers should screen victims of violence for suicidal or homicidal ideation. Ask the abused patient if she is thinking of harming herself or others. If the patient feels at risk for suicide or feels the potential to harm others, provide a safe environment and an emergency psychiatric evaluation. The health care provider has an ethical and legal duty to keep the patient and others safe.

RESOURCES AND REFERRAL

Some health care settings have in-house advocacy programs or services that provide comprehensive care to victims of violence. If the health care organization provides services, then become familiar with the hours of care and how the patient accesses the services:

- Does the program operate during business hours, on weekends, and on holidays?
- Does the patient need to call to make an appointment?
- Does the advocate come directly to the emergency department and provide on-site services during the visit?

If services are not available in the health care setting, resources may be available in the community. Community-based battered women's service groups provide a wide range of services, including counseling and advocacy for victims of intimate partner violence. Patients should be given referral information that links them to qualified experts in intimate partner violence. Appropriate referrals and resources—counseling, internal and external agencies, and a list of therapists who have experience with victims of violence—can be discussed during the visit.

In addition to providing internal and external resources, the National Domestic Violence Hotline number is available: 1-800-799-SAFE, or 1-800-799-7233. The National Domestic Violence Hotline provides crisis intervention, information about intimate partner violence, and referrals to local providers and victims of violence. The hotline helps to link those in need to agencies that can provide more in-depth help, and it will distribute educational information to those who request it. Experts or advocates who provide expert assistance to victims of violence work closely with the client to provide comprehensive services.

One of the areas on which advocates focus on is the development of a safety plan. Basic elements of safety planning are the following:

- Personal safety with the abuser
- Getting ready to leave
- Understanding how to leave an abusive relationship safely
- What to do after leaving the abusive relationship

The following are several examples of safety plan guidelines for the patient:

- Review and list several safe places that she can go if she decides to leave home.
- Have important phone numbers available, and know how to access emergency help, such as 911.
- Talk to a trusted person about the violence, and ask that person to call the police if any suspicious events or sounds take place in or around the home.
- Leave extra car keys, clothes, money, and copies of important documents with a trusted person.
- Review escape routes with a support person.
- Review safe places to go and persons to call with older children in the family.
- Discuss safety measures, such as changing phone numbers and locks on the windows and doors.
- Review safety procedures when going to and from work.

Many states have agencies that provide resources to victims of abuse, including the elderly, disabled persons, and children. Most police departments have officers who are specially trained to respond to victims of violence. When providing this information, health care providers should tell women that the services are confidential and usually free. If there is a charge, it is usually nominal.

LEGAL INTERVENTION

Civil protection orders or restraining orders are available to battered women in every state. The civil order can be used to provide legal protection for battered women and their children. This protective order prohibits the abuser from further acts of violence. Most orders can be obtained through the county or district attorney in the town or city in which the victim resides. Health care providers should be aware of the state laws and understand what is available for their patients who are abused.

Violence against specific age groups or special populations is addressed in the laws of each state. Abuse of the elderly, disabled, and children usually requires reporting by health care personnel. Again, clinical personnel should check state laws.

Personnel should document the treatment, referrals, and safety planning provided while caring for patients. If the patient declines services, include in your documentation that services were reviewed with the patient. The choice is the patient's, and only she can decide when the time is right and safe to leave the violent relationship. Advocates are specially trained to work closely with battered women to assist in future planning.

SUMMARY

The nurse's main role is to support the patient and provide linkage with special intimate partner violence services. Complex issues and challenges arise when providing care for persons who experience intimate partner violence. Remember, the patient is not responsible for the abuse. Nurses working in collaboration with health care organizations and the advocacy community can improve care. An advocacy model that links the health care system with domestic violence advocates provides the optimal integrated community response. Many states have a domestic violence coalition or resource center that can provide information, training, and support for health care providers.

The nurse may be the first person to encounter a victim of violence and must be prepared to offer support and intervention. Intimate partner violence often can be a hidden trauma, and nurses are in an ideal position to help. The goal of nursing is to promote health and provide holistic care. Nurse's actions and support can be life changing and lifesaving for victims of intimate partner violence.

References

1. US Department of Justice: *Extent, nature and consequences of intimate partner violence (NJC 181867),* Washington, DC, 2000, Office of Justice Programs.
2. Melnick D, Maio R, Blow R et al: Prevalence of domestic violence and associated factors among women in trauma services, *J Trauma* 53(1):330-337, 2002.
3. McNutt LA, Carlson BE, Persaud M et al: Cumulative abuses and experiences, physical health and health behaviors, *Ann Epidemiol* 12(2):123-130, 2002.
4. Campbell J, Jones AS, Dienemann J et al: Intimate partner violence and physical health consequences, *Arch Intern Med* 162(10):1157-1163, 2002.
5. National Center for Injury Prevention and Control: *Costs of intimate partner violence against women in the United States,* Atlanta, 2003, Centers for Disease Control and Prevention.
6. Horan I, Cheng D: Enhanced surveillance for pregnancy-associated mortality—Maryland, 1993-1998, *JAMA* 285(11):1455-1459, 2001.
7. McFarlane J, Parker B, Soeken K et al: Assessing for abuse during pregnancy: severity and frequency of injuries and associated entry into prenatal care, *JAMA* 267:3176-3178, 1992.
8. Kearney MH, Haggerty LA, Munro BH et al: Birth outcomes and maternal morbidity in abused pregnant women with public versus private health insurance, *J Nurs Scholarsh* 35(4):345-349, 2003.
9. D'Avolio DA, Hawkins JW, Haggerty LA et al: Screening for abuse: barriers and opportunities, *Health Care Women Int,* 22:349-362, 2001.
10. Joint Commission on Accreditation of Healthcare Organizations: *Accreditation manual for hospitals,* vol 1, *Standards,* Oakbrook Terrace, Ill, 1995, The Commission.
11. Kruf EG, Dalberg LL, Mercy JA et al, editors: *World report on violence and health,* Geneva, 2002, World Health Organization.

Suggested Readings

Campbell J, Humphreys J, editors: *Family violence and nursing practice,* Philadelphia, 2003, Lippincott, William & Wilkins.

Warshaw C, Ganley AL: *Improving the health care response to domestic violence: a resource manual for health care providers,* San Francisco, 1998, Family Violence Prevention Fund.

CHAPTER 24

TRAUMA IN THE ELDERLY

DIANNE M. DANIS

As a result of increasingly better living conditions, lifestyles, and medical advances over the last 200 years, there has been a dramatic increase in the number of citizens over the age of 65 in the United States (Figure 24-1) and in most of the industrialized nations of the world. In 2000, 35 million elderly* accounted for 12.4% of the U.S. population; in 2020, the elderly are projected to constitute 16.3% of the population, and in 2050, they are projected to constitute 20.7% of the population.[1] Medical expenditures in older adults related to injuries were estimated in 2000 to be more than $29 billion.[2]

With increasing health, mobility, and activity in a person's later years, we are seeing an increasing number of elderly trauma patients. In fact, the "typical" trauma patient is no longer the young male. Women over 65 accounted for 28% of hospital admissions from 1996 to 2000, whereas men younger than 40 represented 26%.[3] Although the principles of trauma resuscitation are the same for patients of all ages, with older patients it is essential that we understand the physiologic changes of aging, anticipate different reactions to the stress of injury and therapy, obtain detailed histories to get a complete picture of what may be a complicated set of circumstances, and tailor our approach given the clinical and historical information that we have collected.

MORBIDITY AND MORTALITY IN THE ELDERLY TRAUMA VICTIM

In 2003, among adults 65 years and older, there were 583,240 deaths, 40,728 hospitalized or transferred patients, and 2,292,157 persons treated and released from a hospital subsequent to injury.[4] Although older adults suffer fewer injuries than younger persons, the mortality rate from trauma is highest in the elderly. Further, the elderly require acute hospitalization after trauma at about twice the rate of other age groups.[5] Researchers have calculated that for every year after age 65, the likelihood of dying increases by 6.8%.[6] The elderly, compared with other age groups in the year 2001 had the following statistics[7]:

- Persons aged 85 and older had the highest *case fatality rate* (proportion of injured persons who die from the injury) of all age groups.
- Those aged 85 and older had the highest *death rate* (number of deaths per 100,000 population) from injuries overall.

---

*The age defined as "old" varies from publication to publication and from study to study. One schema uses the following descriptors: young old, 65 to 74; middle old, 75 to 84; oldest old, over 85; centenarian, over 100. This chapter uses 65 years of age and older to define old unless specified otherwise. Similarly, many terms are used to describe this population: *elder, elderly, older adult, senior, geriatric;* the terms are used interchangeably in this chapter.

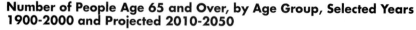

Number of People Age 65 and Over, by Age Group, Selected Years 1900-2000 and Projected 2010-2050

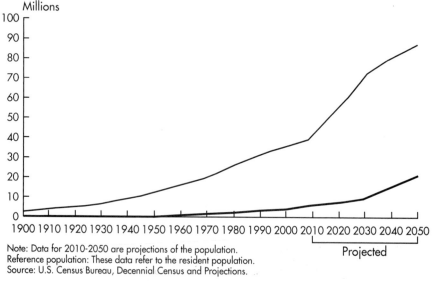

Note: Data for 2010-2050 are projections of the population.
Reference population: These data refer to the resident population.
Source: U.S. Census Bureau, Decennial Census and Projections.

Figure 24–I. Number of persons age 65 and over, by age group, selected years 1900-2000, and projected 2010-2050. *(From Federal Interagency Forum on Aging-Related Statistics: Older Americans 2004: key indicators of well-being, Washington, DC, 2004, US Government Printing Office. Retrieved February 18, 2005, from www.agingstats.gov/chartbook2004/ population.html)*

- Death rates from unintentional injuries were highest among persons aged 75 or older (more than 3 times higher than any other age group).
- Nonfatal injury rates were lowest among persons 65 to 74 years old.

Figures 24-2 to 24-4 display injury and death curves over the life span.

In the elderly, increased vulnerability to trauma seems to have many causes. As we age, body structures such as the bones become weaker. Physiologically, we have less of a reserve with which to cope with injury. We develop chronic diseases that complicate recovery. Also, by some indications the trauma system is not yet designed to care optimally for older persons. A number of research studies have identified undertriage of the elderly to trauma centers. The American College of Surgeons trauma center standards state that in patients over the age of 55, transport or transfer to a trauma center should be considered, but few emergency medical services regions have formalized this recommendation, and many trauma centers do not use age as a criterion for trauma team activation. Trauma clinicians may not have mastered the blend of early aggressive therapeutic intervention along with careful attention to managing chronic diseases and preventing complications that seems to yield the best outcomes in these challenging patients. An important emphasis is that although mortality is high, recovery is still possible for most injured elders.

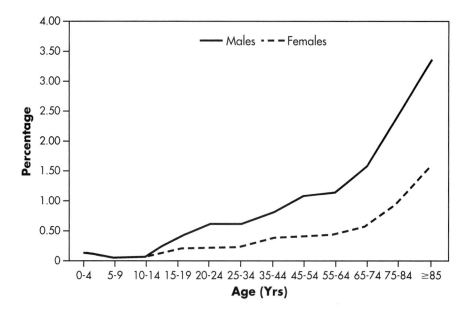

Figure 24–2. Case fatality rate, by age and sex, United States, 2001. Case fatality rate = [Fatal injuries/(Fatal injuries + Nonfatal injuries)] × 100. *(From Vyrostek SB, Annest JL, Ryan GW: Surveillance for fatal and nonfatal injuries: United States, 2001, MMWR Surveill Summ 53[SS-7]:1-57, 2004.)*

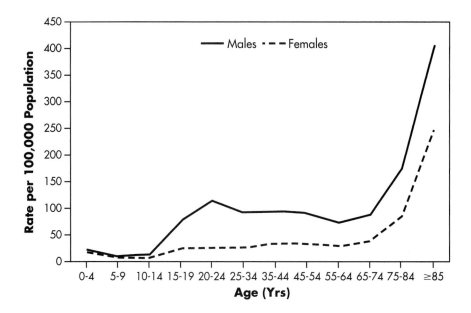

Figure 24–3. Fatal injury rate, by age and sex, United States, 2001. *(From Vyrostek SB, Annest JL, Ryan GW: Surveillance for fatal and nonfatal injuries: United States, 2001, MMWR Surveill Summ 53[SS-7]:1-57, 2004.)*

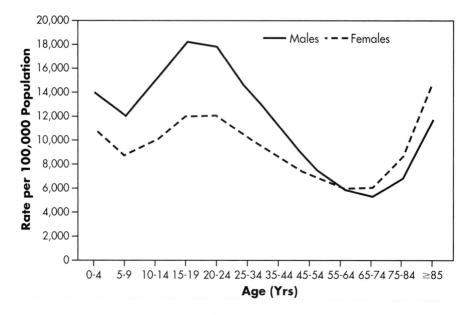

Figure 24–4. Nonfatal injury rate, by age and sex, United States, 2001. *(From Vyrostek SB, Annest JL, Ryan GW: Surveillance for fatal and nonfatal injuries: United States, 2001, MMWR Surveill Summ 53[SS-7]:1-57, 2004.)*

MECHANISMS AND PATTERNS OF INJURY

The elderly experience predominantly unintentional injuries from blunt trauma, specifically falls, motor vehicle crashes (MVCs), and pedestrian injuries. Although the most common mechanism is falls, MVCs are more lethal. Penetrating injury rates are low, but firearm-related suicide rates are highest among males aged 65 and older. Causes differ among different age groups and between men and women[7]:

- In men 65 to 74, the top three causes of fatal injury are suicide by firearm, motor vehicle crash, and fall. For those aged 75 to 84, the top three are fall, suicide by firearm, and motor vehicle crash. For those aged 85 and older, the top three causes were fall, unspecified unintentional injury, and motor vehicle crash.
- In women 65 to 74, the top three causes of fatal injury are motor vehicle crash, fall, and unspecified unintentional injury. For those aged 75 to 84, the top three are fall, motor vehicle crash, and unspecified. For those aged 85 and older, the top three causes are fall, unspecified, and suffocation/inhalation.

In nonfatal injuries, falls are number one for all elder age groups and for men and women. The next most common causes are being struck by or against an object or person and MVCs. About 45% of the injuries occur at home[7]:

- For men aged 65 and older, the most common injuries are laceration/puncture, contusion/abrasion, and fracture in that order. Men injure the head/neck, arm/hand, and the lower trunk.
- For women aged 65 and older, the most common injuries are fracture, contusion/abrasion, and laceration/puncture. Women injure the head/neck, arm/hand, and leg/foot.

Falls

Falls in the elderly are typified by low-energy, low-level, or same-level incidents. Nevertheless, the impact of these falls is significant. In 2002 in the United States, there were almost 13,000 deaths from falls in those aged 65 and older, and there were approximately 1.6 million nonfatal falls.[4] Studies have estimated that about one in three of noninstitutionalized elderly over age 65 fall annually; over age 75, approximately one in two will fall. In nursing homes and hospitals, the rate almost triples.[8]

The older adult is at increased risk for falling because of many factors, the most prominent of which are functional decline (e.g., in strength, balance, and visual acuity), polypharmacy, previous falls, and environmental factors (such as lack of handrails). As the number of risk factors multiply, the risk of falling increases. Injuries to watch for after falls include brain injuries, spine and spinal cord injuries, hip/pelvis fractures, upper extremity fractures, and soft tissue injuries. Older patients who fall should have a thorough medical workup in addition to their trauma evaluation.

Motor Vehicle Crashes

MVCs are a serious problem in the elderly population. The numbers of elderly drivers are increasing, and they are driving more miles. In 2002, older drivers were 16% of the driving population; the percentage is expected to increase to 25% by 2030.[9] In 2003, there were 5309 elderly victims of MVCs.[10] The data are complex. The overall number of elder crashes is low, but the death rate is high, and crashes per mile driven are high. Part, perhaps most, of the higher death rate can be attributed to the poorer outcomes in elderly trauma victims. Fatal crash rates begin to rise at age 75—to higher levels than all other age groups except teenagers—and steeply increase at age 85 and older. At all ages, men have higher death rates; in the elderly, male death rates are 2 to 3 times higher than for women.

Crash patterns are different with older drivers: they are more likely to occur at intersections and twice as likely to involve left-hand turns. Two-vehicle collisions are more common than single-vehicle crashes. The resulting crash pattern is a side-impact collision into the driver's side, which is of great concern. The crash pattern may be a result of the older driver's decreased visual and auditory ability and delayed reaction times. Side-impact crashes are deadly because occupants have so little protection (it is too early to assess the effect of side-impact airbags). Compared with other age groups, older drivers are more likely to be driving close to home, during the daytime, and during weekdays when they crash; and they are less likely to be intoxicated and more likely to be wearing seat belts.

In terms of injuries, chest injuries and fractures occur more commonly in the elderly. Side-impact crashes may cause a constellation of injuries, including severe head injury; cervical spine dislocations and ligamentous injuries; rib fractures including flail chest; pulmonary contusions; cardiac and aortic injuries; ruptured diaphragm; spleen or liver lacerations; and extremity fractures on the side of impact, including femur and acetabular fractures. In evaluating older patients involved in MVCs, one should always consider the possibility of a precipitating (or resultant) medical event, such as syncope, cardiac event, or stroke.

Pedestrian Injuries

In 2002, in adults aged 65 and older, there were 1,182 pedestrian deaths and approximately 14,500 injuries.[4] Pedestrian death rates are highest in those 80 years of age and older. In men the rate increases steadily with age, until at age 80 and older the rate is 3 times higher. In women the rate is lower and increases more slowly and then decreases slightly after age 85.[9] A proportionately larger percentage of these incidents occurs at intersections, even though intersections are intended to be safe crossing points. Again, age-related deficits contribute to these incidents. Elders may not hear oncoming cars, are less able to "look both ways," cross streets much more slowly than most red lights allow, and may not be able to react quickly enough to move out of the way of oncoming traffic. Injuries from pedestrian incidents are similar to those of other age groups except that they tend to result in more severe lower extremity injuries than in the general population.

NORMAL PHYSIOLOGIC CHANGES WITH ADVANCING AGE

Commonly, those age 65 and older are considered "elderly," though trauma outcome studies have demonstrated that trauma-related mortality begins to increase at age 55. As the population continues to age, more attention is being paid to the subset of 85 and over—the "oldest old"— because at this age mortality and morbidity sharply increase. When looking at individuals, however, defining "aged" is really impossible, for some 70-year-olds may be physiologically younger than a 55-year-old. The rate at which a person ages depends on many things. Family background, life history, medical history, medication and drug and alcohol use, nutrition, and social well-being contribute to the onset and degree of physiologic changes of aging. The overall health of the geriatric patient is determined by preexisting illness and the extent of physiologic degeneration. The ability to withstand the stress of critical illness is related to the normal biologic degenerative process, which decreases the functional reserve of the organs.

The physiologic changes that we should anticipate as a normal part of aging include the following:

Respiratory Changes
- Oxygen saturation decreases, and partial pressure of arterial oxygen decreases.
- Carbon dioxide exchange does not appear to deteriorate with age (therefore, respiratory acidosis should always be considered to represent an abnormal finding.)
- Lung field size and compliance are decreased and may alter the ability to provide adequate ventilation.
- Blood flow to the lung is decreased.
- Muscles used for respiration become weaker.
- Kyphosis, thorax shortening, and increased chest wall stiffness increase respiratory effort.
- Vital capacity is diminished, and gas exchange impaired.
- Gag and cough reflexes are decreased and increase the risk of aspiration and pneumonia.

Cardiovascular Changes
- Vasculature becomes less elastic, and sympathetic response is slowed.
- Cardiac contractility decreases and causes a lower stroke volume and cardiac output. Cardiac output may be up to 50% less than that of a young adult.
- Likelihood of atherosclerosis increases and can significantly impair the elderly trauma patient's response to shock.
- Compensatory mechanisms tend to be less effective.

Neurologic and Cognitive Changes
- Cerebral blood flow decreases.
- Volume of brain tissue decreases, and amount of intracranial dead space increases (allowing increased hemorrhage before symptoms become evident).
- Intelligence does not change with aging; however, the speed of processing thoughts slows with age.
- Attention span shortens.

- Short-term memory is poor.
- Reaction time is increased.
- Visual acuity decreases, including ability to focus, dark adaptation, glare sensitivity, peripheral vision, and depth perception.
- Hearing decreases.
- Touch/sensation decreases; the patient may have a higher tolerance for pain that may mask minor injuries; the elderly tend to suffer more burns because of this change, because they often cannot feel the burning sensation until injury is significant.
- Sense of smell decreases; patient may not recognize dangerous situations, such as carbon monoxide or smoke in the air, gas leaks, toxic fumes, and other toxic materials.

Renal Changes
- Kidney mass decreases.
- The number of functioning glomerular and renal tubules decreases.
- The ability of the kidney to dilute and concentrate urine decreases.
- The ability of the kidney to excrete acid or alkaline urine or drugs decreases.
- The kidneys are unable to retain water in the presence of hypovolemia.
- Excretion of antidiuretic hormone is decreased, and activation of the renin-angiotensin system is diminished. The elderly patient who develops acute renal failure as a complication of prolonged hypoperfusion from shock has a poorer outcome than a person of lesser years.

Liver Changes
- Total liver blood flow decreases and may contribute to adverse drug reactions, especially with polypharmacy.
- Liver dysfunction may affect metabolism of medications adversely or increase the toxic effects of drugs.
- Compromised liver function may increase the risk of coagulopathy because several factors important in blood clotting are produced in the liver.

Gastrointestinal System Changes
- Diminished ability to swallow, lessened gag reflex, impaired esophageal motility, and delayed stomach emptying of liquids may predispose the elderly to aspiration.

Metabolic and Nutritional Changes
- Basal metabolic rate decreases.
- Heat production and heat conservation decreases.
- Likelihood of malnutrition increases.
- Likelihood of dehydration increases.
- Total plasma albumin decreases.
- Likelihood of anemia increases.

Immune System Changes
- Antibody production decreases in response to antigens.
- Inflammatory response decreases, and the incidence of multiple organ dysfunction syndrome increases.
- Sepsis from infectious complications increases.

Musculoskeletal Changes
- Osteoporotic changes occur.
- Joint stiffness resulting from arthritic and other inflammatory conditions occurs; this can affect the flexibility of the patient significantly and may contribute to the cause of the injury and create a situation in which routine splinting and securing techniques may not be acceptable.

- Bone density and mass are lost at a rate of 3% to 9% per decade.
- Muscle mass and strength are lost.
- Joints and ligaments become less elastic.
- Minimal to moderate trauma can result in fractures and dislocations.
- Cervical degenerative changes begin at age 40; chronic changes may make x-ray films more difficult to interpret for signs of trauma.

Integumentary Changes
- Subcutaneous tissue decreases.
- Skin fragility increases.
- Blood supply to skin decreases.

Health Changes
- The number of chronic diseases increases, with 65% of patients having one or more.
- Use of multiple medications increases.
- Anticoagulation therapy creates increased risk of bleeding after trauma.

Social Changes
- Fewer social supports are available.
- Sleep pattern is altered.
- Risk for depression increases.
- Risk for elder abuse increases.

Nursing diagnoses relevant to elderly trauma patients are listed in the nursing diagnosis box.

SPECIAL CONCERNS IN RESUSCITATION OF THE ELDERLY TRAUMA PATIENT

Resuscitation of the older trauma patient follows the same principles as in any other trauma patient, only with a special awareness of the potential implications of caring for the elderly. This

---

HIGH-FREQUENCY NURSING DIAGNOSES FOR ELDERLY TRAUMA PATIENTS

- Impaired gas exchange
- Impaired cardiac output
- Acute pain
- Fear or Anxiety
- Ineffective health maintenance
- Self-care deficit
- Risk for impaired skin integrity
- Risk for injury
- Risk for trauma
- Risk for falls
- Caregiver role strain
- *Nursing diagnoses specific to injury*

From NANDA International: *NANDA nursing diagnoses: definitions & classification, 2005-2006*, Philadelphia, 2006, The Association.

section describes initial assessment and therapeutic interventions according to the Emergency Nurses Association Trauma Nursing Core Course prioritized A to I algorithm.[11]

Generally speaking, experts believe that aggressive early resuscitation is indicated and results in better long-term outcomes. This entails a very low threshold for instituting hemodynamic monitoring and for rapid admission to an intensive care unit. The Eastern Association for the Surgery of Trauma evidence-based guidelines (Box 24-1) state that "Any geriatric patient with physiologic compromise, significant injury (Abbreviated Injury Scale [AIS] score greater than 3), and high-risk mechanism of injury, uncertain cardiovascular status, or chronic cardiovascular or renal disease, should undergo invasive hemodynamic monitoring using a pulmonary artery catheter."[12] Noninvasive hemodynamic and tissue perfusion monitors have been designed that may prove useful in the emergency department. The benefit of hemodynamic monitoring is in identifying impaired perfusion and decreased cardiac output that are not clinically apparent. This allows management of underlying volume deficits and pharmacologic support of cardiac function.

Fluid resuscitation in the elderly presents a particularly difficult problem because we know from experience that they do not tolerate hypovolemia well, they do not compensate for fluid

---

Box 24-1	**OVERVIEW OF EAST PRACTICE MANAGEMENT GUIDELINES FOR GERIATRIC TRAUMA**

Triage Issues in Geriatric Trauma: Recommendations

1. Advanced patient age should lower the threshold for field triage directly to a trauma center (Level II).
2. All other factors being equal, advanced patient age, in and of itself, is not predictive of poor outcomes after trauma, and therefore should NOT be used as the sole criterion for denying or limiting care in this patient population (Level III).
3. The presence of preexisting conditions in elderly trauma patients adversely affects outcome. However, this effect becomes progressively pronounced with advancing age (Level III).
4. In patients 65 years of age and older, a Glasgow Coma Scale score of 8 is associated with a dismal prognosis (Level III; should be applied cautiously in individual patients).
5. Postinjury complications in the elderly trauma patient negatively affect survival and contribute to longer lengths of stay (Level III).
6. With the exception of patients who are moribund on arrival, an initial aggressive approach should be pursued with the elderly trauma patient (Level III).
7. In patients 55 years of age and older, an admission base deficit of −6 or lower is associated with a 66% mortality. Patients in this category may benefit from inpatient triage to a high-severity nursing unit (Level III).
8. In patients 65 years of age and older, a trauma score of less than 7 is associated with a 100% mortality (Level III; should be applied cautiously in individual patients).
9. In patients 65 years of age and older, an admission respiratory rate of less than 10 is associated with a 100% mortality (Level III; should be applied cautiously in individual patients).
10. Compared with younger trauma patients, patients 55 years of age and older are at considerably increased risk for undertriage to trauma centers (Level III).

Continued

Box 24-1 OVERVIEW OF EAST PRACTICE MANAGEMENT
GUIDELINES FOR GERIATRIC TRAUMA—cont'd

Parameters for Resuscitation of the Geriatric Trauma Patient:
Recommendations

1. Any geriatric patient with physiologic compromise, significant injury (Abbreviated Injury Scale score greater than 3) and high-risk mechanism of injury, uncertain cardiovascular status, or chronic cardiovascular or renal disease should undergo invasive hemodynamic monitoring using a pulmonary artery catheter (Level II).
2. Attempts should be made to optimize patient to a cardiac index of 4 L/min/m² and/or an oxygen consumption index of 170 mL/min/m² (Level III).
3. Base deficit measurements may provide useful information in determining status of resuscitation and risk of mortality (Level III).

Level I Recommendation: The recommendation is convincingly justifiable based on available scientific information alone; usually based on Class I data (prospective randomized controlled studies); sometimes strong Class II (clinical studies with prospective data collection and retrospective analyses based on clearly reliable data) evidence. (This guideline contains no Level I recommendations.)
Level II Recommendation: The recommendation is reasonably justifiable by available scientific evidence and strongly supported by expert critical care opinion; usually supported by Class II data or a preponderance of Class III (studies based on retrospectively collected data) evidence.
Level III Recommendation: The recommendation is supported by available data, but adequate scientific evidence is lacking; generally supported by Class III data; useful for educational purposes and in guiding future studies.

(Guidelines modified from Jacobs DG, Plaisier BR, Barie PS et al for the EAST Practice Management Guidelines Work Group: Practice management guidelines for geriatric trauma: The EAST Practice Management Guidelines Work Group, *J Trauma* 54:391-416, 2003; and Level I, II, and III Recommendations from Eastern Association for the Surgery of Trauma (EAST) Ad Hoc Committee on Practice Management Guideline Development: *Utilizing evidence based outcome measures to develop practice management guidelines: a primer,* 2000. Retrieved February 18, 2005 from www.east.org/tpg/chap1)

loss well, and they also are unable to tolerate fluid overload well. A traumatically injured patient who is resuscitated from shock but develops pulmonary edema and cardiac problems from fluid overload is a difficult one to manage. Emphasis must be put on *careful* monitoring of the patient's fluid status by the trauma team throughout the resuscitation.

PRIMARY ASSESSMENT

A. *Airway* (with simultaneous cervical spine stabilization and/or immobilization)
- Special concern for the cervical spine must be exercised with positioning for transporting and airway protection. The spine may need to be padded to obtain proper alignment if the patient is kyphotic.

- The oral cavity should be inspected to ascertain the presence and location of dentures. If bag-valve-mask ventilation is necessary, the procedure may be more effective if dentures are left in place.
- If the older patient is to be intubated, preintubation medication dosages may need to be reduced.
- Avoid hyperextension of the neck during endotracheal intubation because doing so may compromise the airway. Tissues of the airway are fragile and prone to injury with intubation.
- Asepsis is important to minimize the risk of pneumonia.

B. *Breathing*
- Serial monitoring to identify trends is important.
- Decrease in chest expansion ability, vital capacity, and ability to cough can be expected, and should not be mistaken for chronic obstructive pulmonary disease.
- Decreased pulmonary reserve limits the ability to produce the expected tachypneic response to stress; this may mask impending respiratory failure.
- Even marginal hypoxia may be harmful with decreased pulmonary reserve; administer high-flow oxygen regardless of whether the patient might have chronic obstructive pulmonary disease.
- Mechanical ventilation should be started early to support ventilation.

C. *Circulation*
- The expected tachycardic response to shock may not appear in older patients because of their inability to generate a catecholamine response or the use of beta-blocker or calcium channel blockers. A "normal" heart rate actually may be tachycardia in the elderly.
- Although dysrhythmias may be more common in the elderly, clinical personnel first must rule out hypoxemia and cardiac injury as the cause and not assume that they were preexisting conditions.
- Blood pressure may not be an accurate clinical indicator. In a patient with underlying hypertension, normotension actually may be relative hypotension.
- Lack of vessel resiliency impairs the ability to shunt blood to vital organs. The usual peripheral vasoconstriction will not be present.
- Consider dual diagnosis if the patient demonstrates signs of cardiac dysfunction: Did myocardial infarction occur and cause the accident? Did low-flow state induce myocardial infarction?
- Prolonged hypovolemia is more detrimental to the patient than fluid overload. Fluids should not be withheld, but repeated boluses with careful monitoring may be safer than continuous rapid fluid resuscitation.
- A base deficit of −6 or below is associated with a 66% mortality rate; these patients should be strongly considered for intensive care unit admission.[12]
- Close monitoring is needed to identify trends and response to resuscitation. A very low threshold should be maintained for the initiation of invasive hemodynamic monitoring and for intensive care unit admission.

D. *Disability* (neurologic status)
- Sensory overload, short-term memory loss, or dementia may alter evaluation of cognitive function. Never assume that altered neurologic status is baseline; always consider the possibility of other factors including trauma, hypoxia, shock, or hypoglycemia.
- A Glasgow Coma Scale score of 8 or below is associated with poor outcomes; however, this should not preclude an initial period of aggressive management.
- Although epidural hematomas are less common because the dura adhere more closely to the skull with age, subdural hematomas are more common. The brain atrophies and shrinks

with age, stretching the fragile veins bridging the subdural space, thus increasing the risk of venous rupture, even with relatively minor mechanisms. Low falls are the most common cause of subdural hematomas in this age group. The shrinking brain creates an enlarged subdural space, allowing significant bleeding to occur before the injury becomes apparent. The mortality rate in elders with subdural hematoma is almost 4 times higher than in younger patients.

- Incomplete spinal cord injuries are more common in the elderly, especially central cord syndrome. Central cord injury is thought to occur after a hyperextension injury, and the elderly are at higher risk because spinal canal stenosis leaves less room for the spinal cord and renders it more vulnerable to injury. Central cord syndrome is manifested by upper extremity weakness greater than lower extremity weakness. This presentation can be subtle and is overlooked or discounted easily.

SECONDARY ASSESSMENT

E. *Expose/Environmental Control* (remove clothing and keep patient warm)
Because of possible injury or expected changes to the thermoregulation system and because of peripheral vascular changes, the elderly patient may become chilled sooner than would a younger adult. Dehydration and poor nutrition and inactivity may exacerbate this problem. Mildly hypothermic geriatric patients may be confused and less communicative than usual. They may display a flat affect, appear senile, and exhibit poor judgment and coordination. Providing warm blankets when care allows not only will prevent heat loss but also will make the patient feel more secure and well cared for. (See also the heat loss–reducing techniques described in Chapter 28 of this manual.)

F. *Full Set of Vital Signs/Five Interventions/Facilitate Family Presence*
- Full set of vital signs should include blood pressure in both arms and temperature.
- The five interventions are electrocardiographic monitoring, pulse oximetry, urinary catheterization, gastric tube insertion, and laboratory study monitoring.
- Urinary catheterization is essential as an assessment tool, but in the elderly it carries a higher risk of infection; asepsis must be strict.
- Family presence not only will be reassuring but also may assist in determining whether the patient's mental status has changed.

G. *Give Comfort Measures*
Verbal reassurance and touch can help patients cope with a frightening experience. To compensate for visual or hearing deficits, stand close to and face the patient and speak slowly and clearly. If the patient has a "good" ear, stand on that side of the bed to talk. Allow plenty of time for patients to process information and questions.

H. *History and Head-to-Toe Assessment*
Obtaining adequate information from witnesses at the scene and from ambulance personnel is essential in evaluating the patient's response to injury and to prehospital treatment. In addition, it is important to find and obtain information from relatives or caretakers, primary care providers, or the medical record. A review of the patient's health history should include details of the precipitating event(s), preexisting medical conditions, current health status, medications and compliance, baseline neurologic status, baseline functional status, advance directives and do not resuscitate status, and living situation and support system. Certain preexisting conditions have been implicated in various studies to increased mortality in patients with trauma. These conditions include cardiac disease, pulmonary disease, neurologic disease and dementia,

hepatic insufficiency, renal insufficiency, diabetes mellitus, coagulopathy, and active cancer. Anticoagulation therapy is a red flag, especially in the presence of head injury; clinicians should be prepared to check laboratory studies rapidly and have fresh frozen plasma thawed.

The head-to-toe assessment includes the following:

- *Head:* Pupil assessment may not be useful in patients with cataracts or glaucoma. Look for dentures, glasses, or hearing aids.
- *Neck:* Assessment of the spine and spinal cord is a real challenge in the older adult. Patients may have fractures without pain or they may report pain that turns out to be associated with a chronic condition. Palpable deformities may be due to degenerative joint disease or old injuries. Because almost all older adults will have degenerative joint disease, cervical spine radiographs often are difficult to interpret, thus necessitating computed tomography scans. Spinal injuries in the elderly commonly are associated with falls. Higher-level fractures are more common than in the younger age group because of aging-associated vertebral ankylosis. For that reason, C2 fractures, particularly odontoid fractures, are more common.

The elderly are more likely to have bone spurs projecting from their cervical vertebrae; these may traumatize the internal carotid artery if it is stretched or hyperextended over the vertebrae and may result in compromised cerebral perfusion and neurologic deficits. The elderly may have no external sign of this injury or may exhibit signs of blunt neck trauma.

- *Chest:* Because of their fragile skeletal structures, the elderly have increased susceptibility to rib/sternal fractures and underlying pulmonary contusions. The use of seat belts has been linked to rib fractures in elderly MVC victims. Seat belts still have a protective function, but clinicians should be aware of the possibility of underlying injury. The incidence of pneumonia, acute respiratory distress syndrome, and death is higher in elderly patients with rib fractures than in other age groups; complications and mortality rates increase as the number of fractured ribs increases, but even one to two fractures increase the mortality rate to more than 10%. Close pulmonary monitoring is essential.
- *Abdomen*
  - Abdominal injuries are less common, but the mortality rate is almost 5 times as high in older adults.
  - Inappropriately high urine output with hypovolemia caused by inadequate compensation may be present; therefore, the clinician cannot rely on urine output to reflect fluid status accurately.
  - If planning a contrast computed tomography scan, be sure to evaluate renal status first.
- *Pelvis:* The hip is the most common bone fractured after a fall. By the year 2040, projections are for half a million hip fractures annually. About half of all hospitalizations for injury in women aged 75 and older are because of a hip fracture (40% in men).[3] The prognosis after hip fracture is sobering, with up to a 30% mortality rate within the first year after injury.[13]

Geriatric trauma patients are more likely to sustain lateral-compression type pelvic fractures. Though lateral-compression fractures generally are considered less severe than anterior-posterior fractures, elderly patients with these fractures are more likely to require transfusions and angiographic control of bleeding than would be expected.[14]

- *Extremities:* In general, the risk of fracture is increased even with minor trauma. While assessing the extremities, be alert for signs of peripheral edema or dehydration, markers of preexisting conditions that might complicate trauma resuscitation.

I. *Inspect Posterior Surfaces*
When logrolling the patient, check for impending skin breakdown, remove the backboard if at all possible, and consider padding bony prominences. Assessment of the spine may be difficult in the patient with degenerative joint disease.

SPECIAL CONSIDERATIONS

Polypharmacy

The use of multiple medications has created a mounting problem in the elderly as they attempt to prevent or halt functional decline with medicines. Often the patient will "doctor shop" and may be taking a number of unsupervised medications, prescription and over the counter. A thorough medication history is important to obtain, especially for the past 24 hours, to be able reliably to administer necessary medications for resuscitation and to be able to anticipate interactions among medications. Obtaining this information may be difficult with an elderly patient who has sustained a traumatic injury. If the patient is unable to provide this information, attempt to obtain previous hospital records and the documentation of the ambulance personnel. Also ask the family about the patient's use of medications. Consultation with a pharmacist during the resuscitation may be necessary to sort out the interactions of many drugs. If at all possible, a pharmacist should be made available to the trauma team.

Pain Control

The elderly are at risk for experiencing suboptimal pain control. They tend to expect pain and may underreport pain or may be afraid to ask for medication. The control of pain is important not only because it is a comfort measure but also because it reduces cardiac oxygen demand and improves respiratory function in patients with chest trauma. Not all elderly patients are able to use traditional pain scales to identify their level of pain; these scales may need to be supplemented by careful observation of facial expressions and other signs. The dosage of pain medication may need to be reduced but should not be withheld. Careful titration and administration of small increments of medication is often the safest approach.

Elder Abuse

The National Center on Elder Abuse defines elder abuse as "any knowing, intentional, or negligent act by a caregiver or any other person that causes harm or a serious risk of harm to a vulnerable adult."[15] Abuse may be physical, emotional, or sexual; exploitation, neglect, or abandonment. Estimates of incidence vary, ranging from 1 million to 2 million victims annually, but it is generally agreed that elder abuse is underreported in our society and that it appears to be increasing. Experts believe that approximately two thirds of abusers are family members, typically spouses or adult children.[16] Elders also may be abused by paid caregivers or in institutional settings.

The trauma history may reveal the possibility of abuse. Clues include a story inconsistent with the injuries sustained, vague or contradictory accounts of how the injury occurred, or a delay in seeking care for the injury. As with assessment of other types of abuse, the potential victim should be interviewed out of the presence of relatives or other caregivers. The interview can be started with general questions such as, "Do you feel safe at home?" or "Has anyone been hurting you lately?" Caregivers should be questioned about frustration or stress associated with their caregiving responsibilities. Interactions between the elder and the caregiver should be observed carefully. Caregivers who are reluctant to allow patients to be interviewed alone, caregivers who persist in speaking for the patient, and patients reluctant to speak in the presence of the caregiver are situations of concern. Another red flag is the history of multiple injury episodes.

The head-to-toe assessment might identify signs of abuse. These include injuries in various stages of healing, burns, rope burns or other signs of restraint, bite marks, welts, and other injuries suggestive of deliberate force. Possible signs of neglect include malnutrition, dehydration, pressure ulcers, and poor hygiene. Abuse is often a difficult diagnosis, and consultation with other members of the health care team is important. Most states mandate reporting of elder mistreatment. An excellent source of more information about elder abuse is the *Violence Prevention Internet Guide* with links to educational resources, publications, and other resources.[17] See also Chapter 23 in this manual.

Advance Directives

Information about advance directives, including living wills and health care proxies, and preexisting do not resuscitate orders should be sought as part of the health history. Although these documents most likely will not be relevant during the initial resuscitation, they may be vital in determining a longer-term plan of care.

INJURY PREVENTION

Emergency and trauma nurses should be involved in injury prevention efforts aimed at the elderly population. Prevention measures often are categorized as educational, environmental, or enforcement. All types of strategies can be valuable, though outcome evaluation data on most educational programs have yet to be as well developed as the effects of environmental or enforcement programs. Selected interventions, programs, and resources are described in the following sections.

Falls

The first preventive intervention is to identify patients at risk for falls, and trauma clinicians can play a key role in this. All patients who arrive at the emergency department after a fall (without a clear nonmedical explanation) should be considered at risk of further falls, as should those who report multiple falls in the past year (with or without injury) or who have impaired gait/balance. The "Get Up and Go" test is an easy and accurate method of assessing gait and balance. The test starts with the patient sitting in a chair, and the clinician observes while the patient stands up without using the arms, walks several steps away from the chair, turns around, and returns. The patient who does this without difficulty has passed the test.[18]

At-risk patients should be referred for a formal fall evaluation by an appropriate clinician. A medical workup should be carried out to eliminate treatable causes, such as syncope or dysrhythmia. Patients taking medications that place them at high risk for falls may benefit from evaluation of their medication regimen. Some may need referral for home safety evaluation, assistive devices, or a "lifeline" alert system. Long-term exercise programs appear to increase balance and strength and to reduce the incidence of falls. A variety of educational programs are suitable for one-to-one or group teaching (Table 24-1).

Motor Vehicle Crashes

The question of whether or when elderly driving should be restricted or prohibited is extremely controversial. From society's perspective, the issue will become more and more serious as the population ages. The ability to live independently often is tied to continuing to drive. Most communities do not have adequate alternate transportation options. Family members may be reluctant to confront an elder with deteriorating function. Elders also may be in denial or sufficiently impaired to be unable to recognize that they are in danger. Those who oppose mandates say that older drivers self-restrict driving patterns and that we do not have sufficient

Table 24–1   Selected Injury Prevention Educational Programs

Sponsor	Title	Content	Source
Fall Prevention			
National Center for Injury Prevention and Control	*A Tool Kit to Prevent Senior Falls*	Fact sheets, brochures, fall prevention checklist	www.cdc.gov/ncipc/ pub-res/toolkit.htm
Emergency Nurses Association	*Take CARE I—Safe Medication Use and Falls Prevention for Mature Adults*	Slide presentation, suggested narrative; also covers safe medication use	www.ena.org/ipinstitute/ institutehealthy_aging/ default.asp
National Fire Protection Association and Centers for Disease Control and Prevention	*Remembering When: A Fire and Fall Prevention Program for Older Adults*	Slide presentation, handouts, lesson plans, checklists, fact sheets, brochures, resource lists, trivia game; also covers fire prevention	www.nfpa.org/ categoryList.asp? categoryID=203
Driving Safety			
Emergency Nurses Association	*Take CARE II—Safe Mobility for Older Adults: Safe Driving Decisions and Pedestrian Safety*	Slide presentation, suggested narrative; also covers pedestrian safety	www.ena.org/ipinstitute/ institute/healthy_aging/ default.asp
The National Highway Traffic Safety Administration	*Driving Safely While Aging Gracefully* and *Safe Driving for Older Adults*	Brochures	www.nhtsa.dot.gov/ people/injury/olddrive/ Driving%20Safely%20 Aging%20Web/ index.htm
AARP	The *Driver Safety Program* (formerly known as 55 Alive).	Classroom driver refresher course	www.aarp.org
AAA	*Lifelong Safe Mobility*	Driving improvement classroom education, brochures, online driving safety quiz, "Roadwise Review" CD-ROM that allows seniors to self-test eight predictors of crash risk	www.aaapublicaffairs.com

T a b l e 24–I   Selected Injury Prevention Educational Programs—cont'd

Sponsor	Title	Content	Source
Pedestrian Safety			
American Trauma Society	*Watch Your Step!*	Slide presentation, suggested narrative, handout, before and after quizzes, safety checklist, risk assessment, related articles, resources	www.amtrauma.org
National Highway Traffic Safety Administration	*Stepping Out: Mature Adults Be Healthy, Walk Safely*	Brochure	www.nhtsa.dot.gov/ people/injury/ olddrive/ steppingOut/ index.html
Emergency Nurses Association	*Take CARE II—Safe Mobility for Older Adults: Safe Driving Decisions and Pedestrian Safety*	Slide presentation, suggested narrative; also covers driver safety	www.ena.org/ipinstitute/ institute/ healthy_aging/ default.asp

Note: Information taken from sponsor websites.

instruments to identify those truly at risk of experiencing an MVC. Others advocate routine driver testing, driving restrictions, or reverse graduated licenses, using an approach analogous to that used with young drivers. Familiarity with the laws of the driver's state is important because state laws vary. Although this issue continues to be debated and researched, other important prevention activities should be used.

For individual drivers, visual perception, cognition, and motor response should be assessed because all have a role in driving ability. Left-turn crashes are red flags of diminished driving ability. Citations for failures to yield the right of way or ignoring traffic signals are other red flags. Medical conditions that may impair driving ability include visual deficits, diabetes mellitus, seizure disorder, Alzheimer's disease, stroke, cardiovascular disease, arthritis and other musculoskeletal conditions, sleep disorders, depression, and alcohol and illicit drug or prescription medication use.[19] Visual acuity is key to safe driving. Regular vision testing should be part of any elder's preventive health regimen. A "useful field of view" vision test is available that focuses on ability to identify important visual cues in cluttered visual fields (such as intersections). This test is one of the few that have been shown to relate to the risk of an MVC.

Though not widespread, programs exist that provide individualized assessment of driving ability; the best are multifaceted programs that include cognitive assessment, useful field of view and other physical testing, and on-the-road driving assessment, coupled with counseling regarding driving restrictions and/or alternatives. Educational programs available include driver "refresher" courses, slide/lecture presentations, and online and printed materials (Table 24-1).

Environmental modifications are an important method of prevention, especially in the area of car design. For example, the growing availability of side-impact airbags may reduce injuries from side-impact crashes. Much attention is being devoted to the improvement of seat belts and minimizing injuries created by seat belts by strategies such as belt force limiters (belts that have some give after a certain force has been reached), widening the belts, adding belt "air bags," or changing to four-point restraints. Road redesign programs at intersections can help to improve these danger zones. Suggested modifications include improved signage, more use of four-way stop intersections, creating roundabouts (rotaries), adding a short all-red phase to traffic signals, and adding protected left-turn signals (green arrows allowing left turns only when all other traffic is stopped).

Pedestrian Injuries

Interventional strategies for pedestrian safety are usually educational or environmental. Older adults can be educated about their risk of injury while walking and about safety tips for walkers. The following tips are from the brochure *Stepping Out: Mature Adults Be Healthy, Walk Safely*, published by the National Highway Traffic Safety Administration.[20]

- Wear sturdy shoes that will provide proper footing.
- Use paths and sidewalks whenever available.
- Remember that cars and other objects can obscure a driver's view.
- Plan routes to avoid hazardous crossings.
- Stop and look for traffic in all directions before crossing the street: left, right, and left again.
- Do not rely only on traffic signs and signals.
- Wait for a "fresh green" (walk signal) when crossing at signals.
- Allow plenty of time to cross streets.
- Be especially careful at intersections.
- Watch carefully for turning vehicles.
- Be especially careful in parking lots.
- Walk with a friend.

Other educational programs that can be used in the acute care setting or in the community are listed in Table 24-1.

Environmental strategies are important. They include analyzing "hot spots" for pedestrian injuries and implementing targeted prevention strategies, such as lengthening walk signals, improving intersection signage, adding pedestrian islands, and eliminating the right-on-red option.

ADDITIONAL RESOURCES

Readers seeking to learn more about geriatric trauma and nursing care of the elderly in general have increasing numbers of resources available. See Suggested Readings for several readings related to trauma. More general resources include the Emergency Nurses Association GENE course (Geriatric Emergency Nursing Education) and the website GeroNurseOnline (*www.geronurseonline.org*).

References

1. US Census Bureau: *U.S. interim projections by age, sex, race, and Hispanic origin,* 2004, Retrieved from www.census.gov/ipc/www/usinterimproj/.
2. Medical expenditures attributable to injuries: United States, 2000, *MMWR* 53(1):1-4, 2004.
3. Shinoda-Tagawa T, Clark DE: Trends in hospitalization after injury; older women are displacing young men, *Inj Prev* 9:214-219, 2003.
4. Centers for Disease Control and Prevention: *Web-based Injury Statistics Query and Reporting System (WISQARS)* [Online], Atlanta, 2003, National Center for Injury Prevention and Control, Centers for Disease Control and Prevention. Retrieved December 8, 2004, from www.cdc.gov/ncipc/wisqars. Database query.
5. McMahon DJ, Shaprio M, Kauder D: The injured elderly in the trauma intensive care unit, *Surg Clin North Am* 80:1005-1019, 2000.
6. Grossman MD, Miller D, Scaff DW et al: When is an elder old? Effect of preexisting conditions on mortality in geriatric trauma, *J Trauma* 52:242-246, 2002.
7. Vyrostek SB, Annest JL, Ryan GW: Surveillance for fatal and nonfatal injuries: United States, 2001, *MMWR Surveill Summ* 53(SS-7):1-57, 2004.
8. Rubenstein LZ, Josephson KR: The epidemiology of falls and syncope, *Clin Geriatr Med* 18(2):141-158, 2002.
9. Insurance Institute for Highway Safety: *Fatality facts: older people 2002,* Arlington, Va, 2003, The Institute.
10. National Highway Traffic Safety Administration: *Traffic safety facts 2003: older population,* Washington DC, 2004, The Administration.
11. Emergency Nurses Association: *Trauma nursing core course,* Des Plaines, Ill, 2000, The Association.
12. Jacobs DG, Plaisier BR, Barie PS et al for the EAST Practice Management Guidelines Work Group: Practice management guidelines for geriatric trauma: The EAST Practice Management Guidelines Work Group, *J Trauma* 43:410, 2003.
13. Atwell SL: Trauma in the elderly. In McQuillian K, Von Rueden K, Hartsock R et al, editors: *Trauma nursing: from resuscitation through rehabilitation,* ed 3, Philadelphia, 2002, Saunders.
14. Henry SM, Pollak AN, Jones AL et al: Pelvic fractures in geriatric patients: a distinct clinical entity, *J Trauma* 53:15-20, 2002.
15. National Center on Elder Abuse: *Frequently asked questions* [about elder abuse]. Retrieved February 12, 2005, from www.elderabusecenter.org/default.cfm?p=faqs.cfm
16. National Center on Elder Abuse: *The basics.* Retrieved February 12, 2005, www.elderabusecenter.org/default.cfm?p=basics.cfm
17. Sise B: *Violence prevention Internet guide: a resource for trauma care professionals,* American Association for the Surgery of Trauma. Retrieved February 12, 2005, from www.aast.org/VPG/index.html
18. American Geriatrics Society, British Geriatrics Society, and American Academy of Orthopaedic Surgeons Panel on Falls Prevention: Guideline for the prevention of falls in older persons, *J Am Geriatr Soc* 49:664-672, 2001.
19. Carr D, Rebok GW: The older driver. In Gallo JJ, Fulmer T, Paveza GJ et al, editors: *Handbook of geriatric assessment,* ed 3, Boston, 2003, Jones & Bartlett.
20. National Highway Traffic Safety Administration: *Stepping out: mature adults be healthy, walk safely,* Washington DC, 2003, The Administration.

Suggested Readings

Jacobs DG, Plaisier BR, Barie PS et al for the EAST Practice Management Guidelines Work Group: Practice management guidelines for geriatric trauma: The EAST Practice Management Guidelines Work Group, *J Trauma* 43:391-416, 2003.

Pudelek B: Geriatric trauma: special needs for a special population, *AACN Clin Issues* 13:61-72, 2002.

Stevenson J: When the trauma patient is elderly, *J Perianesth Nurs* 19:392-400, 2004.

CHAPTER 25

BURN TRAUMA

MARY-LIZ BILODEAU

Evaluation of the patient with a major burn injury is initially the same as for any other trauma victim. The patient should be evaluated for life-threatening conditions and problems with ABCs: airway, breathing, and circulation. A careful primary survey also should aid in the identification of other life-threatening injuries. A secondary head-to-toe assessment is necessary to diagnose other injuries such as fractures, abdominal injuries, and closed head injuries. The burn wound itself should receive low priority during the initial survey except that all clothing and jewelry should be removed, and if the wound is the result of a chemical burn, it should be thoroughly irrigated with water to stop the burning process. Clinical personnel should exercise caution so that they do not get the chemical on themselves and thus sustain an injury.

ETIOLOGY AND INCIDENCE

Burn injuries occur because of exposure to flame, flash, hot liquids, hot objects, chemicals, electrical current, or radiation (Figure 25-1). No national reporting system for burn injuries exists, so most of the available data come from the National Fire Data Center, under the

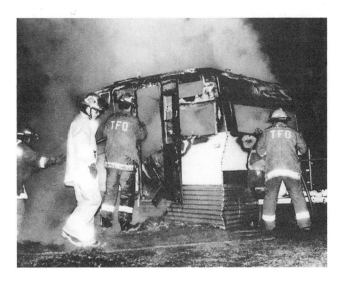

Figure 25-1. Burn injuries occur as a result of exposure to flame and smoke. *(Courtesy Tacoma Fire Department.)*

auspices of the National Fire Prevention and Control Administration. The 2002 data report that more than 3,000 civilians lost their lives as a result of fire. As many as 18,400 civilians sustained injury as a result of fire. Most of the data are related to fires and the injuries they cause and do not include data on burn injuries related to scalds, chemicals, and electrical current. Although fires, especially residential fires, cause most burn-related deaths, scald injuries are the single most common type of burn injury, accounting for 40% to 50% of patients seen in most burn centers. The most common cause of death in the first 48 hours after burn injury is from respiratory complications related to smoke inhalation. After 48 hours, sepsis becomes the most common cause of death.

ASSESSMENT OF DEPTH AND EXTENT OF BURN

Depth of Burn

The depth of the burn injury is referred to as first, second, or third degree or partial-thickness or full-thickness injury (Table 25-1). Initial identification of the depth of injury is often difficult. Unless the burn area is superficial, as with a first-degree burn, or deep, as with a full-thickness burn, there is little need to identify the depth of injury during the initial survey and the initial therapeutic interventions. The depth of the injury actually may increase over time as edema forms, resulting in compromised circulation to the area of the injured tissue. The extent of the burn area is usually complete at about 48 hours, and at 48 to 72 hours a more accurate determination of depth of the burn can be made.

Extent of Burn

The extent of injury for thermal and chemical injuries is assessed by using guides such as the rule of nines (Figure 25-2) or the Lund and Browder charts (Figures 25-3 and 25-4). For the rule of nines, it is important to remember that the formula must be modified for children. As noted in Figure 25-2, B, the head and neck of an infant represent 19% of the body surface area (BSA), and the legs represent a correspondingly smaller percentage of BSA (that is, 13% for each lower extremity). To correct for age, subtract 1% from the head for each year of age through 10 years and add 0.5% to each lower extremity. To obtain a more accurate estimate of the extent of burn, calculate the area burned and the area not burned. Then compare the two estimates. If the total is more or less than 100%, the areas should be reestimated. When estimating burn size, assess the posterior aspects of the body and the anterior aspects. When an electrical injury has occurred, it is much more difficult to assess the extent of injury because surface damage may be minimal, whereas deeper injuries that cannot be visualized may be extensive. Thus when describing an electrical injury, it is more important to describe the injury anatomically and by the amount of voltage (if known), rather than to try to calculate a percentage of burn.

Severity of Burn

The severity of a burn injury is based on an assessment of the extent and depth of injury, as well as the age of the patient, the presence of concomitant injuries, smoke inhalation, and preexisting diseases. The American Burn Association categories for burn injuries are listed in Table 25-2.

Care of patients with burns is determined by the severity of the burn and the availability of specialized care facilities. Initial assessment and stabilization of the patient who has been burned must be available in any community hospital with 24-hour emergency capabilities. Patients with minor burns may be treated as outpatients or admitted to the community hospital.

T a b l e 25-1   Classification of Burn Injury

Depth of Burn	Sensitivity	Appearance	Healing Time and Results	Treatment
Partial Thickness				
First Degree				
Epidermal	Hyperalgesia	Erythema	3-5 days; no scarring	Moisturizers
Superficial dermal	Hyperalgesia to pink	Blisters, red, moist	6-10 days; minimal scarring	Topical antibacterial agents or biologic dressings required
Second Degree				
Moderate dermal	Normal algesia	Blisters, pink, moist	10-18 days; some scarring	Topical antibacterial agents or biologic dressings required
Deep dermal	Hypoalgesia or analgesia	Blisters, opaque, with less moisture	>21 days; maximal scarring if not excised and grafted	Topical antibacterial agents and early excision and grafting
Full Thickness				
Third Degree				
Loss of all dermal elements with extension into fat, muscle, and bone	Analgesia	White, opaque, brown, or black, occasionally deep red; very dry, leathery; may or may not have blisters or thrombosed veins	Never heals if area is larger than 3 cm^2; the longer the wound is open, the more hypertrophic the scar	Topical antibacterial agents and early excision and grafting

Patients with moderate burns may be treated in a community hospital with appropriate staff and facilities to deliver burn care or in a hospital with a specialized burn care facility. Patients with major burns should be cared for in a hospital where specialized burn care is available. Transfer agreements with hospitals with special burn care units should be developed in advance to facilitate timely and uneventful transfer of the burn patient. Nursing diagnoses frequently used with burn victims are listed in the nursing diagnosis box.

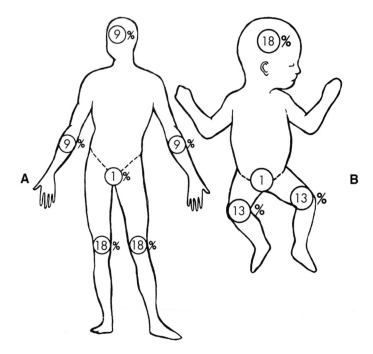

Figure 25–2. Rule of nines. **A,** Adults. **B,** Children.

HIGH-FREQUENCY NURSING DIAGNOSES FOR PATIENTS WITH BURN INJURY

- Ineffective airway clearance
- Ineffective breathing pattern
- Impaired gas exchange
- Fluid volume deficit
- Ineffective tissue perfusion: peripheral, generalized
- Acute pain
- Hypothermia
- Fear
- Knowledge deficit: burn injury aftercare
- Risk for infection
- Disturbed body image

From NANDA International: *NANDA nursing diagnoses: definitions & classification, 2005-2006,* Philadelphia, 2006, The Association.

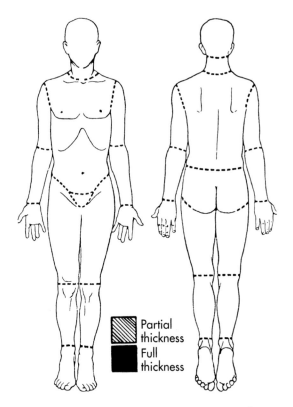

Partial thickness

Full thickness

Percent surface area burned

Area	1 year	1-4 years	5-9 years	10-14 years	Y-15 years	Adult	2°	3°
Head	19	17	13	11	9	7		
Neck	2	2	2	2	2	2		
Ant. trunk	13	13	13	13	13	13		
Post. trunk	13	13	13	13	13	13		
R. buttock	2½	2½	2½	2½	2½	2½		
L. buttock	2½	2½	2½	2½	2½	2½		
Genitalia	1	1	1	1	1	1		
R. u. arm	4	4	4	4	4	4		
L. u. arm	4	4	4	4	4	4		
R. l. arm	3	3	3	3	3	3		
L. l. arm	3	3	3	3	3	3		
R. hand	2½	2½	2½	2½	2½	2½		
L. hand	2½	2½	2½	2½	2½	2½		
R. thigh	5½	6½	8	8½	9	9½		
L. thigh	5½	6½	8	8½	9	9½		
R. leg	5	5	5½	6	6½	7		
L. leg	5	5	5½	6	6½	7		
R. foot	3½	3½	3½	3½	3½	3½		
L. foot	3½	3½	3½	3½	3½	3½		
Total								

Figure 25–3. Lund and Browder formula. *(From Artz CP, Moncrief JA: The treatment of burns, ed 2, Philadelphia, 1969, Saunders.)*

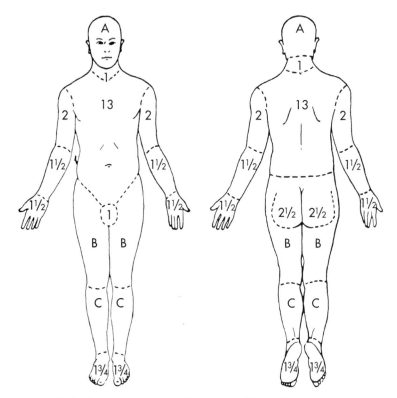

Relative percentage of areas affected by growth

	Age in years					
	0	**1**	**5**	**10**	**15**	**Adult**
A—½ of head	9½	8½	6½	5½	4½	3½
B—½ of one thigh	2¾	3¼	4	4¼	4½	4¾
C—½ of one leg	2½	2½	2¾	3	3¼	3½

Figure 25–4. Lund and Browder formula.

PHYSIOLOGIC RESPONSE TO BURN INJURY

Initial Circulatory Changes

When major electrical burn injuries and thermal or chemical injuries greater than 15% to 20% of BSA occur, fluid shifts may cause hypovolemic states. Circulatory fluid deficits are directly proportional to the extent of the burn injury: the more extensive the injury, the greater the amount of fluid that will shift from the intracellular to the extracellular space. The more fluid that shifts, the more severe the metabolic derangements can be. Figure 25-5 presents a graphic description of this physiologic response.

When injury to the skin occurs, the normal host defense response is activated. This involves the release of histamines and other vasoactive substances that cause an increase in capillary

Table 25-2   Categories of Burn Injuries

	Major Burn* (BSA)	Moderate Burn† (BSA)	Minor Burn† (BSA)
Adults			
Second degree	>25%	15%-25%	<15%
Third degree	>10%	3%-10%	<3%
Children			
Second degree	>20%	10%-20%	<10%
Third degree	>10%	3%-10%	<3%

Data from the American Burn Association: Specific optimum criteria for hospital resources for care of patients with burn injuries, eighth annual meeting, San Antonio, Texas, April 1976.
*In adults and children, burns involving hands, face, feet, or perineum; or burn injuries complicated by smoke inhalation, major associated trauma; or preexisting illnesses, as a percentage of body surface area (BSA).
†Not involving face, hands, feet, or perineum.

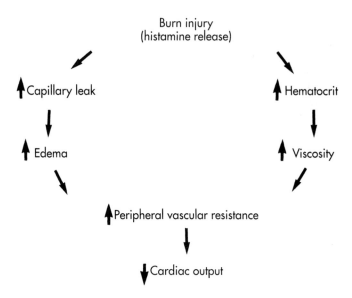

Figure 25-5. Physiologic response to burn injury.

permeability and localization of white blood cells and plasma proteins in the area to fight infection. If the wound is greater than about 15% of BSA, the capillary leak may involve other areas of the body besides the injured area. As a result, the patient develops generalized edema that causes a loss of intravascular volume. Because of translocation of the fluid portion of blood *(plasma)* from the intravascular to the interstitial space, the patient develops a resultant increase in hematocrit, and the blood becomes more viscous. The compensatory response of the body to this functional fluid loss is to increase peripheral resistance so that blood will be shunted from the peripheral to the central circulation. This causes the cool, pale, clammy extremities that are evident in burn patients. This response maintains central circulation for a short time, but eventually the patient develops a decrease in cardiac output and exhibits signs of hypovolemia if appropriate fluid resuscitation is not begun.

Response of the Lung to Smoke Inhalation

Inhalation injury or smoke inhalation is a syndrome composed of three distinct problems: carbon monoxide intoxication, upper airway obstruction, and a chemical injury to the lower airways and lung parenchyma.

Carbon monoxide intoxication is the most common cause of death in victims of fires. Most persons who die in a fire are overcome by carbon monoxide before they sustain a burn injury. In the body, carbon monoxide has 200 times the affinity for hemoglobin than does oxygen, thus causing inadequate tissue oxygen delivery. Carbon monoxide also combines with myoglobin in muscle cells, resulting in muscle weakness. These two factors, tissue hypoxia resulting in mental confusion and muscle weakness, are said to be the major reasons most fire fatalities occur. In addition, carbon monoxide combines with the cytochrome oxidase system of the brain and may result in prolonged coma in some fire victims.

Upper airway obstruction is the result of intrinsic or extrinsic edema that may lead to airway occlusion at or above the vocal cords (Figure 25-6). This injury is primarily a thermal injury, resulting in tissue damage in the posterior pharynx. Actual thermal injury below the vocal cords is rare because the posterior pharynx is an efficient heat exchange system. True thermal injury below the vocal cords is usually the result of injury from superheated steam, in which water vapor carries heat into the lungs, or of injuries that occur in an oxygen-enriched atmosphere or one in which the victim was inhaling gases that exploded during inhalation anesthesia. A true thermal injury to the lungs is almost always fatal. A thermal injury to the upper airway usually is associated with facial burns. With this type of injury, edema progresses rapidly, causing total occlusion of the airway in a short time (minutes to hours). Early management for airway edema is intubation.

Chemical injury to the lower airways occurs when smoke has been inhaled. Chemical injury from acids and aldehydes in the smoke may damage the lung parenchyma. These chemicals are attached to carbon particles in the smoke, and because they are heavier than air, the chemicals readily are inhaled and find their way down the bronchi into the alveoli. This chemical injury results in hemorrhagic tracheobronchitis, increased edema formation, decreased surfactant levels, and decreased pulmonary macrophage function. This in turn leads to the rapid development of acute respiratory distress syndrome in 24 to 48 hours. Severe inhalation injury may increase the patient's fluid needs in the first 24 hours by as much as 50% of calculated values.

GENERAL MANAGEMENT CONSIDERATIONS

The patient initially should be assessed using the ABC assessment tool for trauma. Then assessment for specific burn injuries should be performed.

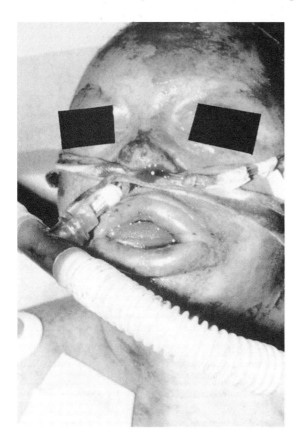

Figure 25-6. Patient with face burns and inhalation injury.

Airway

ASSESSMENT

- History of smoke inhalation/high index of suspicion
- Visual inspection of the oropharynx and vocal cords for redness, blisters, and carbonaceous particles
- Increasing restlessness
- Complaints of difficulty breathing or swallowing
- Increasing difficulty handling secretions
- Increasing hoarseness
- Rapid, shallow respiration

NOTE: Blood gas values, although appropriate for assessing oxygenation problems related to chemical injury to lower airway, reveal little about impending airway obstruction.

THERAPEUTIC INTERVENTIONS

- Early intubation (before complete occlusion)
- A tracheostomy can and should be avoided initially because edema in the neck area makes this procedure especially difficult.

Breathing

Circumferential Chest Wall Burns

ASSESSMENT

Initially, the major, specific, burn-related problem that may impair breathing is a circumferential, full-thickness burn of the thorax. This may limit chest wall excursion and prevent adequate gas exchange.

Assess the patient for the following:

- Visual inspection of chest
- Tight, leathery eschar circumferentially around chest
- Inadequate expansion of chest
- Rapid, shallow respirations
- Restlessness/confusion
- Decreased oxygenation
- Decreased tidal volume

THERAPEUTIC INTERVENTIONS

Escharotomies of the chest are surgical incisions made along the lateral borders of the chest halfway between the midaxillary line and the midnipple line. If the abdomen also is involved, an incision can be made over the diaphragm to connect the two lateral incisions.

Escharotomies are made deep enough only to release the eschar and expose the underlying subcutaneous tissue. This procedure should result in immediate improvement in the excursion of the chest wall. These incisions cause bleeding. Clinical personnel should have an electrocautery unit or 10 to 20 small hemostats available to control the bleeding.

General anesthesia is not necessary because the incisions are made only in the area of the full-thickness burn. Narcotic analgesia given intravenously is sufficient to relieve any pain.

Carbon Monoxide Intoxication

ASSESSMENT

- Decreased respirations or apnea at scene
- Cherry red, normal skin
- Confusion or coma
- Increased level of carboxyhemoglobin in the blood
- Carbonaceous sputum

THERAPEUTIC INTERVENTIONS

- Administer oxygen at 100% or at as high a percentage as possible.
- If the patient is not breathing, intubate and ventilate.

- If unconsciousness continues after 1 to 1½ hours with adequate resuscitation and no evidence of head injury, hyperbaric oxygen therapy may be a consideration.
- Obtain a chest x-ray film.

Chemical Injury or Acute Respiratory Distress Syndrome
ASSESSMENT

- Acute respiratory distress syndrome is usually not a problem for at least 8 hours after injury.

Assess for the following:

- Decreased oxygenation
- Increased secretions
- Rapid respirations
- Increased patchy infiltrates on x-ray film

THERAPEUTIC INTERVENTIONS

- Intubation and ventilation
- Positive end-expiratory pressure
- Bronchodilators, as indicated
- *No steroids* (steroids given to patients with burns plus smoke inhalation increase morbidity and mortality at least threefold)
- Sedation and skeletal muscle relaxation

Clinical personnel should assess for other trauma-related causes for problems in breathing, especially pneumothorax or hemothorax, tension pneumothorax, and flail chest. These problems should be expected when burn victims have been in car accidents or explosions or have jumped or fallen. A history of chronic pulmonary problems that may complicate therapy also should be noted.

Circulation
ASSESSMENT

These assessment parameters should be followed closely. If present, they indicate a low-flow state.

- Tachycardia
- Hypotension
- Tachypnea
- Central venous pressure less than 3 cm H_2O
- Oliguria
- Hematocrit greater than 50 mg/dL
- Diminished capillary refill
- Restlessness or confusion
- Nausea
- Vomiting
- Ileus

THERAPEUTIC INTERVENTIONS

- Start one or two large-bore intravenous lines (one if less than 40% BSA; two if greater than 40% BSA or if patient is to be transferred).
- Avoid leg veins when possible in adults because of increased risk of thrombophlebitis.
- Administer fluid replacement by one of many accepted formulas; more popular are Baxter formula and modified Parkland formula.

Parkland Formula

Administer the Parkland formula as follows:

- *First 24 hours:* 2 to 4 mL lactated Ringer's solution per kilogram body mass per percent BSA
  - One half the first 8 hours
  - One fourth the second 8 hours
  - One fourth the third 8 hours

Time is calculated from time of injury, not the time intravenous therapy was initiated.

- *Second 24 hours:*
  - 5% dextrose in water with potassium in sufficient quantities to maintain normal electrolyte balance
  - Plasma or plasma expander to maintain adequate volume with normal pulse, blood pressure, and urine output

Modified Brooke Formula

Administer the modified Brooke formula as follows:

First 24 hours: 2 mL lactated Ringer's solution per kilogram body mass per percent BSA
- One half the first 8 hours
- One fourth the second 8 hours
- One fourth the third 8 hours

Time is calculated from time of injury, not the time that intravenous therapy was initiated.
Second 24 hours: Same as Parkland formula

NOTE: The Parkland and modified Brooke formulas and other formulas are intended only as a guideline for fluid replacement and may need to be adjusted up or down according to the patient's response to resuscitation. Assessment components include the following:

- Pulse in upper limits of normal range for age
- Urine output of 30 to 50 mL/hr for adults; 20 to 30 mL/hr for children; 1 to 1.5 mL/kg body mass for infants
- Mentally alert
- Absence of ileus or nausea

NOTE: A potential complication of resuscitation is abdominal compartment syndrome. This syndrome occurs when the inflexibility of eschar does not allow for the progression of edema formation, resulting in compression of abdominal organs and vessels. Signs of abdominal compartment syndrome include a decreasing urine output, increasing difficulty with ventilation, increasing acidosis in the setting of full-thickness burns to the abdomen. Measuring bladder pressure provides some evidence of the degree of compression. Abdominal compartment syndrome is an emergency requiring surgical decompression of the abdomen to prevent permanent damage. Abdominal compartment syndrome generally does not occur during the first 12 hours after injury. However, the index of suspicion must be high in the setting of full-thickness burns to the abdomen and high resuscitation volumes.

For electrical injuries, there is no formula for fluid resuscitation. Lactated Ringer's solution is administered rapidly, 1 to 2 L/hr in the average adult, until the patient shows signs of adequate resuscitation.

Additional therapeutic interventions include the following:

- Urine output usually is maintained at 2 to 3 times normal to facilitate excretion of myoglobin.
- Once urine output is established, mannitol may be given to increase urine flow and aid excretion of myoglobin.
- Acidosis (pH 6.8 to 7) is an early complication and may require repeated administration of sodium bicarbonate to prevent dysrhythmias until fluid therapy can correct acidosis.
- Draw blood for a complete blood count, electrolytes, and type and crossmatch.
- Place a Foley catheter.
- Send urine for urinalysis and myoglobin level.
- Monitor hourly urine output.
- Monitor urine sugar and acetone every 2 to 4 hours.
- Monitor cardiac rhythm.
- Obtain a 12-lead electrocardiogram.

Prevention of Infection
Aseptic Technique
Follow these guidelines:

- All personnel should wear gloves, mask, cap, and gown.
- Treat all invasive procedures as sterile procedures.
- Keep wounds covered with clean sheets while other care is provided.

Antibiotics
Follow these guidelines:

- Topical antibiotics should be applied as soon as possible after wound is débrided.
- Systemic antibiotics rarely are indicated even in severe burns until the patient has a culture-proven infection. Exceptions to this may be young children, elderly patients, diabetic persons, or patients with immune deficiency diseases.

Tetanus Prophylaxis
Follow these guidelines:

- For all burns, give tetanus immunization if previous immunization has been given more than 5 years ago.
- In patients who have never been immunized or in whom there is no clear history of immunization, give tetanus immune globulin (HyperTET) in addition.

Management of Pain
ASSESSMENT

- Patient complains of pain specific to burn injury or other injuries.
- Patient is restless and tachycardic with rapid respirations (rule out other potential causes).
- Ask patient to rate pain on an established scale.

THERAPEUTIC INTERVENTIONS

- Administer morphine.
  - Small doses (3 to 5 mg in adults)
  - Frequently (every 20 to 40 minutes)
- Always administer intravenous analgesia in burns greater than 15% of BSA because intramuscular absorption is unreliable in these cases.
- Explain procedures.
- Administer an anxiolytic drug such as diazepam (Valium) if patient is severely agitated for no apparent reason.

NOTE: Burn wounds are exquisitely painful, especially partial-thickness injuries. Careful titration of morphine, as needed or as a morphine drip, can be used effectively to control pain initially.

Obtain History

Obtain the following information:

- How did injury occur (flame, scald, or other)?
- Was smoke involved? Was it in closed space?
- Who was involved? What happened to others?
- What was patient doing before the accident? (This information may lead to early diagnosis of stroke or myocardial infarction.)
- What previous medical problems or allergies did patient have?

Burn Wound Care

Burn wound care can wait until the patient's condition is stabilized.

Circumferential Full-Thickness Injuries
ASSESSMENT

- Assess all full-thickness, circumferential burns for circulatory problems.
- Check distal pulses with Doppler ultrasonography.
- Assess capillary refill.
- Note paresthesia.

THERAPEUTIC INTERVENTIONS

- If patient develops signs of circulatory compromise, escharotomy will be performed (Figure 25-7 shows placement of surgical incisions).

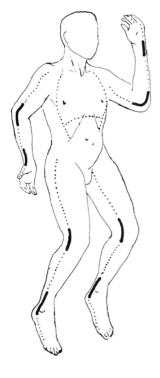

Figure 25–7. Placement of escharotomies.

- Be prepared for significant bleeding with an electrocautery unit or 10 to 20 small hemostats to control bleeding (Figure 25-8).
- Once procedure is completed, apply a topical antibacterial to the open wound, dress with a light pressure dressing, and keep arms and legs slightly elevated.

Thermal Burns: Flames, Flashes, Scalds, and Hot Objects

For thermal burns, perform the following interventions (Figure 25-9):

- Cleanse wounds with sterile or clean water and clean cloths or coarse mesh gauze dressings.
- Keep blisters intact; unroof blisters only when they have broken spontaneously.
- Shave all hairy areas of burns and adjacent areas.
- Cover wound immediately with prescribed topical antibacterial agent and apply a dressing.
- Elevate extremities slightly to reduce swelling.

Chemical Burns

For chemical burns, perform the following interventions:

- Thoroughly rinse chemical wounds immediately with tap water or saline to remove the chemical. Remember to remove clothing and jewelry and to rinse the nonburned areas because some areas of chemical exposure may not begin to hurt, blister, or even become red immediately.
- Then treat the wound as if it were a thermal burn.
- Chemical burns of the eyes are ophthalmologic emergencies.

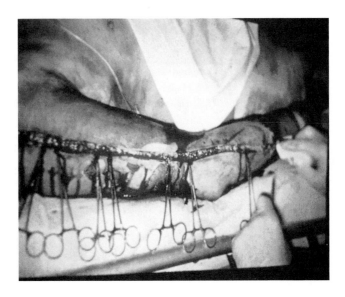

Figure 25-8. Control of bleeding from escharotomy.

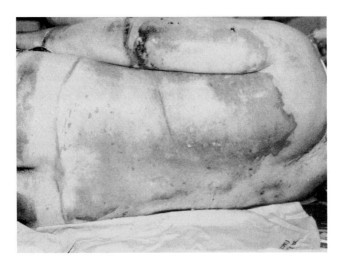

Figure 25-9. Flame burns to back.

As with other chemical wounds, thoroughly rinse the eye with copious amounts of water or saline. If the patient is wearing contact lenses, wash the eye before trying to remove lenses. Then if the lens does not come out during irrigation, carefully remove the lens with a lens removal suction cup. If the lens is adherent, leave it in place for the ophthalmologist to remove and continue irrigation of the eye. When the lens is removed, the eye should be irrigated thoroughly again.

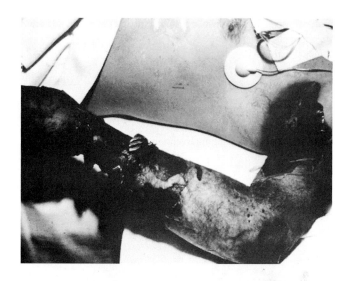

Figure 25–10. Electrical injury.

Electrical Injuries

For electrical burns, perform the following interventions:

- Electrical wounds are different from thermal or chemical wounds because there may be little superficial tissue loss with massive muscle injury underlying normal-looking skin (Figure 25-10).
- These wounds should be cleansed gently with water or saline.
- Rarely is there any need to débride the wound immediately.
- These wounds should be handled minimally. Cadaver-like limbs should not be moved about or manipulated because large patent vessels may be torn and massive hemorrhage may occur.
- Topical agents, such as silver sulfadiazine (Silvadene) and/or silver nitrate, should be used to cover the wound.
- Light dressings may be applied to cover these often grotesque wounds, taking care not to impair observation of extremities for development of compartment syndrome.
- Because of possible muscle damage, injured extremities should be observed for compartment syndrome (see Chapter 20).
- Symptoms may include the following:
  - Pain disproportionate to the injury
  - Pallor
  - Paresthesia
  - Decreased motor function
  - Decreased pulse (late sign)
  - Elevated muscle compartment pressures
- Fasciotomies are performed to relieve compartment syndrome.

Fasciotomies usually are carried out under general anesthesia so that all compartments can be explored completely. Fasciotomy can be a painful procedure because the incisions often are made through normal skin.

- Fasciotomies are left open, covered with a topical antibacterial agent, and dressed with a light dressing postoperatively.
- Elevate the affected extremity.

Tar or Asphalt Burns

Tar wounds may be deep or superficial, depending on the temperature of the tar, which may range from 150° to 600° F or higher (Figure 25-11).

For tar burns, perform the following interventions:

- Cool tar with cool liquids.
- Do not try to peel off tar.

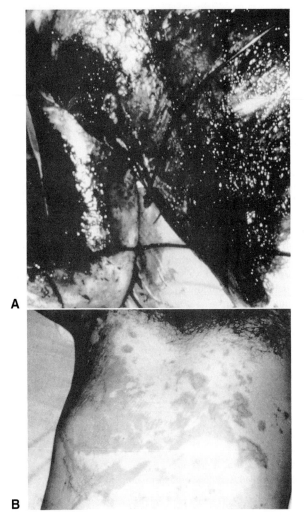

Figure 25-11. **A,** Tar burns to chest before removal of tar. **B,** Tar burns after removal of tar.

- Remove tar by loosening it with the following:
  - Mineral oil
  - Petroleum jelly (Vaseline)
  - Solvent, such as Medi-Sol

Removal of tar can be accomplished in areas of noncircumferential burns by applying oil or ointment and a light dressing and removing the dressing after 4 to 12 hours and reapplying the oil or ointment and a dressing.

- For circumferential areas, the oil or ointment can be applied with light dressings and changed every 20 to 30 minutes until the tar is removed.
- Then the wound can be treated as a thermal or chemical wound.

INTERFACILITY TRANSFER

Once the injury has been identified as a significant burn, the team should consider transfer to a regional burn center. Patients should be considered for transfer based on their age, the percentage of BSA of burn, and any associated factor that would decrease their chances for optimal outcome (Box 25-1). Prehospital providers and community emergency department personnel should establish a network with their regional burn center to ensure a consistent approach to clinical management from injury to definitive care.

Box 25-1 **TRANSFER CRITERIA FOR BURN PATIENTS TO A BURN CENTER**

Second-degree burns: 10% to 20% total body surface area
　　Children less than 10 years old
　　Adults more than 50 years old
Second- and third-degree burns: 20% total body surface area
　　All age groups
Third-degree burns: greater than 10%
　　All age groups
Second- and third-degree burns and chemical burns to the following areas:
　　Face
　　Hands
　　Feet
　　Genitalia
　　Perineum
　　Major joints
Electrical burns, including lightning strikes
Burns with associated factors:
　　Major trauma
　　Inhalation injury
　　Comorbid/preexisting medical problems

Suggested Readings

Ahrns K: Trends in burn resuscitation: shifting the focus from fluids to adequate endpoint monitoring, edema control, and adjuvant therapies, *Crit Care Nurs Clin North Am* 16:75-98, 2004.

Hemdon D: *Total burn care,* ed 2, Philadelphia, 2002, Saunders.

LaBorde P: Burn epidemiology: the patient, the nation, the statistics and the data sources, *Crit Care Nurs Clin North Am* 16:13-25, 2004.

CHAPTER 26

THE OBESE TRAUMA PATIENT

ALICE A. GERVASINI

The number of overweight and obese adults and children in this country has increased dramatically over the last 20 years. The health effects for those significantly overweight are varied but impressive and result in increased morbidity and mortality. Trauma is the fifth leading cause of death in the United States. For the traumatized obese patient the incidence of death and complications is 8 times higher. The rationale for this significant increase focuses on the unique anatomic and physiologic differences of the obese patient, associated co-morbidities, and the ability of trauma systems to meet their needs. As true with any trauma patient, the presence of comorbidities contributes to longer hospital stays and poorer outcomes. Currently, trauma remains a public health problem, and trauma systems and centers need to establish consistency in their ability to meet the challenge of managing the traumatized obese patient.

DEFINITION

Practice standards and management strategies recommend that height and weight be recorded for all trauma patients. A body mass index should be calculated and recorded on the chart. The body mass index is the ratio of mass in kilograms to height in meters squared. The National Heart, Lung, and Blood Institute at the National Institutes of Health has established standards for determining categories of weight ranges (Table 26-1).

Table 26-1 Definition of Weight Groupings by Body Mass Index

Weight Category	Body Mass Index
Underweight	<18.5 kg/m^2
Normal weight	18.5-24.9 kg/m^2
Overweight	25-29.9 kg/m^2
Obesity	30-39.9 kg/m^2
Morbid obesity	≥40 kg/m^2

ANATOMY AND PHYSIOLOGY

To manage the obese trauma patient successfully, the clinician needs to understand the anatomic and physiologic uniqueness of this population (Table 26-2) and to identify measures to support and minimize the negative effects. These parameters vary depending on the age, weight category, and existing comorbidities. Common comorbidities in the obese patient population include the following:

- Obesity hypoventilation syndrome
- Coronary artery disease
- Congestive heart failure
- Hypertension
- Insulin resistance and type 2 diabetes mellitus
- Osteoarthritis and degenerative joint disease
- Gastroesophageal reflux disease
- Urinary incontinence

Physiologic compromise generally increases as weight categories increase. All trauma patients should be assessed using the same standard approach of primary and secondary survey.

Table 26-2   Unique Features of Obese Patients

System	Anatomic Differences	Physiologic Differences
Pulmonary	Large neck circumference ↓ excursion of the diaphragm because of presence of abdominal fat ↑ depository of fat around the ribs and diaphragm ↑ chest wall diameter	↑ work of breathing ↓ chest wall compliance ↑ minute ventilation ↓ total lung capacity ↓ functional residual capacity ↓ expiratory reserve ↑ ventilation-perfusion mismatch ↑ airway resistance
Cardiovascular	↑ body mass index as an independent risk factor for cardiac disease ↑ in circulating volume in response to elevated percentage of adipose tissue Polycythemia in response to chronic hypoxemia	Pulmonary hypertension ↑ cardiac output ↑ blood pressure ↑ incidence of congestive heart failure Left ventricular hypertrophy ↑ preload
Gastrointestinal	General sphincter weakness resulting in gastroesophageal reflux	↑ potential for aspiration
Integumentary	Friability of the skin, especially in the folds ↓ vascularity in adipose tissue	↑ potential for fungal and yeast infections in areas of skin folds ↑ incidence of delayed wound healing ↑ potential for skin breakdown and/or venous stasis ulcers

The approach should not vary, and the uniqueness of any individual should be taken into consideration throughout the assessment.

ASSESSMENT/DIAGNOSTIC RECOMMENDATIONS

The initial assessment for trauma patients is standardized, including a primary survey with management of all identified issues (airway, breathing, circulation) and a head-to-toe secondary survey (see Chapter 11). The variation that is required in the primary and secondary survey of the traumatized obese patient involves adapting traditional approaches to minimize the potential negative effects contributed by the challenges of increased body habitus or existing comorbidities. Nursing diagnoses frequently used with the obese trauma patient are listed in the nursing diagnosis box.

Positioning

Generally, trauma patients are transported from the field immobilized on a backboard in a supine position. The obese trauma patient likely will not be able to tolerate this position for any length of time. When supine, pressure from the intraabdominal contents on the diaphragm impedes the downward excursion, resulting in poor gas exchange. In the presence of gastro-esophageal reflux disease, there is an increased potential of aspiration when supine. To minimize these effects, the patient should be put in the reverse Trendelenburg's position to at least a 45-degree angle throughout the transport and initial resuscitation. All trauma patients should be removed from the backboard as soon as possible to decrease the incidence of skin breakdown. Specialty equipment includes backboards and stretchers that are wide enough and strong enough to accommodate the increased weight of the patient. Appropriate personnel need to be available to ensure a safe environment for the patient and to minimize injury to those transporting the patient.

Airway and Breathing

Cervical spine immobilization is not always amenable to the use of extrication collars. Sizing is often difficult to match with the obese patient, and therefore immobilization of the head to the backboard using tape and standard block immobilizers is better. For those patients with

---

HIGH-FREQUENCY NURSING DIAGNOSES FOR OBESE TRAUMA PATIENTS

- Impaired gas exchange
- Impaired physical mobility
- Risk for impaired skin integrity
- Self-care deficit
- Ineffective health maintenance
- Risk for injury
- *Nursing diagnoses specific to injury*

From NANDA International: *NANDA nursing diagnoses: definitions & classification, 2005-2006,* Philadelphia, 2006, The Association.

sleep apnea, there is a greater potential for airway obstruction when supine, and therefore they benefit from the reverse Trendelenburg's position. Ventilation also is impaired when the obese patient is supine, and depending on the degree of respiratory compromise, the patient may benefit from biphasic positive airway pressure. Bag-valve masking requires high pressures to overcome the weight of the chest and abdomen when the patient is supine. If there is significant respiratory compromise, the clinician needs to remember that landmarks and redundant skin folds may make accomplishing endotracheal intubation or a surgical airway difficult. In those cases that require chest tube insertion, consider accessing the chest one or two intercostal spaces above normal landmarks to avoid violating an elevated diaphragm.

Fluid Resuscitation

Intravenous access should be obtained using standard large-bore catheters. Depending on body habitus and excessive skin folds, access to peripheral and central venous sites may be difficult. Consideration for vessel depth may require longer catheters or access via a surgical cutdown. When determining the need for intravenous fluid administration, a careful approach to resuscitation of the obese trauma patient is required to minimize exacerbation of congestive heart failure or pulmonary edema. The goal for fluid management should be to maintain euvolemia.

Fixation/Splinting

Because of body habitus, it might be difficult to assess the patient for musculoskeletal defects and vascular compromise. Dislocations and fracture patterns are often difficult to assess and reduce. Standard prefabricated splints do not provide adequate stabilization for this population. Suspected areas of concern should be supported with splints made specifically for the patient to maintain stabilization and position of function. Pulses should be assessed before and after splint application. Skin assessment for new and old areas of concern should be detailed in the documentation of the secondary survey.

Pharmacologic Issues

Consultation from the clinical pharmacologist when dosing medications for the obese trauma patient may be beneficial. In general, there are few recommendations for specific medications when dosing for those with increased body mass indexes. Generally, obese patients have a higher fat-to-muscle ratio, with muscle tissue holding more water than fat tissue. When giving drugs that are hydrophilic, the clinician must remember that distribution throughout both tissues is unreliable. Also, when giving drugs that are lipophilic, the clinician needs to be aware of the potential need for higher doses and the risk of prolonged effect because the drug is stored in the fat tissue and is released over time. Review of drug delivery routes is also important, with intravenous and enteric routes being the preferred choice. Subcutaneous and intramuscular routes are inconsistent in drug absorption and may result in the ineffective action of the drug with the inability to achieve therapeutic levels.

Diagnostic Workup

Following the physical assessment, further delineation of injury patterns through diagnostic tests is critical for the trauma patient. Currently, a significant challenge exists for use of state-of-the-art technology for the obese trauma patient. Tests that have become the cornerstone of diagnostics for injury patterns are not reliable and have obesity-related limitations.

Diagnostic tests include the following:

- *Focused assessment sonography for trauma:* Ultrasound is unreliable when used on patients with extensive abdominal fat.
- *X-ray films:* Standard plain films are compromised by the layers of body fat that they need to penetrate; along with the larger surface areas involved, standard film cassettes may not be sufficient to image specific body parts (chest/abdomen/pelvis).
- *Computed tomography scans:* Clinicians need to assess accurately not only body weight but also shoulder, chest, and abdominal girth; scan tables need to move freely for the test and have weight limits, unique to each product, that often only allow for patients under 350 lb; the second consideration is the diameter of the gantry into which the patient moves while on the computed tomography table; if the patient's girth exceeds gantry size, then the scan cannot be done.
- *Magnetic resonance imaging:* Similar to the restrictions of the computed tomography equipment, the table and opening of the magnetic resonance imaging equipment may prohibit access to this test; table weight limits need to be assessed, as well as the patient's girth compared with the diameter of the machine opening.
- *Angiography:* Although not limited by a machine opening, the angiography table also needs to be able to move freely, and access to this technology is limited by the table weight limits unique to each product.

RECOMMENDATIONS

From impact to definitive care, standards and strategies for the management of trauma patients are critical. Each institution needs to establish guidelines to address various patient populations. System and clinical considerations for management of the obese trauma patient include the following:

- *Equipment:* immediate access to weight- and size-appropriate stretchers, patient gowns, bedside commodes, transfer aids that minimize shearing of the skin, blood pressure cuffs, longer-length catheters and endotracheal tubes, biphasic positive airway pressure/continuous positive airway pressure, wheelchairs, walkers, canes, splint material, bedpans, and floor-mounted toilets
- *Protocols:* predetermined approach to monitor blood pressure (using appropriate cuff but measuring on the forearm or calf); assessment guidelines when standard diagnostic technology is inadequate; weight-based dosages for routine medications; positioning guidelines when supine during assessment phase, diagnostic screening (reverse Trendelenburg's position), and perioperative (Trendelenburg's position for abdominal procedures, reverse Trendelenburg's position for thoracic procedures)
- *Missed injuries:* With the variability in diagnostic work up and application of studies, it is not uncommon that injuries that potentially would be identified early in the course of the assessment will be missed and identified later in the obese trauma patient. As true for all trauma patients, a tertiary survey is critical to complete within 24 hours of injury. This survey is a complete review of mechanism of injury, primary and secondary survey, and the incorporation of all final readings on diagnostic studies and lab results. The clinician needs to maintain an index of suspicion for injuries in the absence of films/studies.

An organized, professional approach to management strategies for trauma patients is critical and will result in optimal outcomes. Trauma systems and centers need to be prepared to apply these strategies to address the challenge of managing the obese trauma patient.

Suggested Readings

Boatright JR: Transporting the morbidly obese patient: framing an EMS challenge, *J Emerg Nurs* 28(4):326-329, 2002.

Brodsky JB, Lemmens JH, Brock-Utne JG et al: Morbid obesity and tracheal intubation, *Anesth Analg* 94:732-736, 2002.

Bushard S: Trauma patients who are morbidly obese, *AORN J* 76(4):585-589, 2002.

Charlebois D, Wilmoth D: Critical care of patients with obesity, *Crit Care Nurse* 24(4):19-27, 2004.

Davidson JE, Kruse MW, Cox DH et al: Critical care of the morbidly obese, *Crit Care Nurs Q* 26(2):105-116, 2003.

Nasraway SA, Albert M, Donnelly AM et al: Morbid obesity is an independent determinant of death among surgical critically ill patients, *Crit Care Med* 34(4):964-970, 2006.

National Heart, Lung, and Blood Institute: *Body mass index table.* Retrieved November 5, 2006, from www.nhlbi.nih.gov/guidelines/obesity/bmi_tbl.htm

Padberg F, Cerveira JJ, Lal BK et al: Does severe venous insufficiency have a different etiology in the morbidly obese? Is it venous? *J Vasc Surg* 37:79-85, 2003.

Snyder JM, Arita A, Inampudi C et al: Intra-operative ultrasound guidance of vena caval umbrella placement in a super obese patient, *Obes Surg* 12:679-681, 2002.

Ziglar MK: Obesity and the trauma patient: challenges and guidelines for care, *J Trauma Nurs* 13(1):22-27, 2006.

CHAPTER 27

THE AGITATED TRAUMA PATIENT

ANNE P. MANTON

The agitated trauma patient presents the trauma care provider with a particular challenge. Agitation can interfere seriously with necessary elements of assessment and intervention. However, in the approach to care of the trauma patient, there can be no rush to judgment about the source of the agitation or about the most appropriate intervention. As always, emergency care clinicians are responsible for identifying the contributing factors, initiating the most appropriate interventions, and evaluating the patient's response to those interventions.

Agitation can be thought of as a continuum from moderate restlessness to uncooperativeness to manifest aggression with many points in between. The cause of agitation in the trauma patient may be physiologic, psychological, or psychiatric. Identification and treatment—or ruling out—of physiologic causes of agitation first is of utmost importance.

ASSESSMENT OF AGITATION

Even with an agitated trauma patient, trauma assessment and intervention should follow the standard ABC (airway, breathing, circulation) protocol. Key data obtained during this process will assist in analysis of the source of the agitation.

Airway, Breathing, Circulation, and Vital Signs

Assess the patient for abnormal function of the pulmonary and circulatory systems that may contribute to agitation:

- *Tachypnea:* Rapid breathing may represent respiratory distress, but fearful patients also hyperventilate. Additional assessment parameters—such as oxygen saturation, auscultation of breath sounds, and color of mucous membranes—will assist with the differential diagnosis.
- *Oxygenation:* Low oxygen saturation levels may point to hypoxia as a cause of agitation.
- *Tachycardia:* Rapid heartbeat may result from hypovolemia but also may reflect pain, anxiety, or an interaction of physiologic and psychological variables, such as the coexistence of hypovolemia and anxiety. Tachycardia also may be related to alcohol withdrawal.
- *Blood pressure:* Hypotension, and thus decreased cerebral perfusion, may contribute to agitation. Blood pressure may be elevated with head injury or alcohol withdrawal.
- *Temperature:* Elevated temperature in an agitated trauma patient may indicate alcohol withdrawal or thyrotoxic crisis (thyroid storm) as potential causes of agitation.
- *Pain:* Pain is frequently the source of agitation.

Disability (Neurologic Assessment)

Assess the patient for neurologic dysfunction that may contribute to agitation:

- Subtle changes in the level of consciousness may signal decreased cerebral perfusion or increased intracranial pressure. Agitation may represent a change in the patient's level of consciousness or awareness.
- Glasgow Coma Scale score: An abnormal score suggests traumatic brain injury or alcohol or drug overdose.
- Pupillary response: The presence of a sluggish or unequal response of pupils to light may indicate that increased intracranial pressure is the root of the patient's agitation. Pupils that are equal in size but pinpoint or dilated may be a sign of drug ingestion.

History

Assess the patient's health and medication history for factors contributing to agitation:

- Injury history: A prime consideration in the care of the agitated trauma patient is whether the behavioral changes began before or after the trauma. History of airway obstruction or head injury is also significant. Prehospital personnel also should be asked about indicators of a suicide attempt or circumstances involving violent crime.
- Health history: Psychiatric or substance abuse history is important to obtain. Psychiatric hospitalizations, suicide attempts, past aggressive or violent behavior, and current source of treatment (if any) help in the assessment and management of the agitation. Medical conditions such as diabetes mellitus or other endocrine disorders might cause agitation.
- Medications: first determine whether the patient has any known allergies. Then assess the patient's use of prescription and nonprescription medication. For patients who have been prescribed psychiatric medications, determine whether the patient has followed the prescribed medication regimen. Evaluate the patient for a history of alcohol abuse, including when alcohol was last used. Determine whether the patient ever experienced withdrawal symptoms. Explore the patient's usual and recent use of street drugs, identifying the type of drug used and the usual effect.

HIGH-FREQUENCY NURSING DIAGNOSES FOR AGITATED TRAUMA PATIENTS

- Acute confusion
- Ineffective tissue perfusion: cerebral
- Acute pain
- Fear or Anxiety
- Ineffective coping
- Disturbed thought processes
- Risk for violence: other directed
- Risk for violence: self-directed
- Risk for suicide
- *Nursing diagnoses specific to injury*

From NANDA International: *NANDA nursing diagnoses: definitions & classification, 2005-2006,* Philadelphia, 2006, The Association.

Head-to-Toe Assessment

A great deal of evidence can be gleaned during the head-to-toe assessment, such as the following:

- Signs of airway obstruction, inadequate ventilation, or shock
- Signs of head trauma
- The presence of pain-causing injuries
- Previous suicide attempts (healed wrist lacerations)
- The odor of alcohol
- Signs of neglect or disorganization that might suggest the possibility of mental illness
- Alcohol, prescription medications, or other drugs among the patient's belongings

For a list of nursing diagnoses frequently used for the agitated trauma patient, see the nursing diagnosis box.

PHYSIOLOGIC CAUSES OF AGITATION

Hypoxia

Restlessness is an early symptom of decreased oxygen supply to the brain. As hypoxia increases, restlessness may progress to agitation. Hypoxia should be a primary concern in the agitated trauma patient. Assessment for hypoxia is an essential component of the initial assessment of trauma patients, and the patient's oxygenation status should be monitored continuously. If hypoxia is present, oxygen should be administered, and then the cause should be determined. Hypoxia may be related to inadequate airway patency, chest injury, or inadequate circulation. Once the source of hypoxia is identified, it can be treated appropriately.

Head Injury

Head injury is another frequent physiologic cause of agitation in the trauma patient. Agitation may be a sign of an unrecognized head injury, especially when other injuries may be more visible or dramatic. Mental status changes related to head injury may be subtle but can be lethal if not recognized. New or increasing restlessness in a patient with known traumatic brain injury may be a sign of increasing intracranial pressure. The patient's level of consciousness is part of the initial assessment and also should be monitored and recorded frequently using the Glasgow Coma Scale and other neurologic indicators.

Interventions for the agitated, head-injured patient present a challenge to emergency providers because the patient's behavior may interfere with treatment, yet treating the agitation may impair the provider's ability to perform a proper neurologic assessment. Before using physical restraints or sedation, the nurse should attempt to calm the patient with reassurance, comfort measures, and the reduction of external stimuli. Sedation, if used, must be used cautiously because neurologic evaluation is affected and changes in the patient's neurologic status may not be as readily apparent. Additionally, the administration of sedation may compromise the patient's respiratory status. If sedation is used to control agitation, short-acting agents such as lorazepam (Ativan) should be administered at the lowest possible dose to achieve control. For patients with significant brain injuries and significant agitation, the administration of a sedative and a short-acting neuromuscular paralytic agent or the use of propofol (Diprivan) may be the best option. The use of physical restraints should be a last resort because a patient's resistance may lead to increased intracranial pressure. Physical restraints may be necessary as a safety measure, but in this case they should be used with sedation. Other interventions that may assist the agitated head-injured patient may include the administration of oxygen and elevation of the head if not contraindicated by other traumatic injuries.

Pain

One of the most common causes of agitation in trauma patients is pain. The suddenness of a traumatic injury and the ensuing pain can result in agitation when the patient does not understand why the pain cannot be eradicated. The trauma nurse must assess the patient's level of pain, using a pain rating scale when possible, and elicit the patient's description of the pain. Restlessness also can be a valuable clue to pain in the patient who cannot talk because of injury, sedation, or endotracheal intubation.

The emergency nurse plays a key role in the management of pain in the agitated trauma patient. The value of establishing rapport and trust between patient and nurse cannot be overstated. The prescriber should determine the risk versus the benefit of pain medication, keeping in mind that there are few situations in which pain medication is absolutely contraindicated. If ordered, the medication should be administered as soon as possible. If it is determined that pain medication poses an unacceptable risk, this should be explained to the patient (and family if present). The level of pain needs to be reassessed frequently for variation in quality and/or response to medication. Nonpharmacologic interventions, such as the application of ice, positioning, family presence, or information giving, also should be used when possible.

Refer to Chapter 13 for more information on pain assessment and management.

Substance Use/Abuse

One of the most common causes of agitation in the trauma patient is the use of alcohol or drugs. Often use of these substances is the major contributing factor in the trauma event. Drugs and alcohol can lead to uninhibited behavior and loss of the sense of social propriety, which may cause the patient to become agitated. Agitation also can be experienced as the drugs are wearing off.

Alcohol continues to be the most common substance used by patients who use the emergency department for services, including trauma. Alcohol intoxication frequently is associated with agitation. Other drugs that may lead to agitation in the trauma patient include stimulants such as methylphenidate (Ritalin, Concerta), cocaine, phencyclidine, MDMA (3,4-methylenedioxymethamphetamine, Ecstasy), methamphetamine, and hallucinogenics. The presence of alcohol or other drugs should be evaluated by toxicologic screening in all agitated trauma patients, especially if more obvious causes of agitation, such as hypoxia, have been ruled out. Interventions include treating the toxic effects of the drug.

Patients experiencing alcohol withdrawal or at risk for withdrawal, which can ensue in as short a period as a few hours after drinking, should be monitored and managed using a protocol such as the Clinical Institute Withdrawal Assessment for Alcohol, Revised (CIWA-Ar) protocol.[1] Signs and symptoms of early withdrawal include anxiety, tremor, nausea/vomiting, and elevated temperature.

The CIWA-Ar assessment tool measures the severity of alcohol withdrawal by recording pulse rate (taken for 1 minute) and blood pressure and by rating 10 signs and symptoms: nausea and vomiting, tremor, paroxysmal sweating, tactile disturbances, auditory disturbances, visual disturbances, anxiety, agitation, headache, and orientation. The maximum possible score is 67; however, patients with a score of greater than 10 usually are treated pharmacologically for alcohol withdrawal. The CIWA-Ar protocol recommends medication administration, such as benzodiazepines, according to the patient's assessment score. CIWA-Ar scoring should be repeated at regular intervals to monitor the patient's progress and ensure appropriate treatment.

Early alcohol withdrawal syndrome may exist simultaneously with an elevated blood alcohol level. A decrease in a patient's usually high blood alcohol level or abrupt cessation of alcohol intake may precipitate alcohol withdrawal syndrome even in the presence of blood alcohol levels that correspond with intoxication. Withdrawal initially is managed with benzodiazepines. Chlordiazepoxide (Librium) is the most commonly used drug for alcohol withdrawal, but diazepam (Valium) often is used for patients with a history of seizures, and lorazepam (Ativan) is used for patients with severe liver disease. The selection and use of benzodiazepines must be considered in the context of the patient's trauma status.

Emergency care providers should be vigilant about ensuring their own safety because patients who are substance abusers are prone to violent behavior. The trauma patient should be assessed in the early stages of agitation so that measures can be taken to deescalate or resolve the cause of agitation to prevent violence. The best predictor of agitation that will escalate to violence is a history of previous violence. Emergency care providers should institute precautions, use a calm and soothing voice but maintain a safe distance from the patient, allow the patient choices and participation in decision making if possible, use deescalation techniques, provide adequate security personnel if indicated, consider sedation, and as a last resort, apply physical restraints. The safety and well-being of the staff and other patients is paramount.

Metabolic Imbalance

Metabolic imbalance also can be a source of agitation in the trauma patient. Hypoglycemia can be associated with altered levels of consciousness and may have been a contributing factor to the traumatic event. In addition, agitation is not uncommon in hypoglycemia. Blood glucose levels should be included as part of the initial assessment of trauma patients. Although a glucose level lower than 60 mg/dL is considered hypoglycemia, signs and symptoms of hypoglycemia can occur at higher blood glucose levels depending on the patient's baseline levels. If the patient's history is unavailable and the blood glucose level is less than, or even within, the accepted normal range, intravenous administration of glucose might be considered. If hypoglycemia is the cause of the agitation, prompt improvement will be noted after the intravenous administration of glucose. If the patient has an insulin pump, and hypoglycemia is suspected, the pump should be stopped.

Although rare, hyperthyroid disease is another metabolic disorder that may be the cause of a trauma patient's agitation. When the history yields information suggestive of behavioral change *before* the trauma and other more common explanations for agitation have been ruled out, hyperthyroidism (thyroid storm) might be considered.

Electrolyte and acid-base imbalances may precipitate agitation and should be considered in instances of agitation in the trauma patient. Once identified, measures should be taken to correct the imbalance.

PSYCHOLOGIC CAUSES OF AGITATION

Fear and Anxiety

Because trauma occurs suddenly, unexpectedly, and usually unpredictably, trauma clinicians should expect that fear and anxiety will be a predominant cause of agitation in the trauma patient. Because most injuries are undiagnosed initially, fear of pain, dysfunction, or disfigurement is valid. Psychological responses to such stressors vary widely, and agitation may result. For the person suddenly thrust into the vulnerable role of "trauma patient," surrounded by strangers and undergoing physical examination and procedures, agitation may be a defensive response to fear and anxiety. In fact, this may be particularly true if the patient's trauma resulted from an assault. The emergency care staff should use an empathetic, concerned yet assured and in-control approach to the patient, offer reassurance as appropriate, build rapport and trust, give information about procedures, and provide comfort measures to the extent possible. For victims of violence, assurance of safety is important. These interventions sound simple, yet in the midst of caring for a trauma patient, emergency care staff may unknowingly react to the patient's behavior in a manner that increases fear and agitation. Family and significant others may provide substantial support to patients experiencing fear or anxiety.

Guilt

Trauma care providers should explore the circumstances surrounding the trauma event to determine whether guilt is an issue. Were there others involved? Does the patient feel responsible for injury to others or property? Did the trauma occur as a result of an inappropriate action by the patient? Although these issues likely will not be resolved in the emergency department, awareness of the source of agitation can provide the nurse with the information on which to base interventions to moderate the agitation.

Ineffective Coping

Trauma often plunges a patient into a life crisis. The coping skills of most persons are adequate to deal with day-to-day events. However, when a trauma occurs, the impact of the event may exceed their usual coping ability. Moreover, some patients may never have developed even basic coping skills. Agitation may represent a patient's feeling of loss of control. Emergency nursing care should focus on providing calm and consistency, demonstrating respect for the patient as a capable person by giving information and including the patient in decision making (when feasible), and establishing a trusting relationship. This approach can be a valuable adjunct to the physical and physiologic aspects of trauma care. The presence of family or friends also may enhance the agitated trauma patient's coping ability.

PSYCHIATRIC CAUSES OF AGITATION

Underlying acute or chronic psychiatric disorders are not unusual for trauma patients. Because the chronically mentally ill commonly live on the street or in shelters, they are frequently victims of assault. Also, patients with acute and chronic psychiatric disorders have a tendency to act in an impulsive manner, which may lead to a traumatic event. Agitation is a component of many acute and chronic psychiatric diagnoses and is particularly likely to be apparent in the situation of trauma care.

NOTE: It is essential that clinicians NOT assume agitation in the trauma patient with a psychiatric disorder is CAUSED BY the psychiatric diagnosis until physiologic causes for the agitation have been ruled out.

Mood Disorders: Mania

The trauma patient with an established diagnosis of bipolar disorder or schizoaffective disorder may exhibit agitation in the emergency care setting. In fact, the impulsivity and lack of insight that is integral to manic states may have contributed to the traumatic event. The possibility of a dual diagnosis also needs to be considered in patients with these psychiatric diagnoses because the incidence of concurrent substance abuse is high. This potential must be taken into consideration and addressed as a coexisting source of agitation.

An important first step in treating a trauma patient with agitation believed to be related to a psychiatric diagnosis is to determine, if possible, the patient's current medication regimen and level of compliance. Use of medications already found to be efficacious for a particular patient is a good initial strategy. In the absence of such information, the most likely choice of medication to reduce agitation in a manic episode is an atypical antipsychotic (e.g., risperidone [Risperdal], olanzapine, or ziprasidone). These medications have been found to act as quickly as haloperidol, and they have a better safety profile. Because agitation can progress quickly to aggression and then violence in these patients, it may be prudent also to administer a short-acting benzodiazepine, such as lorazepam or clonazepam.

Mood Disorders: Depression

Although depressed patients often are thought of as being quiet and withdrawn, patients who are depressed also can be irritable or agitated. Depression interferes with sleep and concentration and therefore might be a causative factor in the trauma incident. Depression and anxiety are highly comorbid, and agitation in the circumstance of trauma may represent anxiety. For the trauma patient with a diagnosis of depressive disorder, management of agitation is best handled in the emergency setting with a short-acting benzodiazepine at the lowest dose needed to reduce agitation, once physiologic causes of the agitation have been ruled out.

In the instance of an agitated patient with depressive disorder, nursing support and comfort measures will assist in reducing agitation. Use of a calm, controlled but caring approach and establishing trust in the nurse-patient relationship will help to minimize agitation as well.

Suicide Attempt

A suicide attempt can lead to a trauma event in a number of ways, including single-occupant motor vehicle crashes, jumping from substantial heights, self-inflicted gunshot injuries, and so-called suicide by cop (creating a situation in which a police officer is forced to shoot the instigator). Clinicians should always consider the possibility that trauma was the result of a suicide attempt. The agitation observed in these patients may be the expression of underlying mental illness, frustration with the current situation, or the influence of alcohol or other drugs. In serious suicide attempts, agitation should be taken seriously as well. Is agitation a manifestation of the patient rejecting treatment? If the patient is considered still to be actively suicidal, the agitation may progress to aggressive attempts to interrupt or obstruct treatment. If so, the patient may need to be sedated in order for treatment to be carried out. Again, a short-acting benzodiazepine is a first-line intervention. If the agitation evolves toward aggression, other drugs such as atypical antipsychotics also may be used. Mental health specialists should be consulted to evaluate the patient.

Paranoia

The major issues in managing the agitated trauma patient with paranoia is establishing trust, assuring the patient that she or he will be safe, and incorporating the patient in care decisions to the extent possible. When patient involvement in decision making is not possible, the emergency care staff should provide timely information.

The patient with paranoia is fearful. If fear progresses beyond a level the patient can tolerate, he or she may become aggressive or even violent as a perceived act of self-defense.

If paranoia is associated with a diagnosed psychiatric condition, such as schizophrenia, care providers should make concerted attempts to determine the patient's usual medication regimen, compliance, and control of symptoms. If the patient's current medication information is unavailable, and the patient's paranoia and agitation are increasing, atypical antipsychotic agents (risperidone [Risperdal], olanzapine, or ziprasidone) should be administered, possibly in combination with a short-acting benzodiazepine.

SUMMARY

Agitation in the trauma patient can have many causes, thus thorough patient assessment to identify the underlying cause is critical. The trauma care practitioner should assess the patient with an open and inquisitive mind. Inaccurate assessment of agitation leads to inadequate or incorrect interventions. At best, this can lead to agitation that remains unresolved or worsens, thus creating an unnecessary burden for the emergency staff. At worst, it could compromise the patient's care and lead to a poor treatment outcome.

Physiologic causes for agitation should be explored and treated or ruled out first—even when the patient is known to have an existing psychiatric diagnosis. Only when it is clear that the basis of agitation is not physiologic should the psychological or psychiatric causes be explored.

Creating a therapeutic, trusting relationship between the nurse and patient is of critical importance. The ways in which trauma patients react to their situation are unpredictable. The trauma patient must deal with issues of safety, pain, potential disfigurement, loss of function, and even survival. Regardless of the nature of the trauma incident, it is a situation that presents a crisis for the patient and likely for family as well. Emergency nurses can help.

At times, agitated trauma patients need to be medicated/sedated in order for care to be delivered effectively. All other measures to reduce or eliminate the patient's agitation should be taken first. Sedation should never be the first solution to agitation. However, when pharmacologic intervention is necessary, doses should be as low as possible to achieve the desired outcome, and evaluation of response should be ongoing. Patient and staff safety is always the top priority.

Reference

1. Sullivan JT, Sykora K, Schneiderman J et al: Assessment of alcohol withdrawal: the revised Clinical Institute Withdrawal Assessment for Alcohol scale (CIWA-Ar), *Br J Addict* 84:1353-1357, 1989.

Suggested Readings

Antai-Ontong D: *Psychiatric emergencies: how to accurately assess and manage a patient in crisis,* Eau Claire, Wis, 2001, PESI Healthcare.

Beebe JM: Substance abuse and trauma care. In McQuillan KA, VonRueden KT, Hartsock RL et al, editors: *Trauma nursing from resuscitation through rehabilitation,* ed 3, Philadelphia, 2002, WB Saunders.

Farrar JA: Psychosocial impact of trauma. In McQuillan KA, VonRueden KT, Hartsock RL et al, editors: *Trauma nursing from resuscitation through rehabilitation,* ed 3, Philadelphia, 2002, WB Saunders.

Lisanti P: Adult health: acute care. In Naegle MA, D'Avanzo CE, editors: *Addictions & substance abuse: strategies for advanced practice nursing,* Upper Saddle River, NJ, 2001, Prentice Hall.

Petit JR: *Handbook of emergency psychiatry,* Philadelphia, 2004, Lippincott, Williams & Wilkins.

CLINICAL SKILLS AND PROCEDURES

CHAPTER 28

SKILLS FOR TRAUMA MANAGEMENT

PATRICIA MAHER HARRISON

MANAGEMENT OF THE DIFFICULT AIRWAY

The primary goal in the management of trauma patients is to ensure that they have a secure airway and adequate ventilation. For those patients who need supplemental oxygen and assistance with ventilation, bag-mask ventilation with 100% oxygen is the first step in managing the airway. For some patients, this strategy may be successful in itself to ensure good oxygen saturation en route to the trauma center. In those patients who are not managed successfully by this strategy alone, they will need to progress to standard intubation practices. For those clinical situations in which standard bag-mask ventilation and intubation are unsuccessful, patients will benefit from nonsurgical adjuncts to managing the difficult airway, laryngeal mask airway, and/or surgical interventions through a needle or surgical cricothyrotomy.

LARYNGEAL MASK AIRWAY

An adjunct approach to managing the difficult airway may be through the use of a laryngeal mask airway (LMA). When used in elective airway management, the LMA may be used as the sole therapy. In trauma cases the LMA is never used alone or in place of intubation or cricothyrotomy. The LMA is used in place of bag-mask ventilation in those patients with clinical features such that an adequate seal for the ventilating mask is impossible. The LMA then would be one step in the progression to establishing a secure airway. The LMA provides no protection against aspiration of gastric contents, and therefore steps should be taken to ensure a smooth, rapid transition to definitive airway strategies.

NEEDLE CRICOTHYROTOMY

Needle cricothyrotomy or transtracheal jet ventilation is a procedure that can provide not only lifesaving oxygenation but also ventilation until a more adequate airway is established. The technique involves inserting an over-the-needle catheter into the trachea and ventilating the patient's lungs. The most frequent complication of needle cricothyrotomy or transtracheal jet ventilation is subcutaneous emphysema, occurring 2% to 10% of the time. This complication can be minimized by firmly securing the hub of the catheter to the neck. Other complications include tracheal mucosal ulceration, bleeding, and vocal changes.

A needle cricothyrotomy can provide ventilation for 30 to 40 minutes and is an advanced airway skill reserved for emergent airway management when other methods of airway management have failed. Needle cricothyrotomy most frequently is used for children less than 12 years old because of the low tidal volumes generated by the catheter and jet insufflation technique.

Indications

Needle cricothyrotomy is indicated for complete upper airway obstruction resulting from the following:

- Pharyngeal and epiglottic edema or obstruction
- Facial trauma and/or neck trauma with airway compromise
- Inability to remove foreign body with abdominal thrusts or forceps
- Inability to obtain and maintain adequate airway with conventional means
- Inability to ventilate by bag-mask

Contraindications

Significant laryngeal injury or total airway obstruction is a contraindication (because this can lead to barotrauma).

Equipment

The following equipment is required:

- 12- or 14-gauge, 8.5-cm over-the-needle catheter
- 5- to 10-mL syringe
- 3-mm pediatric endotracheal tube adapter
- Oxygen tubing
- Skin prep solution (swab or kit)
- Y connector
- Tape
- Bag-valve resuscitator
- Suction with appropriate catheter(s)

Procedure

Use the following procedure:

1. Place the patient supine with the neck in a neutral position.
2. Palpate cricothyroid membrane (located on the anterior neck between inferior margin of the thyroid cartilage and superior margin of the cricoid cartilage; Figure 28-1).
3. Prep the area.
4. Open sterile packages on a sterile field.
5. Put on sterile gloves.
6. Assemble the 10-, 12-, or 14-gauge catheter with a 5- or 10-mL syringe.
7. Identify the cricothyroid membrane (as in step 2), and stabilize the thyroid cartilage with the nondominant hand.
8. Puncture the skin in the midline directly over the cricothyroid membrane.
9. Direct the needle at a 45-degree angle caudally.
10. Carefully insert the needle through the lower half of the membrane, aspirating the syringe as the hand advances (air return into the syringe signifies entry into the lumen of the trachea).
11. Withdraw the stylette while gently advancing the catheter downward.

NOTE: Do not force the catheter, or puncture of the posterior wall of the trachea may occur.

Figure 28–1. Cricothyroid membrane.

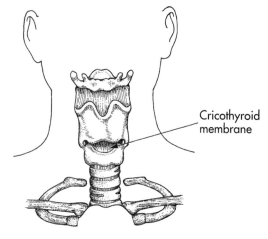

Cricothyroid
membrane

12. Attach catheter hub to a 3-mm pediatric endotracheal tube adapter.
13. Connect Y connector to 3-mm pediatric endotracheal tube adapter.
14. Administer oxygen at 15 L/min (50 psi).
15. Tape the catheter in place.
16. Use a 1:2 technique for jet insufflation; hold finger over open end of Y connector for 1 second, and then leave connector open for 2 seconds for exhalation of air; repeat sequence until a more definitive airway can be established.
17. Observe lung inflations; auscultate for adequate ventilation (other lung injuries may become apparent at this time).

SURGICAL CRICOTHYROTOMY

Surgical cricothyrotomy is the approach of choice for the patient who cannot be intubated or ventilated by any other means in a timely fashion. Surgical cricothyrotomy provides effective airway control and allows for oxygenation and ventilation of the patient's lungs. Relative contraindications include age younger than 5 years and bleeding diathesis; absolute contraindications include significant damage to the cricoid cartilage or larynx. Complications of surgical cricothyrotomy can be divided into early and late. Early complications include failure to place tube or prolonged procedure time, subcutaneous emphysema, and infection. Late complications include voice changes, laryngeal stenosis, and tracheomalacia. This technique is more complicated than a needle cricothyrotomy and should be performed by a clinician specifically trained to establish a surgical cricothyrotomy.

Indications

Indications for surgical cricothyrotomy are the same as for needle cricothyrotomy.

Contraindications

Contraindications are any airway impairment that can be corrected by more conventional means such as suctioning, nasopharyngeal or oropharyngeal airways, endotracheal intubation, or bag-valve-mask ventilation.

Equipment

The following equipment is required:

Appropriate-size endotracheal tube such as tracheostomy tube or cuffed endotracheal tube
10-mL syringe
Hemostats
Retracting device such as tracheal hook, small rake retractors, and/or tracheal spreaders
No. 10 and 11 scalpel blades and handle
Skin prep solution
Suction with appropriate catheters
Tracheal tape or adhesive tape
Bag-valve resuscitator
Sterile 4 × 4-inch sponges

Procedure

Use the following procedure:

1. Position patient supine with the neck in a neutral position.
2. Palpate the cricothyroid membrane (located on the anterior neck between the inferior margin of the thyroid cartilage and the superior margin of the cricoid cartilage).
3. Prep the area.
4. Open sterile packages onto a sterile field.
5. Put on sterile gloves.
6. If the patient is conscious, consider a local anesthetic.
7. Identify the cricothyroid membrane, and stabilize the thyroid cartilage.
8. Make a vertical or horizontal incision through the skin over the cricothyroid membrane and sharply dissect through the cricothyroid membrane.
9. Insert the scalpel handle or available retracting device into the incision and rotate at least 90 degrees to open the airway.
10. Insert the appropriate-sized, cuffed tube into the cricothyroid membrane incision and direct it caudally into the trachea.
11. Inflate the cuff and begin ventilating the patient's lungs.
12. Confirm placement by lung auscultation, and observe for chest expansion, misting in the tube, end-tidal carbon dioxide detection, no gurgling over epigastrium, and chest x-ray film.
13. Secure the tube in place.

SPINAL IMMOBILIZATION

Cervical and complete spinal immobilization must be considered simultaneously with airway management as one of the first priorities of care in the management of the injured patient. Injuries to the cervical, thoracic, and lumbar spine can range from minor muscle strain to life-threatening injuries. In most cases of trauma, cervical spine protection is required until an injury can be ruled out. Injuries to the spine can result in death, quadriplegia, paraplegia, and chronic disability. Half of these injuries occur from motor vehicle and motorcycle collisions, and the other half occur from falls, sporting activities, and intentional trauma. Extreme caution and a high index of suspicion are recommended when handling trauma patients before cervical spine injury has been ruled out.

Initial patient management includes the assessment for the need for spinal immobilization based on mechanism of injury and the clinician's index of suspicion for potential injury. Field or emergency department personnel need to establish manual cervical in-line stabilization while the team is preparing to assess the neck and apply a semirigid or hard cervical collar.

Equipment

The following equipment is required:

Semirigid cervical collar (preferably with window in anterior portion, which allows for evaluation of trachea and carotid pulse) or other commercially available cervical immobilization device
Long spine board with straps
Blankets and towels for padding
2- or 3-inch adhesive tape

Equipment used to immobilize the neck may be as varied as the situation in which the items are being used. If equipment is being applied in the hospital or in the field, many commercial devices are available. However, if cervical spine immobilization is indicated in the absence of this equipment, commonly available materials are adequate for achieving the necessary stabilization.

Procedure

Use the following procedure:

1. Stabilize the patient's head; tell the patient not to move the neck or turn the head.
2. Assess the airway; ensure patency by using jaw thrust or chin lift; do not hyperextend the neck. If endotracheal intubation is necessary, maintain manual in-line stabilization during endotracheal tube placement.
3. Evaluate the cervical spine by observation: palpate each spinous process. Note deformity, crepitus, pain, and instability (talk to the patient; also remember to inform the patient of each step of the procedure to enlist his or her cooperation and to alleviate anxiety and movement).
4. Gently apply in-line manual stabilization by placing one hand on either side of the head and stabilizing head and neck in a neutral vertical position. (Once manual, stabilization must be maintained until complete immobilization of the neck and spine has been achieved.)
5. Direct other members of the team in body positioning, spine board placement, and patient movement. The patient is logrolled with strict in-line manual stabilization onto the spine board. The person maintaining in-line stabilization is the team leader and directs all movement of the patient.
6. When satisfied with absolute immobility of patient's cervical spine, release manual stabilization.
7. Be prepared to logroll the patient using the backboard if vomiting occurs; have suction at hand.
8. Be sensitive to the frightening nature of this procedure; maintain a dialogue with the patient to explain each new move and to evaluate changes in neurovascular status and cognizant function.

Criteria for Evaluating the Cervical Spine

The cervical collar should remain in place if any of the following are true:

- Patient complains of pain, weakness, or parasthesias suggestive of acute cervical injury.
- Patient complains of neck pain, tenderness, spasm, or limited range of motion.

- Patient is unreliable because of altered mental status from injury, alcohol, or other drugs.
- Communication is impaired because of language barrier, aphasia, developmental delay, or dementia.
- Patient has preexisting cervical injury.
- Patient has distracting pain from other injuries or long-bone fractures.
- Patient's neurologic exam reveals deficit.
- Patient is in shock following blunt trauma.

If the foregoing criteria are not present, the clinician may elect to remove the collar and completely examine the patient's neck. The clinician may clear the cervical spine by examination if no signs or symptoms of injury exist.

In the presence of any of the foregoing criteria along with or without physical findings, the patient should have radiographic evaluation. In a patient with a low index of suspicion for injury, plain films including a lateral, an anteroposterior, and an odontoid view of the cervical spine are adequate. If there is an increased index of suspicion for injury, a cervical spine computed tomography scan with three-dimensional reconstruction provides excellent radiographic images to help rule out injury. A completely negative computed tomography scan (bony and soft tissue) along with a negative clinical exam support the removal of the cervical collar. In patients who cannot participate in a clinical exam or those who are comatose or chemically paralyzed, the decision to remove the collar is difficult. Most trauma centers have established protocols to remove collars following negative computed tomography scans with three-dimensional reconstructions, negative cervical spine magnetic resonance imaging scans and/or low index of suspicion for a cervical injury. Currently, there is no consensus on this protocol. Patients who have collars left in place for prolonged periods have increased incidence of skin breakdown, difficulty with clearing their secretions leading to increased incidence of aspiration, and pneumonia. Timely removal of collars is important.

For those patients with a cervical injury, the decisions regarding long-term stabilization are the responsibility of the orthopedic spine surgeon or the neurosurgical spine surgeon. Often the long-term stabilization is determined in the initial phase of care while the patient is still in the emergency department. Depending on the injury, long-term management can be the semirigid hard collar for 6 to 8 weeks, the placement of a halo traction vest, or surgical intervention. If the collar is to be the sole therapy, ensure the collar that is in place is the correct type, is correctly fitted, and is appropriately applied. Halo vest traction is applied by the spine surgeon. The halo ring is applied via screws into the scalp, and then the ring is attached to the vest via four titanium rods. The ring, rods, and vest provide the external fixation such that the neck is completely immobile.

NEEDLE THORACENTESIS AND FLUTTER VALVE

Needle thoracentesis (thoracostomy) is a procedure for the rapidly deteriorating critical patient who has a life-threatening tension pneumothorax. The procedure involves relieving the trapped air in the pleural space and allowing for decompression of positive pressure within the pleural space. You should never see a chest x-ray film of a tension pneumothorax because this condition should be recognized during the primary survey. Decompression may be accomplished with an over-the-needle catheter, allowing the air to escape passively via the catheter or a simple one-way valve (flutter valve) attached to the catheter. When an angiocatheter is used, the needle should never be reinserted into the catheter because of the risk of shearing the catheter tip in the pleural space. Needle thoracostomy is only temporary, and definitive treatment with a chest tube is needed urgently. The catheter tip quickly becomes occluded by blood if a hemothorax is present. Complications include lung puncture or laceration, hematoma, retained catheter fragment, iatrogenic infection, or failure to decompress.

Indication

Tension pneumothorax (absent breath sounds, tracheal deviation) is the indication for needle thoracentesis and flutter valve.

Equipment

The following equipment is required:

- Prep solution
- 14-gauge over-the-needle catheter of adequate length to reach the pleural space
- 3-inch collapsible tubing for flutter valve (Penrose drain or Heimlich valve)
- Suture ties or small rubber band

Procedure

Use the following procedure:

1. Evaluate the patient's respiratory status and skin color: look at chest excursion, auscultate for absence of breath sounds on affected side, observe for tracheal deviation away from affected side, look for distended neck veins to determine the presence of tension pneumothorax.
2. Administer oxygen per bag-mask or non-rebreather mask.
3. If the patient is intubated, confirm correct tube placement and insertion depth before needle decompression.
4. Prep insertion area (second intercostal space, midclavicular line) with antiseptic solution.
5. Insert the needle into the second intercostal space, riding just over the top of the third rib to avoid the intercostal neurovasculature that lies on the inferior borders of the ribs (Figure 28-2).

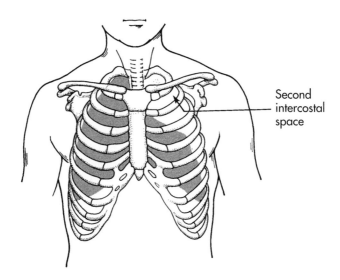

Second
intercostal
space

Figure 28-2. Needle thoracentesis.

6. Puncture the parietal pleura (a hissing sound should confirm proper venting if using a needle and flutter valve).
7. Leave the catheter in place. If using a flutter valve, no dressing is necessary. (Intubated patients receiving positive pressure ventilation do not necessarily require a flutter valve.)
8. Leave the catheter in place until a chest tube is inserted.
9. Obtain a chest radiograph (preferably an upright view) to confirm relief of the tension pneumothorax.

CHEST TUBE PLACEMENT AND CHEST DRAINAGE

Chest tubes are placed so that air and blood can be removed from the intrathoracic cavity. The procedure involves placing a chest tube usually at the nipple level (fifth intercostal space) anterior to the midaxillary line on the affected side so that air or blood/fluid can be drained by gravity drainage or with the assistance of suction.

The accumulation of blood and air in the pleural cavity along with the loss of negative pressure causes the lung to collapse. Once a chest tube is inserted through an intercostal space into the pleural cavity, air, blood, or fluid is drained by gravity or suction into a drainage collection device, and negative pressure is restored. Complications include laceration or puncture of intrathoracic and/or abdominal organs; introduction of pleural infection; damage to the intercostal nerve, artery, or vein; incorrect tube position; or extrathoracic, intrathoracic, and persistent pneumothorax.

Indications

The following are indications for placement of a chest tube:

- Hemothorax
- Pneumothorax
- Tension pneumothorax
- Open pneumothorax
- Pleural effusions
- Chylothorax

Equipment

The following equipment is required:

Closed chest drainage system with autotransfusion capabilities
Prep sponges and solution
Two large, curved Kelly clamps
Syringes, 6 and 10 mL
18- and 25-gauge needles
Scalpel and blade
Lidocaine 1%
Suture to secure chest tube
Suction
Sterile water
Suture for wound approximation
Chest tube (usually 32, 36, or large enough to collect large quantities of blood)
Sterile gloves

Occlusive dressing material
Sterile drape
Needle holder
Benzoin
Wide adhesive tape

Preparation for the Procedure

Preparation for chest tube placement requires the following:

1. Prepare the patient by explaining the procedure.
2. Evaluate the patient's respiratory status. Observe for respiratory rate, respiratory effort, skin color, tracheal deviation, distended neck veins, and chest expansion; and auscultate breath sounds.
3. Monitor the patient's vital signs throughout the procedure.
4. Administer oxygen via the appropriate route.
5. Administer analgesia, as prescribed.
6. Chest drainage systems vary among manufacturers.

The tubing connection to the patient should be clamped before insertion to prevent unnecessary exposure or loss of blood from the pleural space. If there is concern for a hemothorax, the autotransfusion collection system should be set up and ready to collect as the chest tube and drainage system are connected. Once connected to the closed chest drainage system, the tubing should not be "milked" or "stripped."

Procedure

Use the following procedure:

1. The most advantageous and more cosmetically appealing site for chest tube insertion is the midaxillary fifth intercostal space; this position allows for adequate removal of air and/or blood.
2. Assist the physician as necessary with the procedure:
   - Prep and drape the site with sterile towels.
   - Infiltrate the skin and periosteum with lidocaine.
   - Using a scalpel, make a 2- to 3-cm transverse incision through the skin.
   - Using a scalpel, sharply dissect through the subcutaneous tissue over the superior edge of the fifth rib.
   - Carefully puncture the tip of the Kelly clamp, and dissect through the pleura. If there is a pneumothorax, air will rush out through the punctured pleura.
   - Explore the intrathoracic area with a sterile, gloved index finger of the dominant hand to free adhesions, clots, or lung tissue.
   - Place the Kelly clamp over the perforation on the distal end of the chest tube so that the tip is firm. This aids in the insertion of the chest tube through puncture placed in the pleura.
   - Maneuver the distal tip of the tube into the thoracic cavity, ensuring that the tube is advanced past the most proximal fenestration.
3. After the tube is determined to be in the proper place, secure it using suture attached to skin.
4. Close the skin edges with nonabsorbable suture.
5. Apply an occlusive dressing around the tube.

6. Cover the dressing with wide adhesive tape.
7. Attach the tube to a closed chest drainage system. The chest drainage system should be adaptable for autotransfusion.
8. Maintain the chest drainage system below the level of the chest to facilitate the flow of drainage and prevent reflux into the chest.
9. Record the amount of blood that returns initially and any subsequent drainage on the collection chamber and the trauma flow sheet.
10. Obtain a chest x-ray film to ensure proper positioning of the chest tube.

Troubleshooting

The assessment of air leaks allows the clinician to monitor lung expansion, tube placement, the integrity of the closed chest drainage system, and potential injury of the trachea or esophagus. The water-seal chamber directly reflects the change of pressure within the pleural space. Fluid in the water-seal chamber normally fluctuates with inspiration and exhalation.

Initially, fluctuation of fluid in the water-seal chamber reflects the removal of air from the pleural space. Any ongoing fluctuations or vigorous bubbling suggests potential tracheal or bronchial injury, leak in the chest drainage system itself, or improper tube placement.

To help determine the location of a leak, first occlude the chest drainage tubing proximally to the patient. Immediate cessation of bubbling in the water-seal chamber indicates a problem with tube placement, the dressing site, or ongoing leak from the pleural space. Working distally from the chest tube toward the chest drainage device, intermittent occluding of the system will isolate the problem between the area occluded and the drainage system. Any continued bubbling at the end of the tubing indicates a leak within the closed chest drainage system.

Loss of chest tube patency indicates a mechanical or blood clot occlusion. Examine the tubing to determine any kinks in the line. Suspected clots may be dislodged by gently squeezing the drainage tubing in a proximal to distal direction from the patient. The only indication for squeezing the drainage tubing is to dislodge a suspected clot.

AUTOTRANSFUSION

Autotransfusion is the collection and reinfusion of a patient's shed blood from his or her pleural cavity. The blood is collected in an autotransfusion collection device and then is reinfused into the patient. In the absence of type-specific or crossmatched blood, autotransfusion is readily available, warm, and perfectly crossmatched.

Several types of autotransfusion setups are available. The clinician should be familiar with the type of equipment used at his or her own facility.

Patients with injuries that include thoracoabdominal communication, such as with a diaphragmatic tear, are candidates for autotransfusion in the emergent setting. Any collected blood with obvious fecal material, clots, or coagulopathies should NOT be reinfused. The reinfusion of contaminated blood may result in an adverse effect, such as sepsis or worsening of a coagulopathic state. Autotransfused blood needs to be returned to the patient in a timely fashion (see guidelines for your product). All blood is infused through a filtered system.

Indications

The following are indications for autotransfusion:

- Massive hemothorax
- Myocardial rupture

- Great vessel rupture
- Other chest trauma in the following situations:
  - Nonavailability of banked blood
  - History of transfusion reactions
  - Refusal of blood for religious reasons

Contraindications

The following are contraindications for autotransfusion:

- Wounds more than 4 hours old
- Contamination of blood by outside sources, gastrointestinal tract contents, or cancer cells
- Mediastinal, pericardial, pulmonary, or systemic infection
- Coagulopathies

Procedure

The autotransfusion procedure varies depending on the type and brand of equipment used (Figure 28-3). However, some basic principles apply, regardless of which type of equipment is used:

- Set up the equipment as if doing regular chest drainage.
- Blood that is collected in the autotransfusion unit must be reinfused within 4 hours from the start of the collection.
- When the collected blood is being transfused, be sure to switch the patient's chest tube to another autotransfusion unit or to a regular blood chest drainage unit.
- Attach a blood filter to the bag of collected blood before reinfusion.

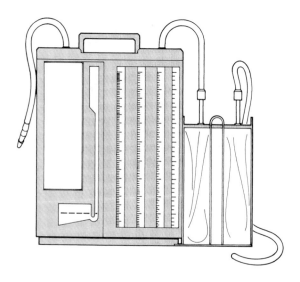

Figure 28–3. Autotransfusion equipment.

EMERGENCY THORACOTOMY

Patients with penetrating thoracic injuries who lose pulses en route or in the emergency department may be candidates for immediate resuscitative thoracotomy. A qualified surgeon must be present at the time of the patient's arrival to determine the need and potential success of an emergency department resuscitative thoracotomy. A left anterior thoracotomy is performed to gain access. Restoration of intravascular volume is continued, and endotracheal intubation and mechanical ventilation are imperative. Patients sustaining blunt trauma who arrive pulseless but with myocardial electrical activity are generally not candidates for resuscitative thoracotomy. The therapeutic goals effects of a thoracotomy are (1) evacuation of pericardial blood causing tamponade; (2) direct control of exsanguinating intrathoracic hemorrhage; (3) open cardiac massage; and (4) cross-clamping of the descending aorta to slow blood loss below the diaphragm and increase perfusion to the brain and heart.

Equipment

The following equipment is required:

Surgical prep solution
Scalpel and blades
Large, heavy scissors
Bone cutters
Two large Kelly clamps
Suture material
Rib spreaders
Two aortic clamps
Two needle holders
Four mosquito clips
Sterile gloves
Prep solution
Large-bore suction needles

Criteria

Criteria for performance of emergency thoractomy are the following:

- Loss of vital signs (respiratory effort, auscultated heartbeat, motor function, or pupillary activity) en route to the hospital or in the emergency department and/or less than 5 minutes of cardiopulmonary resuscitation that is unresponsive to volume resuscitation, airway management, or chest decompression
- Cardiac-specific, penetrating injury
- Persistent pericardial tamponade unrelieved with pericardiocentesis
- Adequate support services to manage the patient once resuscitated (i.e., appropriately trained surgical staff, operating room, and ongoing critical care capabilities)

PERICARDIAL WINDOW/PERICARDIOCENTESIS

The accumulation of blood in the pericardial sac with impairment of the diastolic filling of the heart should be suspected in any blunt trauma patient with disproportion between hemodynamic status and the apparent blood loss. Pericardiocentesis is indicated for a pericardial tamponade with decompensation. Current recommendations support a surgical approach to this problem via a pericardial window with the full back up of surgical support in the operating room should the clinical condition deteriorate or require emergent surgical repair. A *pericardial window* is a small incision made just under the xiphoid process. The tissue is dissected until the apex of the heart can be visualized directly. A segment of pericardium is lifted with forceps; and a small, square incision is made, creating a window from which pericardial fluid can drain.

INTRAOSSEOUS INFUSION

An *intraosseous infusion* is the administration of intravenous fluids and drugs directly into the bone marrow.

Intraosseous Cannulation

The intraosseous administration of fluids and medications is a safe and effective procedure in children and adults. This procedure has been used successfully in the prehospital and emergency settings. The procedure may be used when the patient is in hypovolemic shock, cardiopulmonary arrest, or status epilepticus or has lack of venous access because of burns or obesity. Intraosseous infusion also can be used when administration of fluids or drugs is critical to survival and the establishment of an IV cannot be accomplished. Catecholamines, colloids, crystalloids, blood products, antibiotics, calcium, heparin, lidocaine, atropine, sodium bicarbonate, and digitalis have been infused successfully by the intraosseous route. Complications include extravasation or subcutaneous fluid administration, tibial fracture, compartment syndrome, osteomyelitis, cellulitis, and fatty embolism.

Contraindications

The following are contraindications for intraosseous infusion:

- Fractured or previously penetrated bone
- Cellulitis or burn at the site of insertion
- History of osteogenesis imperfecta or osteoporosis

Equipment

The following equipment is required:

- Skin prep solution
- Intraosseous needle
- Sterile gloves

Procedure

Use the following procedure:

1. Locate the anterior medial surface of the tibia 1 to 3 cm below the tibial tuberosity (Figure 28-4, *A*). Other (optional) sites are the distal anterior femur (Figure 28-4, *B*), distal tibia (Figure 28-4, *C*), the medial malleolus, sternum, and the iliac crest.
2. Prep the area.
3. Using an osseous needle, advance the intraosseous needle through the skin, fascia, and bony cortex with a rotating, boring motion. It will become apparent that the needle is in the bone marrow when a popping sensation occurs, followed by a sudden absence of resistance, when the needle can stand upright without manual support, and when fluid flows freely through the needle.

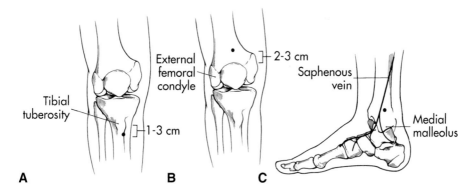

Figure 28-4. Recommended sites for intraosseous infusion. **A,** Proximal tibia. **B,** Distal femur. **C,** Distal tibia. *(From Emergency Nurses Association:* Sheehy's emergency nursing: principles and practice, *ed 5, St Louis, 2003, Mosby.)*

4. Aspirate, using a syringe. If bone marrow is returned, the needle has been placed correctly. If bone marrow is not returned, try running fluid into the needle.
5. After needle is in place, tape it and infuse solutions or medications.
6. Observe for infiltration on local irritation.

BEDSIDE ASSESSMENT FOR INTRAABDOMINAL HEMORRHAGE

Rapid assessment for intraabdominal hemorrhage is critical in the trauma patient who has experienced blunt or penetrating injury. The identification of intraabdominal blood can be accomplished at the bedside using a noninvasive ultrasound procedure or a minimally invasive abdominal aspiration/lavage.

FOCUSED ABDOMINAL SONOGRAM FOR TRAUMA

Focused abdominal sonogram for trauma (FAST) uses a bedside ultrasound machine systematically to assess for fluid collection in four key areas of the chest/abdomen/pelvis. A FAST is a rapid diagnostic procedure that may be used to determine intraperitoneal hemorrhage when results of a physical examination are equivocal or when the patient is unstable with unidentified blood loss, is unable to participate in abdominal evaluation, or requires emergency surgery with general anesthesia for other injuries. FAST can be done on all patients, although the ability to obtain a good study is decreased in the morbidly obese patient. The physician places the transducer (1) midline under the xiphoid process to assess for pericardial fluid; (2) on the right side of the abdomen over the intercostal space, between the anterior and midaxillary line at the level of the seventh and eighth ribs to assess for fluid in Morrison's pouch; (3) on the left midaxillary line subcostal margin to assess for fluid around and/or between the spleen and left kidney; and (4) midline above the symphysis pubis to assess for fluid around loops of bowel in the pelvis.

A FAST examination will not identify the origin of the hemorrhage but will identify the presence of intraabdominal blood. Generally, there needs to be at least 500 mL of blood present to be detected, although the accuracy of the ultrasound interpretation is operator dependent. Advantages of the FAST include the noninvasive process, ease of exam, and the ability to repeat the exam as often as clinically needed.

Diagnostic Peritoneal Aspiration/Lavage

A minimally invasive approach to identifying the presence of blood in the abdomen is accomplished through the diagnostic peritoneal aspiration or lavage procedure. In centers where the FAST is readily available, diagnostic peritoneal aspiration or lavage rarely is done. Diagnostic peritoneal aspiration or lavage is sensitive and relatively accurate for the presence of abdominal injury but not specific with regard to the type or extent of organ injury.

Diagnostic peritoneal aspiration involves the placement of a catheter through the abdomen, into the peritoneum, and evaluating the gross aspirate. In a hemodynamically unstable patient, if the aspiration involves freely flowing blood, the clinician may stop at this point and make the determination to go urgently tò the operating room. If the aspirate is clear, a lavage is initiated with the infusion of crystalloid fluid (500 to 1000 mL). When retrieved, the fluid is analyzed for the presence of red blood cells, white blood cells, amylase, bacteria, and fecal matter. Complications may include infection, hematoma, wound dehiscence, systemic infection, hollow visceral injury, vascular penetration, preperitoneal placement, or diaphragmatic tear.

Extremity Splinting

Splints often are used for temporary immobilization of any orthopedic injury, including fractures and soft tissue injuries, until a definitive procedure is performed. Splints also serve as protection of an injured extremity when occult injury is suspected although radiographs do not reveal a fracture. Splinting reduces pain and may limit or prevent further bleeding and vascular or neurologic damage associated with movement at the site of injury. Splinting also may prevent a closed injury from converting into an open injury. Complications include skin breakdown from pressure over bony prominences or maceration in areas of excessive pressure, compartment syndrome resulting from edema from the splint, and Ace wrap. General principles include the following:

- Immobilize (splint) joint above and below injury.
- Elevate injured part above level of heart.
- Apply ice for first 48 hours; then apply heat.
- Continuously reevaluate neurovascular status distal to injury.
- Splint extremity in position of function, if possible.

Indications

The following are indications for splinting:

- Known or suspected extremity trauma that causes the patient pain or dysfunction or demonstrates swelling, ecchymosis, neurovascular compromise, or deformity
- Trauma that causes bleeding or effusion of fluid into a joint, rendering it symptomatic, as mentioned previously

Contraindications

The following are contraindications for splinting:

- Necessity for open reduction of an unstable or open fracture
- Concern for compartment syndrome in the affected extremity and skin at high risk for infection (i.e., with abrasions or ulcerations)

Caution should be used when applying a splint in these circumstances.

Equipment (Options)

The following equipment is required:

- Hard splints (padded boards, metal splints)
- Air splints (inflatable plastic bladders or negative-pressure bead splints)
- Traction splints (provide traction and immobilization)
- Plaster splints (custom made specifically for the type of injury encountered)
- 2-inch adhesive tape
- Kerlix, roller gauze, or elastic wrap
- Generous amounts of padding

Procedure

Use the following procedure:

1. Evaluate the neurovascular status of the extremity.
2. Keep the patient informed throughout the procedure.
3. Choose the type of splint appropriate for the injury (it must be large enough to splint the joint above and the joint below the injury).
4. Secure the splint on the extremity in a position of function or least manipulation, padding bony prominences well.
5. When lifting an injured limb onto a splint, be certain to support both ends of the injured limb (distal and proximal) adequately to reduce mobility (this takes two hands).
6. Leave part of the extremity distal to the injury (e.g., fingers on a forearm injury) exposed to allow for reassessment of the neurovascular status.
7. Elevate injured part, preferably above the level of the heart, to reduce edema.
8. Apply well-insulated ice pack to the injury.
9. Repeat neurovascular evaluations for color, pain, temperature, swelling, capillary refill, sensation, and function frequently.

TRACTION SPLINTING DEVICES

Several devices are used for splinting injured femurs that offer not only immobilization but also a means of applying traction to the distal part of the leg, reducing muscle spasm, pain, and deformity.

Indications

The following are indications for use of traction splinting:

- Midshaft femur fracture
- Proximal tibia fracture

Contraindications

The following are contraindications for use of traction splinting:

- Hip fractures
- Pelvic injuries
- Middle or lower tibial fractures

- Ankle or foot injuries
- Most knee injuries

Procedure

The procedure outlined is for the HARE traction splint. Other similar devices are available. Clinical personnel should refer to product literature for specific directions for use.

　　Use the following procedure:

1. Remove traction splint from the case, and loosen collet sleeves to release for lengthening.
2. Position traction splint parallel to injured leg; adjust length to allow 8 to 10 inches past the foot, measuring from the position of the ischial tuberosity.
3. Tighten collet sleeves to lock.
4. Fold down heel stand until it locks at 90-degree angle; position it about 5 inches from end of splint (flexion of the fracture and pain result from not using this stand to provide elevation of the foot).
5. Position Velcro support straps according to patient's size, with two above the knee and two below; to keep the Velcro out of the way until needed, wrap it under the splint and hook it on itself (Velcro tends to stick to blankets, carpet, and the like).
6. Place the ankle straps under the patient's ankle, padding heel and ankle as necessary to ensure fit.
7. Place one hand under the ankle and one hand under the knee, and apply gentle, manual traction such as for the traction splint (when manual traction is on, it must not be released until the entire traction splint has been applied and secured; Figure 28-5).
8. Have an assistant place the splint under the injured leg with the half-ring positioned just below the buttock, against the ischial tuberosity; continue to maintain manual traction.
9. When the leg is lowered onto the splint, attach the ankle hitch into the S hook; twist knurled knob on splint to apply traction, and tighten until the strap is snug. Ask the patient for feedback regarding pain relief and comfort.

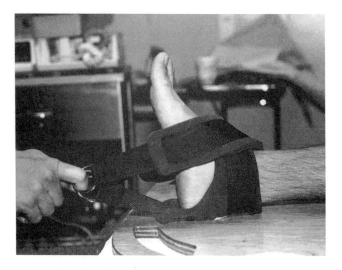

Figure 28–5. Traction harness for traction splinting devices must be evaluated for fit, function, and provision of adequate blood flow to the foot.

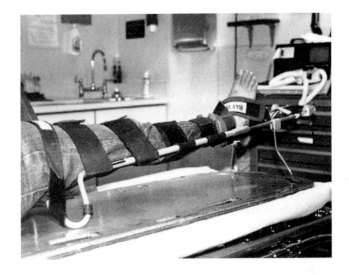

Figure 28-6. Traction splinting device correctly applied to patient's leg.

10. Fasten the Velcro straps around the leg. If the patient has an open wound, dress it with a sterile dressing first; Velcro straps can hold the dressing in place and may be tightened if direct pressure is needed (Figure 28-6).
11. Support the leg in the area beneath the splint to ensure stable positioning.
12. Reassess neurovascular status in the limb; make strap and stabilization adjustments as necessary.
13. Inform and comfort the patient.

When properly applied, the traction device alleviates a great deal of muscle spasm and pain. Patient comfort (or discomfort) is an important indicator of accurate placement and effectiveness of the splint. Clinical personnel should never release the traction on the splint without first providing manual traction to maintain tension on the muscles.

PELVIC STABILIZATION

Pelvic fractures represent a disruption of the bony structure of the pelvis. The fracture pattern is often representative of the mechanism of injury (See Chapter 19). Timely stabilization of pelvic fractures can be beneficial to the support of hemodynamic stability. Pelvic fracture patterns often result in a large volume of blood loss and the sequelea associated with hemodynamic instability. Based on the fracture pattern, the orthopedic surgeon may opt to initiate pelvic stabilization in the emergency department. This process can involve the use of external compression devices such as a sheet tied snugly around the pelvis, commercial products that provide consistent equal pressure around the pelvis, or the application of an external fixator.

HELMET REMOVAL

Various helmets are available for those sports in which head protection is recommended. Motorcycling, bicycling, kayaking, ice hockey, football, and auto racing are just a few. The careful removal of this gear is imperative for protection of the cervical spine.

Procedure

A quick examination of the helmet to determine its construction before attempting removal may save time, effort, and risk to the patient. Some sport helmets have air bladders that can be deflated to make space in the helmet, some have removable parts, and some are made of molded plastic that can be cut safely with a cast saw. Creating enough space to allow hands for cervical spine immobilization is the objective in altering the helmet, and all procedures should be explained to the patient as removal progresses.

Use the following procedure:

1. Never attempt to remove a helmet alone; airway protection can be achieved with most helmets in place, and the potential for complicating an injury with a difficult removal is great.
2. One person should apply in-line stabilization by placing one hand behind the head, resting on the occiput, and the front hand on the angles of the mandible, thumb on one side, fingers on the other (this person is in control of the head and neck).
3. The second person then should remove the helmet by pulling laterally on the sides and sliding it off in caudad maneuver. If the helmet has full face protection, special consideration must be given to the eye and mouth covering, which must be removed first. If it cannot be removed, tilt the helmet (not the head) back to pass the face protector over the patient's nose.

Preventing Heat Loss in Trauma Patients

Hypothermia may be present when a trauma patient arrives or it may develop quickly in the emergency department in the uncovered patient and by rapid administration of room temperature fluids or refrigerated blood. Hypothermia is a potentially lethal complication in the injured patient, and aggressive measures should be taken to prevent the loss of body heat and to restore body temperature to normal. *Preventing* heat loss is much more efficient than attempting to rewarm the patient. Practicing a few techniques can avert a complicated situation. Anticipation of heat loss in *all* trauma patients prepares caregivers for preventing loss of precious body heat. The environments where we resuscitate and manage injured patients directly affect the degree of heat loss. Often, exposure during transport and in radiologic suites may enhance heat loss unless adequate measures are taken to prevent the loss.

The following is a list of methods of preventing heat loss:

- Removal of wet clothing
- Raise the ambient air temperature in the rooms where the patient will be managed
- Use of head coverings (caps made of Mylar or stockinette work well)
- Administration of warm oxygen
- Warm fluid replacement
- Use of warm irrigating solutions for wound cleansing
- Covering the patient with warmed blankets and commercially available devices between exams and procedures
- Administration of fluid and blood through an infuser/warmer

CHAPTER 29

DIAGNOSTIC DATA

DIANNE M. DANIS

Diagnostic data collection is often necessary in order to obtain a complete picture of a trauma patient's injuries and clinical condition. Diagnostic tests play an essential role in the assessment process, but they always need to be evaluated in the context of the patient's entire clinical picture. This chapter reviews key laboratory and imaging studies commonly used in trauma care.

Accurate patient identification must be ensured before performing any diagnostic tests. This is generally not a problem with major trauma patients when clinicians are in constant attendance. For minor trauma and multiple casualties, care must be taken to follow institutional policy and to use at least two patient identifiers when confirming patient identity.

Another important consideration with diagnostic data is the timely communication of critical test results. The Joint Commission on Accreditation of Healthcare Organizations expects hospitals to identify critical test results relevant to their institution. Hospitals also must develop procedures and time parameters for reporting of critical test results.

TRAUMA LABORATORY TESTS

When a trauma patient enters the emergency department, a predetermined set of laboratory tests known as *trauma labs* or *trauma panels* often are performed. Ideally, the laboratory tests ordered should be tailored to the specific needs of the patient. For unstable trauma patients, however, relying on a standard panel is efficient and provides a comprehensive baseline. In most institutions the trauma panel consists of chemistry, hematology, and coagulation profiles and a urinalysis. Blood typing and arterial blood gas studies also are performed for major trauma patients. Alcohol and toxicology studies are often a standard element of trauma labs. In major trauma cases, trauma labs should be flagged to receive expedited treatment. Satellite laboratories and extensive use of point-of-care testing can facilitate the rapid availability of results.

The following sections define the major laboratory tests used in trauma care and the implications of the test results. Neither normal values nor critical test result values are provided: for these, clinicians should consult institutional references. Hospital policy also should be consulted for collection procedures and to ensure that samples are labeled accurately. Standard precautions should always be used when collecting blood and body fluid samples.

Type and Screen or Type and Crossmatch

The type and screen or type and crossmatch of blood is one of the most important laboratory tests performed on the critically injured trauma patient. Type and screen tests are performed to determine the patient's blood group antigen (A, B, AB, or O) and the presence (positive) or absence (negative) of the Rh antigen. Type and crossmatch tests are performed for compatibility between a mixture of the patient's own blood and the donor's blood. Successful type and crossmatch occurs when no hemolysis or clumping occurs in the mixture.

The following is a general rule:

O negative blood = universal donor
AB positive blood = universal recipient

Arterial Blood Gases

Arterial blood gas values are obtained from arterial blood samples. These values help to evaluate the effectiveness of gas exchange at the alveolar capillary cellular membrane level. They also assist in evaluating the efficiency of lung ventilation and perfusion and in determining the acid-base balance of the body.

The partial pressure of arterial oxygen (Po_2) is an indirect measurement of the oxygen content in arterial blood that is available for combining with hemoglobin. Po_2 is a measure of the tension, or pressure, of oxygen, dissolved in the plasma. This pressure determines the force of oxygen necessary to diffuse across the pulmonary alveolar membrane. The arterial oxygen saturation measures the quantity of oxygen that actually is bound to hemoglobin. The potential hydrogen (pH) measures the acidity or alkalinity of arterial blood. The pH is an expression of the hydrogen ion concentration in arterial blood. The Pco_2 measures the partial pressure of carbon dioxide in arterial blood to determine how well the lungs are maintaining acid-base balance (respiratory component of acid-base balance). The lungs do this by "blowing off" or retaining carbon dioxide (acid).

The level of arterial bicarbonate (HCO_3) reflects how well the kidneys are maintaining acid-base balance (metabolic component of acid-base balance). The kidneys do this by retaining or excreting HCO_3 (base).

NOTE: Pco_2 and HCO_3 levels influence pH values. Increased Pco_2 depresses the pH, whereas increased HCO_3 elevates the pH:

- $\uparrow Pco_2 = \downarrow pH$
- $\downarrow Pco_2 = \uparrow pH$
- $\uparrow HCO_3 = \uparrow pH$
- $\downarrow HCO_3 = \downarrow pH$

The base excess/deficit is calculated by using the arterial pH and Pco_2 and blood hematocrit values. The base excess/deficit represents the amount of buffering anions in the blood (metabolic component of acid-base). Positive values indicate a base excess; negative values indicate a base deficit (sometimes called a "negative base excess"). Base deficit can be helpful in evaluating the adequacy of trauma resuscitation because the test results can be available on an almost real-time basis and can be followed over time for extended resuscitations.

Abnormal Base Deficit Value	Possible Causes
$\uparrow$ (> –2 mEq/L)	• Metabolic acidosis
	• Lactic acidosis
	• Hemorrhagic shock

Serum lactate is an end product of carbohydrate metabolism. Excessive amounts of lactate may be produced when anaerobic metabolism occurs because of lack of oxygen. Elevated lactate levels reflect metabolic acidosis, usually lactic acidosis in trauma. Some studies have suggested a relationship between elevated lactate levels and poor outcomes in trauma patients. The test is most useful in critically injured patients where trending results over time suggests whether trauma resuscitation is succeeding. Lactate also may be measured on venous blood samples.

Abnormal Lactate Value	Possible Causes
↑ (> 7 mg/dL)	• Lactic acidosis
	• Hemorrhage/shock
	• Cardiac/respiratory failure
	• Diabetic ketoacidosis

The tables that follow illustrate the typical constellation of arterial blood gas values seen in selected traumatic injuries.

Hypovolemic Shock (Hypoventilation and Hypoperfusion)

Test	Value
Po_2	↓
Oxygen saturation	↓
pH	↓ (late)
Pco_2	↑ (late)
HCO_3	↓

NOTE: Hyperventilation in early shock may increase pH and decrease Pco_2.

Hypoventilation (Airway Obstruction, Chest Trauma, Central Nervous System Trauma)

Test	Value
Po_2	↓
Oxygen saturation	↓
pH	↓
Pco_2	↑
HCO_3	Normal or ↑ (mild)

NOTE: Bicarbonate may be mildly increased to compensate for respiratory acidosis.

Simple Pneumothorax

Test	Value
Po_2	↓
Oxygen saturation	↓
pH	Normal
Pco_2	Normal
HCO_3	Normal

Hyperventilation (Central Nervous Sytem Injury, Pain, Anxiety)

Test	Value
Po_2	Normal
Oxygen saturation	Normal
pH	↑
Pco_2	↓ (mild)
HCO_3	Normal or ↓ (mild)

NOTE: Bicarbonate may be mildly decreased to compensate for respiratory alkalosis.

Complete Blood Count

A complete blood count is obtained (usually from venous blood) to identify the number of red blood cells with indices, white blood cells with differentiation, hematocrit, hemoglobin, and platelets in whole blood.

Red Blood Cells (Erythrocytes)

Red blood cell values vary, depending on the age, sex, and geographic location (in relation to sea level) of the patient.

Abnormal Values	Possible Causes
↑ ↓	• Dehydration • Hemorrhage • Fluid overload (dilutional) • Anemia (iron deficiency) • Pregnancy

Red Blood Cell Indices. Red blood cell indices define the size, weight, and hemoglobin content of red blood cells. The indices include the following:

- Mean corpuscular volume (MCV)
- Mean corpuscular hemoglobin
- Mean corpuscular hemoglobin concentration (MCHC)
- Red cell size distribution width

Red blood cell indices are useful in identifying various types of anemia that may be present in trauma patients.

Abnormal Values	Possible Causes
MCV, MCHC ↓	Iron deficiency anemia
MCV ↑	Alcoholism, ↓ vitamin B_{12} or folic acid

White Blood Cells (Leukocytes)

A white blood cell count is obtained to identify the presence of an infection.

Abnormal Value	Possible Causes
>10,900 cells/µL	• Infection/inflammation
	• Tissue necrosis
	• Immunocompromise

NOTE: For elderly patients with a severe bacterial infection, the white blood cell count may not increase as rapidly or to as high a level as in a younger patient.

White Blood Cell Differential

A white blood cell differential count, often called a "diff," is performed to supplement the white blood cell count and provide additional information about existing infections and their severity, as well as about the ability of the body to resist and fight infection. Each component represents a relative percentage of the total white blood cell count. The differential count includes the following:

- Neutrophils
- Eosinophils
- Basophils
- Monocytes
- Lymphocytes

Abnormal Values	Change	Possible Causes
Neutrophils (pyogenic infect)	↑	• Bacterial infection
		• Stress response
		• Ischemic necrosis
Neutrophils	↓	• Viral infections
Eosinophils (allergic and parasite	↑	• Drug sensitivity
disorders)		• Allergic reaction
	↓	• Stress response
		• Shock
		• Burns

Abnormal Values	Change	Possible Causes
Basophils (parasite infection)	↓	• Stress
Monocytes (severe infection)	↑	• Chronic infection
	↓	• Prednisone treatment
Lymphocytes	↑	• Viral infection
	↓	• Renal failure
		• Steroid therapy

NOTE: Neutrophils are the most numerous and the first activated to fight infections. With overwhelming infections, immature neutrophils (bands) are produced, reflecting a shift to the left on the complete blood count results.

Hematocrit

A hematocrit value is obtained to determine the percentage of red blood cells in whole blood. Hematocrit values parallel red blood cell values. Serial hematocrit values may be obtained at short intervals to detect hemorrhage.

Abnormal Values	Possible Causes
↓	• Hemodilution (from compensated hypovolemia or excessive volume replacement)
	• Anemia
	• Hemorrhage
↑	• Hemoconcentration
	• Burns
	• Dehydration

NOTE: When blood is lost acutely, the number of red blood cells lost is in the same ratio as that of whole blood. Therefore, the percentage of hematocrit in a whole blood sample would remain normal. Only after hemodilution occurs (from shock compensation or crystalloid replacement) does the hematocrit level drop.

Hemoglobin

A hemoglobin value is obtained to measure the amount of hemoglobin in whole blood. The amount of hemoglobin determines the oxygen-carrying capacity of blood. Hemoglobin values closely reflect red blood cell values. Serial hemoglobin values may be obtained at short intervals to detect hemorrhage.

Abnormal Values	Possible Causes
↑	• Hemoconcentration
	• Severe burns
	• Dehydration
↓	• Hemorrhage
	• Anemia
	• Transfusions of incompatible blood

NOTE: When whole blood is lost acutely, the amount of hemoglobin that is lost is proportionate. Only after hemodilution occurs (as a result of shock compensation or crystalloid volume replacement) does the hemoglobin level drop.

Platelets (Thrombocytes)

A platelet count is obtained to evaluate platelet function. In trauma patients, platelets play a major role in coagulation and are essential to achieve hemostasis when bleeding occurs.

Abnormal Values
↑

↓

Possible Causes
- Splenectomy
- Injury
- Infection
- Hemorrhage
- Disseminated intravascular coagulation

Coagulation Studies

Research has shown that within hours after major trauma or severe head trauma, patients can develop disseminated intravascular coagulation (DIC) syndrome leading to serious coagulopathy and death. Coagulation status is also of concern for patients receiving anticoagulation therapy before injury. The collection of early coagulation studies facilitates appropriate and effective treatment. An important consideration is the need for these studies as soon as a patient arrives, because some of the tests take time to perform—the sooner started, the sooner results will be available. Coagulation studies may include the following:

- Prothrombin time
- Activated partial thromboplastin time
- Fibrinogen level
- Platelet count
- Fibrinogen degradation products
- D-dimer

Which specific tests are indicated depend on the patient situation.

Prothrombin Time

A prothrombin time is evaluated in trauma patients to measure clotting time. Clotting time is a function of the effects of factors V, VII, and X; fibrinogen/factor I; and prothrombin/factor III. A prothrombin time is important in determining the ability of the blood to form clots.

Abnormal Values
↑
≥2.5 times normal = abnormal bleeding tendency

Possible Causes
Deficiency of the following:
- Factors V, VII, and/or X
- Fibrinogen
- Prothrombin

NOTE: Clotting times may be prolonged in the presence of liver disease, warfarin (Coumadin) ingestion, DIC, and massive blood transfusions.

Activated Partial Thromboplastin Time

An activated partial thromboplastin time is obtained to screen for problems with intrinsic clotting factors (except factors VII and XIII). The test also can be used to monitor the effectiveness of anticoagulation therapy with heparin. This laboratory test measures the amount of time it takes for fibrin to form a clot. In the trauma patient the activated partial thromboplastin time is used to determine the patient's tendency to bleed.

Abnormal Values	**Possible Causes**
↑	• DIC (after head injury)
	• Heparin therapy
↓	• Early DIC

Fibrinogen

Fibrinogen is a protein in the blood clotting network that rises sharply in response to acute phase injury or tissue necrosis. In trauma patients the fibrinogen level is used to screen for DIC.

Abnormal Value	**Possible Causes**
↑	• Compensated DIC
	• Various cerebral accidents
↓	• DIC
	• Liver disease

Fibrinogen Degradation Products

Fibrin degradation products (FDP) are an end product of fibrinolysis (clot breakdown). When FDPs are present in elevated amounts, an anticoagulant effect can result (DIC). FDP is one of the screening tests for DIC.

D-Dimer (Fragment D-Dimer)

D-dimer is a fibrin degradation fragment that is produced through fibrinolysis in conditions such as DIC. Normal plasma does not contain this fragment. The D-dimer is a specific test used for diagnosing DIC. D-dimer test results usually correlate with FDP results.

Chemistry Profile

In most institutions a modified version of the complete chemistry panel (chem panel) exists. The most commonly ordered chemistries in this panel include serum glucose, potassium, sodium, chloride, carbon dioxide, blood urea nitrogen, and creatinine.

Serum Glucose

Serum glucose is produced from the digestion of carbohydrates and from the liver when it converts glucagon into glucose. Glucose is necessary for cellular metabolism to occur. In trauma patients, this test rules out metabolic causes of decreased level of consciousness, such as hypoglycemia.

Abnormal Values	**Possible Causes**
↓	• Hypoglycemia
↑	• Hyperglycemia/diabetic ketoacidosis
	• Stress response

Potassium

Potassium is a cation and the primary electrolyte in intracellular fluid. Potassium is essential for the maintenance of cellular osmosis and plays a critical role in the electrical conduction of cardiac and skeletal muscle. Potassium is also important to acid-base balance and kidney function.

Abnormal Values	Possible Causes
↑ (hyperkalemia)	• Major burns/cell damage
	• Renal failure
	• Major crush injuries
↓ (hypokalemia)	• Hypovolemia
	• Intravenous fluid therapy without potassium chloride supplementation

NOTE: Hemolysis of the blood specimen results in inaccurately high potassium levels.

Sodium

Sodium, one of the two major extracellular cations, plays a major role in regulating osmotic pressure in extracellular fluid. Sodium also plays a major part in acid-base balance and neuromuscular function.

Abnormal Values	Possible Causes
↑ (hypernatremia)	• Fluid intake/fluid loss
	• Sodium intake
↓ (hyponatremia)	• Sodium loss
	• Severe burns
	• Excess fluid

Chloride

The measurement of serum chloride is important for the assessment of acid-base status. Chloride is a major extracellular anion that plays a role in the maintenance of oncotic pressure and thus blood volume and arterial pressure. Chloride levels are also important in the assessment of the trauma patient's acid-base balance.

Abnormal Values	Possible Causes
↑ (hyperchloremia)	• Dehydration
	• Renal failure
	• Central nervous system trauma with central neurogenic breathing
	• Hyperventilation
↓ (hypochloremia)	• Excess vomiting
	• Excess gastric suctioning
	• Overhydration
	• Burns

Carbon Dioxide Content

Serum carbon dioxide content measures carbonic acid (H_2CO_3), dissolved carbon dioxide, and HCO_3, with HCO_3 by far the largest component; therefore, carbon dioxide content is an indirect measure of HCO_3 and acid-base status.

Abnormal Values	Possible Causes
↓ (metabolic alkalosis)	↑ vomiting
	↑ gastric suctioning
↑ (respiratory acidosis)	↓ ventilation

Blood Urea Nitrogen

A blood urea nitrogen study evaluates renal function and determines the patient's hydration status. Urea is an end product of metabolism and is excreted in urine.

Abnormal Values	Possible Causes
↑	• Shock
	• Dehydration
	• Tissue necrosis
↓	• Overhydration

Serum Creatinine

Creatinine is a by-product of the breakdown of muscle mass for energy necessary for metabolism. The creatinine study in trauma patients detects the amount of muscle damage that has occurred and tests kidney function. This test is a more sensitive test than blood urea nitrogen.

Abnormal Values	Possible Causes
↑	• Shock
	• Dehydration

NOTE: Before using intravenous contrast in computed tomography scans, blood urea nitrogen and serum creatinine levels should be checked to evaluate kidney function. However, scans should NOT be delayed for test results in the trauma patient who is critically injured or unstable.

Urine Tests

Urine tests are indicated in trauma patients to test for genitourinary tract injury, for toxicology screening, and to test for pregnancy.

Urinalysis

The urinalysis in trauma patients checks for genitourinary trauma and specific disease states. The absence of hematuria is reassuring about the absence of serious genitourinary tract injury. However, the presence or degree of hematuria does not correlate with severity of injury.

	Abnormal Values	Possible Causes
Color	Dark or red	• Presence of blood
Specific gravity	>1.02	• Shock
pH	Alkaline >8	• Alkalosis
	Acidic <4.5	• Acidosis

	Abnormal Values	**Possible Causes**
Glucose	Present	• Diabetes
		• Increased intracranial pressure
Protein	Present	• Renal failure
Ketone	Present	• Diabetes/diabetic ketoacidosis
		• Diarrhea/vomiting

Microscopic

White blood cells	4 cells/hpf	• Urinary tract infection
Epithelial	↑	• Renal tubular necrosis
Casts	↑	• Glomerular capsule trauma
Bacteria/yeast/parasites	↑	• Infection

Urine Toxicology

Urine toxicology screens for trauma patients determine possible causes for altered levels of consciousness. Although some toxicology tests require blood, urine usually is preferred. The most common urine drug tests include the following:

- Alcohol
- Amphetamines
- Analgesics
- Barbiturates
- Benzodiazepines
- Cocaine/Crack
- Cyanide
- LSD (lysergic acid diethylamide)
- Major tranquilizers
- Marijuana
- Opiates
- PCP (phencyclidine hydrochloride)
- Sedatives
- Stimulants

Urine and Serum Human Chorionic Gonadotropin

The urine pregnancy test determines whether a female trauma patient is pregnant. This qualitative test measures the presence or absence of human chorionic gonadotropin. Given the wide age range within which girls and women can become pregnant, broad criteria should be used when deciding whether the test is indicated for a particular patient.

NOTES:
- The presence of human chorionic gonadotropin indicates pregnancy.
- Obtain a catheterized specimen if urine is grossly bloody.
- A blood serum human chorionic gonadotropin also may be sent to the lab to test for pregnancy.

Serum Ethanol (Ethyl Alcohol)

Serum ethanol (often called alcohol level or ETOH) detects alcohol levels in trauma patients to determine possible causes for altered levels of consciousness. Serum is the preferred medium for testing serum ethanol levels.

NOTE:

- Alcohols other than ethanol (isopropyl, methanol) also are detected with this test.
- Alcohol also can be identified by using a breath analyzer and in urine.
- Special procedures need to be followed when samples are obtained for legal reasons.

Serum Amylase

Serum amylase is an enzyme that is secreted by the pancreas and is used for carbohydrate catabolism. This test is performed in trauma patients to detect acute pancreatic injuries.

Abnormal Values	Possible Causes
↑	• Pancreatic injury
	• Aortic aneurysm rupture
	• Ethyl alcohol toxicity
↓	• Severe burns

TRAUMA IMAGING STUDIES

This section reviews imaging studies performed for trauma patients. Only key studies and major points related to trauma patients are covered. For more discussion of assessment and diagnosis related to specific injuries, refer to the relevant chapter in this text. For a fuller explanation of imaging studies and clinical implications, the reader should consult other texts.

Trauma imaging studies are immensely valuable in assessing the extent of injury. However, they often necessitate moving unstable patients out of the trauma room or intensive care unit into the less secure environment of the radiology department. Radiology and other imaging areas may not be as well-equipped and configured as trauma resuscitation areas. They may require moving patients inside the imaging machine and may prohibit provider presence in the exam room, thus limiting direct visualization of the patient. For all these reasons, patients receiving imaging studies should be considered at high risk for adverse events, and trauma clinicians should assess these patients closely and frequently.

Initial Trauma Radiographs

Major trauma patients typically undergo a standard series of radiographs in the trauma resuscitation area. These include chest, cervical spine, and pelvis x-ray films. Additional radiographs then are ordered based on suspected injuries. During a trauma resuscitation, films should be obtained rapidly and without delaying patient care. Many trauma protocols require clinicians to don protective lead gowns so that care may be continued while radiographs are in process.

Chest Radiographs

- Initial chest radiograph is usually an anteroposterior supine portable film.
- When possible, an upright film should be obtained.
- The goal is to identify major injuries such as pneumothoraces, hemothoraces, and/or potential aortic injury.

Cervical Spine Radiographs

- The lateral cervical spine view must include all seven cervical vertebrae plus the superior portion of the first thoracic vertebra.

- Not all centers include the cervical spine radiograph in the initial studies because a single view is insufficient to clear the cervical spine.
- The cervical spine radiograph provides information only about bony fractures and/or dislocations visible in the lateral view.

Pelvis Radiographs

- The initial pelvis x-ray film is an anteroposterior view.
- The goal is to identify major pelvis fractures suggestive of significant bleeding and potential hypovolemia.

Ultrasound

Ultrasonography uses high-frequency sound waves targeted at specific body structures. Wave pulses are reflected back from the targeted structures, generating images. Hollow, solid, and fluid-filled structures can be discriminated via ultrasound. Ultrasound is noninvasive, can be performed with a portable machine, and does not involve radiation.

Focused Assessment Sonography in Trauma

- The focused assessment sonography in trauma refers to cardiac and abdominal ultrasonograms performed according to a trauma-focused protocol.
- Focused assessment sonography in trauma is a component of many initial trauma resuscitation protocols.
- The cardiac ultrasound is focused on identifying pericardial fluid and the possibility of cardiac tamponade.
- The abdominal ultrasound is focused on identifying hemoperitoneum.

Transesophageal Echocardiography

- Transesophageal echocardiography (TEE) involves the endoscopic placement of an ultrasonography probe in the distal esophagus or proximal stomach.
- TEE in trauma most commonly is used to evaluate the possibility of thoracic aortic injury.
- TEE is one of several tests used to assess for aortic injury (see following sections on computed tomography and angiography).

Computed Tomography

Computed tomography scans provide three-dimensional cross-sectional views of body structures. More advanced machines, usually called helical or spiral scanners, provide superior speed and image quality and generally are preferred for trauma evaluations. The capability to reformat and provide three-dimensional reconstructions is of great value, especially for facial, spinal, and great vessel injuries. In many cases, image quality also may be enhanced by the use of contrast dye. Computed tomography (CT) scans are used widely in trauma, especially in blunt trauma. They provide accurate and detailed information about almost every type of injury. As yet, unfortunately, no portable CT scanners are available. Therefore a patient's stability must be evaluated before deciding whether a patient can be transported for CT scanning. This section is limited to discussion of head, spine, chest, and abdominal/pelvis scans.

Head/Brain

- Head CT scans are used to identify the following:
  - Skull and facial fractures
  - Subdural and epidural hematomas
  - Cerebral contusions and intracerebral hematomas
  - Intraventricular hemorrhage
  - Cerebral edema, midline shift, and herniation
- Obtaining a head CT scan requires inserting the patient's head into the CT scanner. This limits visibility and presents the risk of unidentified airway compromise from respiratory arrest or vomiting. High vigilance is necessary in order to prevent adverse events.

Spine

- CT scans may be obtained of any section of the spine or of the entire spine.
- Spinal CT identifies bony abnormalities, including spine fractures of all types, and dislocations.
- CT images are generally superior to standard spine x-ray films and in some centers are replacing the traditional spine radiographic series.

Chest

- The chest CT scan provides information about injury to the thoracic skeleton, intrathoracic structures, and the vasculature.
- The chest CT/CT angiography (see the following discussion) has proved its value in the assessment of possible aortic injury under the following circumstances:
  - Helical scanner
  - Contrast-enhanced
  - Study is performed according to proper procedure
  - Study is interpreted by experienced radiologist
- A chest CT scan performed according to the preceding criteria can identify accurately the presence of aortic injury. Aortogram (see the following discussion) remains the gold standard, and aortography may be required for further assessment of patients who have positive CT scans.

Abdomen and Pelvis

- Scans of the abdomen and pelvis provide information about organ, vascular, and bony injury and about the presence of hemoperitoneum.
- CT scanning of the abdomen and pelvis is not an alternative for an emergency laparotomy in patients who have clear clinical indications for surgery. These studies should be reserved for hemodynamically stable patients.
- Scans are particularly helpful with retroperitoneal and pelvic organ injuries that are difficult to evaluate by other means.
- The scans are not 100% accurate and may miss some bowel, pancreas, and diaphragm injuries.
- Single, double, or triple contrast dye administration may be needed in order to achieve maximum diagnostic value when evaluating certain organs.

Computed Tomography Angiography

In computed tomography angiography (CTA), a CT scanner is used to visualize blood flow in arterial and venous vessels throughout the body. Traditional catheter angiography requires accessing a large artery or vein, whereas CTA only requires intravenous injection of contrast material into a small peripheral vein. In trauma, CTA may be used to assess a variety of vessels. CTA has been used increasingly to assess potential blunt or traumatic vascular injuries of the neck.

Angiography (Arteriography)

Angiography entails the injection of radiopaque contrast material into arterial blood vessels. X-ray films or computerized fluoroscopy using digital subtraction angiography produces images of blood flow, vascular anatomy, and trauma. Nearly all blood vessels can be visualized through angiographic technique.

Aortogram

Historically, the aortogram has been considered the gold standard test for identification and assessment of aortic injury. However, the literature now also supports CT and TEE as studies that are useful under certain circumstances (see previous sections in this chapter on chest CT and TEE).

Pelvic Angiography

- Pelvic angiography may be indicated to manage hemorrhage from lacerated or disrupted pelvic cavity vessels usually associated with major pelvic fractures.
- If an injury is identified, interventional therapy such as embolization may be used to halt bleeding.
- Pelvic angiography requires a skilled angiographer and the ability to manage an active resuscitation within the angiography suite.

Magnetic Resonance Imaging

Magnetic resonance imaging (MRI) is an imaging technique derived from exposing a patient to radiofrequency waves in a strong magnetic field. The test is noninvasive and does not involve radiation. However, limitations of the MRI environment make it difficult to provide continuous close clinical care, thus the test should be reserved for stable patients. MRI cannot be performed in patients with metal implants of any type, nor are any metal objects allowed within the MRI room.

Head/Brain

MRI of the brain is helpful in evaluating diffuse axonal injuries.

Spine

- MRI of the spine provides superior images of the soft tissue structures of the spinal cord and of spinal disks.
- Spinal MRI can detect the following:
  - Spinal cord contusion or disruption
  - Spinal cord compression
  - Paraspinal ligament injuries
  - Disk herniation
  - Spinal epidural hematoma

Magnetic Resonance Angiography

Magnetic resonance angiography uses MRI to provide another method of visualizing blood flow through the arteries. In trauma, magnetic resonance angiography sometimes is used to evaluate the cervical carotid artery and intracranial vessels.

Suggested Readings

Committee on Trauma, American College of Surgeons: *Advanced trauma life support for doctors,* ed 7, Chicago, 2004, The College.

Emergency Nurses Association: *Trauma nursing core course provider manual,* ed 5, Des Plaines, Ill, 2000, The Association.

Pagana KD, Pagana TJ: *Mosby's manual of diagnostic and laboratory tests,* ed 2, St Louis, 2002, Mosby.

INDEX

A